Lady Lushes

Critical Issues in Health and Medicine

Edited by Rima D. Apple, University of Wisconsin–Madison, and Janet Golden, Rutgers University, Camden

Growing criticism of the U.S. health care system is coming from consumers, politicians, the media, activists, and healthcare professionals. Critical Issues in Health and Medicine is a collection of books that explores these contemporary dilemmas from a variety of perspectives, among them political, legal, historical, sociological, and comparative, and with attention to crucial dimensions such as race, gender, ethnicity, sexuality, and culture.

For a list of titles in the series, see the last page of the book.

Lady Lushes

Gender, Alcoholism, and Medicine in Modern America

Michelle L. McClellan

Rutgers University Press
New Brunswick, Camden, and Newark, New Jersey, and London

Library of Congress Cataloging-in-Publication Data
Names: McClellan, Michelle L., author.
Title: Lady lushes : gender, alcoholism, and medicine in modern America / Michelle L. McClellan.
Description: New Brunswick : Rutgers University Press, [2017] | Series: Critical issues in health and medicine | Includes bibliographical references and index.
Identifiers: LCCN 2016043247 | ISBN 9780813576985 (hardcover : alk. paper) | ISBN 9780813576978 (pbk. : alk. paper) | ISBN 9780813576992 (e-book (epub)) | ISBN 9780813577005 | ISBN 9780813591131 (e-book (mobi))
Subjects: LCSH: Women—Alcohol use—United States—History. | Women alcoholics—United States—History. | Alcoholism—United States—History.
Classification: LCC HV5137 .M425 2017 | DDC 362.292082/0973—dc23
LC record available at https://lccn.loc.gov/2016043247

A British Cataloging-in-Publication record for this book is available from the British Library.

Copyright © 2017 by Michelle L. McClellan
All rights reserved
No part of this book may be reproduced or utilized in any form or by any means, electronic or mechanical, or by any information storage and retrieval system, without written permission from the publisher. Please contact Rutgers University Press, 106 Somerset Street, New Brunswick, NJ 08901. The only exception to this prohibition is "fair use" as defined by U.S. copyright law.

∞ The paper used in this publication meets the requirements of the American National Standard for Information Sciences—Permanence of Paper for Printed Library Materials, ANSI Z39.48–1992.

www.rutgersuniversitypress.org

Manufactured in the United States of America

To all those women, known and unknown, who have struggled with alcohol in modern America

Contents

	Introduction	1
Chapter 1	The Female Inebriate in the Temperance Paradigm	28
Chapter 2	"Lit Ladies": Women's Drinking during the Progressive Era and Prohibition	49
Chapter 3	"More to Overcome than the Men": Women in Alcoholics Anonymous	75
Chapter 4	Defining a Disease: Gender, Stigma, and the Modern Alcoholism Movement	98
Chapter 5	"A Special Masculine Neurosis": Psychiatrists Look at Alcoholism	119
Chapter 6	"The Doctor Didn't Want to Take an Alcoholic": The Challenge of Medicalization at Midcentury	141
	Epilogue	164
	Acknowledgments	177
	Notes	179
	Bibliography	215
	Index	231

Lady Lushes

Introduction

In 1963, a glamorous blonde woman appeared in the pages of *Reader's Digest*, offering a dramatic life story. After growing up in an elite family in Chicago, Margaret "Marty" Mann had "entered a world that was all champagne and caviar."[1] Following a brief marriage and divorce, she found work and a robust drinking culture in New York City, where she shared an apartment with other young women during the 1920s. Initially, she had a high tolerance for liquor, amazing her companions with her capacity. But then she began to rely on alcohol when facing emotionally stressful events, she began to drink secretly at parties, and her first drink came ever earlier in the day. Then she experienced blackouts. Unable to drink as before, she also found that she could not stop. A fall from a balcony while drunk led to months in the hospital. Upon release, though, she drank still more and could not keep a job. Fearing she was losing her sanity, Mann sought professional help, but at this time many doctors, including psychiatrists, preferred not to treat alcoholics. Finally, one Dr. Henry Tiebout accepted her as a patient at Blythewood Sanitarium in Connecticut. Even there, *Reader's Digest* reported, she had a year's worth of psychiatric counseling with no results.

The turning point came when Dr. Tiebout gave her a copy of the "The Big Book" of Alcoholics Anonymous (AA), urging her to read it because it was "written by people like you." Mann said that she recognized herself in the text even though it focused on the experiences of alcoholic men, and she immediately found inspiration through a sense of belonging, as the *Reader's Digest* profile explained: "These people were drunks; they had suffered just as she had suffered, and they had survived!" Mann learned that her drinking problem had a name—she was neither insane nor immoral, and knowledge replaced confusion and despair: "As she read on, the fog of fear and ignorance began to part, and she learned that alcoholism was a disease!" Shortly after this exposure to a medical understanding of her condition—"an allergy of the body coupled with an obsession of the mind"—Mann experienced a spiritual awakening, leading to a "feeling of serenity and soaring confidence such as she had never known." This combination finally enabled her to conquer her problem—she stopped drinking and gained a "new radiance."[2]

Turning her attention thereafter to helping others, Mann founded the National Council on Alcoholism (NCA; initially organized as the National Committee for Education on Alcoholism) in 1944. Her success in achieving sobriety and rebuilding her life was mirrored in the institutional growth of the NCA. By 1963, the organization boasted a staff of forty-five in its central office, while the Alcohol Information Centers it established across the country employed one hundred and fifty counselors. The NCA helped expand the number of general hospitals that would accept alcoholic patients and created support systems for workers in corporations and industries. Its founder literally embodied the cause: "Out of Marty Mann's suffering has been born a network of hope and help immediately available to any lost or frightened individual."[3]

This tidy and uplifting narrative, published more than two decades after Mann achieved sobriety, advanced Mann's public health agenda only by obscuring years of heartache and struggle. A brilliant strategist, Mann carefully crafted her life story to reinforce her message that alcoholism was a disease that could strike anyone, even a debutante like her. Mann's revelation that she had drunk herself almost to death defied the assumption that only men, whether skid row bums or high-strung writers, would do such a thing. For decades, medical experts, social scientists, and the general public alike believed that male alcoholics greatly outnumbered their female counterparts and that women who became alcoholic were especially debased, often sexually promiscuous and neglectful mothers as well as problem drinkers. In this context, Mann's biography was complicated: Aside from her alcoholism, her status as a divorced career woman with no children contradicted the domestic values so celebrated in mid-twentieth-century America. Still, her poise and beauty provided an implicit challenge to pejorative attitudes about drinking women.

In the *Reader's Digest* profile, as in all her public pronouncements, Mann rarely commented directly on her experiences as a woman. Instead, she claimed the gender-neutral label "alcoholic" and worked tirelessly to promote a view of alcoholism not as a sin or lack of willpower but as a legitimate illness, in men and women alike. As she made a place for herself in the AA fellowship, Mann insisted that the experience of alcoholism overrode other differences, including gender identity. She similarly believed that harnessing the cultural prestige of science and medicine was the most effective way to reduce the stigma faced by *all* alcoholics. Mann combined scientific language with the irrefutable proof of her own experience into a potent form of authority, promising that other alcoholics—male and female—could join her in health and recovery. But many forces worked against the realization of Mann's goals: continuing social and scientific disapproval of drinking women as morally flawed, sexual threats to men; the inability of social scientific and medical researchers to engage gender meaningfully as a theoretically and clinically relevant category of analysis; and the failure of treatment regimes to accommodate alcoholic women's domestic obligations and lack of power in the family. The very existence of female alcoholics raised crucial questions about how to define alcoholism as a disease as well as the salience of gender as an aspect of personal identity and as a social category.

Precisely because alcoholism does not conform to a straightforward model of disease—one caused by an infectious agent and cured by a pill—analyzing it historically yields rich insights into the contested process of medicalization (the expansion of medical and scientific authority into new realms of behavior and cultural practice). For centuries, most Americans have shared a commonsense understanding of the phenomenon we now call "alcoholism" as an uncontrollable craving to drink excessively regardless of negative consequences, a pattern that continues even when the person has expressed a desire to stop. It did not take an advanced degree or technical expertise to observe this troubling behavior in family members, friends, or even public figures—but efforts to understand *why* some people drink this way, and to determine what to do about it, have sparked heated debate and wide-ranging responses including prayer, shunning, incarceration, and legislation as well as medical treatment.

In cultural expectations, in social practices, and in the agenda of reformers, women's traditional job has been to prevent men from drinking—as pious wives who influenced their men through example, as temperance activists who sought to rid American society of saloons, and as understanding spouses who supported men's sobriety in Alcoholic Anonymous and twentieth-century therapeutic regimes.[4] *Lady Lushes* places drinking women center stage to offer new insights regarding the meanings of gender in American society, the limitations of medical expertise in defining diseases, and the sometimes unexpected interactions between gender-role ideology and medical authority.

This book traces two waves of medicalization in which various experts sought to define problem drinking as a disease. The first wave unfolded in the late nineteenth century, centering on a group of physicians called "inebriate specialists," while the second occurred in the three decades after the repeal of Prohibition and featured a loose coalition of scientific researchers, public health advocates, mental heath experts, and the Alcoholics Anonymous fellowship. In many ways, these were very different eras, characterized by profound changes in medical theory and practice, in American attitudes regarding alcohol, and in beliefs and customs governing women's behavior and social roles. Despite these changes, alcohol retained its symbolic power as a way to define and regulate femininity, reinforcing even now the idea that women—including the most privileged women in our society—cannot escape a biological and social vulnerability to alcohol and its effects. Even those women who had the most access to new opportunities in education, employment, and politics found that a double standard persisted when they engaged in recreational drinking or were diagnosed as alcoholics.

The temperance movement, a massive campaign to restrict access to alcoholic beverages, shaped American attitudes regarding women, men, and alcohol so deeply that its legacy can still be felt today, more than seventy-five years after the repeal of national Prohibition. This campaign gained momentum during the nineteenth century, when most Americans viewed women and men as fundamentally different, with biological and social roles that—ideally at least—complemented one another. Given this value system, women's recreational drinking was met with severe censure, with particular ire directed at uncouth working-class girls and decadent upper-class women. But some doctors insisted that middle-class women only relied on alcohol—just as they turned to drugs, tonics, and patent medicines—to cope with the frailty and biological vulnerability inherent in being female. Focusing on women's motivation to drink alcohol allowed experts to distinguish among women even as they underscored differences between women and men. Inebriate experts could also use "respectable" drinking women as the vanguard of a medicalized model of inebriety, insisting that such women's dependence on alcohol was not about recreation or pleasure, but a matter best managed by physicians.

This relatively sympathetic view of at least some drinking women faded as new federal laws and two constitutional amendments reshaped drinking habits and drug use in the United States during the early twentieth century, separating alcohol from other drugs and highlighting alcohol as a source of recreation and pleasure. Overall consumption actually declined during national Prohibition (1920–1933), but the meanings attached to women's drinking changed significantly as increasing numbers of middle-class women drank along with men, thereby forfeiting their position as innocent victims of men's drunken excesses or as delicate patients hooked on alcohol for pain relief. After Prohibition was repealed in 1933, the reinvention of alcohol as a benign consumer good served as a convenient testing ground for evolving gender relations and the growth of medical and scientific authority, particularly during the upheavals of World War II and the reconstitution of domestic life in the postwar era.

In the wake of Repeal, constituencies as diverse as social scientists, psychiatrists, public health advocates, and the new Alcoholics Anonymous fellowship launched a second wave of medicalization (although many of them were unaware of their nineteenth-century predecessors). They narrowed the temperance-era agenda, insisting that those individuals who became dependent on alcohol constituted a distinct category of people who suffered from a disease. Labeling some drinking patterns (and some individuals) "pathological" required simultaneously determining what was acceptable. But drawing that line was especially challenging when it came to women. Even as advertising, alcohol consumption patterns, medical advice, and popular attitudes assimilated social drinking back into mainstream masculinity during the middle decades of the twentieth century, standards for "normal" or appropriate drinking among women remained uncertain, just as women's motivation to drink remained suspect. Furthermore, the intoxicating qualities of alcohol seemed especially dangerous to women who were often considered naïve drinkers regardless of their individual histories. During Prohibition and for decades afterward, social scientists, doctors and psychiatrists, and journalists criticized drinking women for abandoning traditional feminine virtues such as restraint, self-denial, and chastity, for wanting to act like men, and for neglecting their children. At a time when conventional roles seemed dangerously in flux, drinking women threatened to unravel them further. Experts who defined women's drinking as a problem to be solved thus imagined themselves defending an entire social system.

Lady Lushes traces a dramatic shift in how women's alcoholism was defined, from a biological diagnosis stemming from feminine weakness in the late nineteenth century to psychoanalytically inflected accusations of gender maladjustment in the middle decades of the twentieth. I show that this new, ostensibly "modern" language reflected an incomplete transformation from the separate spheres of the nineteenth century and was, if anything, more damning of women who drank to excess. The flapper of the Prohibition era who sampled cocktails in speakeasies, the World War II factory worker who visited a bar after her shift, and the postwar suburban housewife who drank at home alone, all defied conventional rules governing women's comportment, and each faced considerable censure as a result. Even after Repeal, many Americans continued to view women's drinking as a sign of individual misbehavior or worse and as a threat to family stability and social harmony. Such deep-seated disapproval made it more difficult to conceptualize women's excessive drinking as a medical matter, since a drinking woman did not have to be a full-fledged alcoholic to pose a threat.

Because the emerging medical model of alcoholism rested on a distinction between alcoholic and social drinkers, these lingering misgivings about women's consumption sharply limited the therapeutic and social impact of disease model advocates. That it has been so difficult to determine how much is enough reflects wider challenges associated with remaking women's roles, and those of men as well, in twentieth-century America. It also shows that the promise of modern medicine to contain, label, and manage complex human behaviors cannot always be realized.

Women and Alcohol in American History

Today, more than fifty years after Mann's profile appeared in *Reader's Digest*, many Americans remain ambivalent or even confused about what it means to call alcoholism a "disease." And while fewer women than men become alcoholic—the National Institute for Alcohol Abuse and Alcoholism calculates that women constitute approximately one-third of the alcoholic population[5]—women's drinking of any variety raises particular concerns, as demonstrated by warning labels against maternal drinking during pregnancy and accusations that intoxicated victims of sexual assault have only themselves to blame. Even the U.S. government defines acceptable levels of consumption differently for men and women.[6] Recent books such as *Her Best-Kept Secret: Why Women Drink and How They Can Regain Control* and *Drink: The Intimate Relationship between Women and Alcohol* highlight the recurrent idea that women's drinking is linked to the stresses women feel because of too much social change—or not enough.[7] Women write blogs and memoirs in which they explicitly connect their drinking—both recreational and alcoholic—with their domestic lives: for example, *Sippy Cups Are Not for Chardonnay*; *Mommy Doesn't Drink Here Anymore: Getting through the First Year of Sobriety*; and *Diary of an Alcoholic Housewife*.[8] The phenomenon of playdates as cocktail hour provides a sharp contrast—sometimes intentionally so—with conventional wisdom about the need to abstain from alcohol during pregnancy. Meanwhile, current findings in biology and neuroscience make new claims about the importance of sex differences in substance use and addiction: Public health experts admonish us that it takes fewer drinks to count as a "binge" for women as compared to men, while researchers use animal studies to examine how sex hormones influence the progression of drug abuse.⁹ When it comes to drinking customs, the lines we draw between pleasure and pathology have been deeply entwined with our beliefs about what it means to be male and female, masculine and feminine.

To understand why Americans continue to be so conflicted about alcoholism—and about women's drinking, in particular—we must recognize how the temperance movement and national Prohibition left deep-seated legacies in American society and culture. The temperance impulse—a decades-long campaign that began in the nineteenth century to reduce and then restrict Americans' consumption of alcohol and that culminated in a constitutional amendment to prohibit the manufacture and sale of alcohol in the United States—built upon and reinforced perceptions of men and women as fundamentally different. By the end of the century, reformers and politicians increasingly targeted saloons to combat men's drunken excesses and associated vices such as prostitution and gambling. Women—especially native-born Protestants—avoided saloons and public recreational drinking.¹⁰

Drinking patterns and temperance rhetoric thus buttressed the ideology of "separate spheres," a form of family and social organization that manifested the idea that women and men differed in essential ways—in their bodies; in their moral, intellectual, and spiritual natures; and in their social roles. Regarded as naturally purer than their male counterparts, women leveraged this moral authority outward to reform society through the temperance movement and other campaigns, often with the explicit goal of protecting women from men's destructive behavior. But women only achieved this influence, limited as it was, by adhering to the most stringent codes of respectability and morality. In other words, only by abstaining did women earn a voice regarding the alcohol issue.

As the temperance campaign shows, consuming drugs—or maintaining abstinence—is a way to create a social identity, reinforcing divisions along lines of gender, age, ethnicity, and class status. In the nineteenth-century context, women who drank, especially to excess, could be seen as especially degraded and debased because their consumption violated gender-role prescriptions and class-based standards of respectability. Working-class prostitutes and immigrant girls might consume alcohol in saloons, while debutantes might indulge in liquor while in cabarets, but middle-class observers considered such drinking further evidence that women like these were outside the bounds of "true" womanhood.

In contrast, women who turned to alcohol for medicinal reasons did not contradict a gendered standard but instead fulfilled it, demonstrating frailty and ill health that were consistent with idealized femininity. Middle-class women could justify alcohol use if they had medical need, especially that which might result from repeated pregnancies or other "female complaints." This kind of consumption did not look like public recreation or pleasure seeking; rather, alcohol used in this way was understood as a medicine, grouped with commercial nostrums and even narcotics, all of which women might turn to in order to cope with the pain and discomfort associated with being female.[11] This pattern of use could bring its own problems, including dependence and potential harm to offspring, especially feared when alcohol itself was regarded by many Americans as a poison. But women's motivation to drink in this manner seemed consistent with the feminine role, not a violation of it. In fact, some physicians and reformers in the late nineteenth century called for sympathetic treatment, not censure, for women (especially those women who were otherwise respectable) who became dependent on alcohol as a result of a misguided but legitimate attempt to control pain.

These vastly different views of drinking women—as especially debased or as vulnerable individuals who deserved sympathy for their suffering—remind us that the legal status or cultural acceptance of a particular substance is often less about its pharmacological effects than the meaning ascribed to those effects and the social position of the individuals and groups who use that substance.[12] Vice reformers, doctors, social scientists, and public health experts have long recognized that many people enjoy or overuse more than one substance, and they—as well as users—have identified common elements such as intoxication, craving, and loss of control that can characterize experiences with different drugs. Despite these commonalities in psychoactive effects and in the experiences of users, laws and social sanction have differentiated among various substances and their users. In the modern United States, elaborate legal, medical, and economic regimes monitor and control access to, and use of, a variety of drugs, with many distinctions made about who can consume them and under what circumstances. Legal and medical classification schemes have generally become more specialized, parsing out distinctions between legitimate drugs that are used medicinally, illicit substances, and products that are considered consumer goods (despite what may be negative health consequences).[13]

The history of alcohol in the United States illustrates these trends, illuminating how changes in the legal rules and cultural conventions regarding psychoactive substances—especially distinctions between recreational and therapeutic use—had profound implications for evolving definitions of addiction and for the gendered and racialized associations attached to various drugs. The nineteenth-century United States featured a robust and largely unregulated market in alcohol and other drugs, driven by such developments as technological innovations including the mechanical cigarette machine and the hypodermic syringe, business practices that linked brewers and saloons, and aggressive advertising that pushed "soothing syrups" for children and tonics and elixirs for women.[14] Early twentieth-century federal laws and constitutional amendments changed this landscape. The Pure Food and Drug Act (1906) created new standards for labeling and advertising, the Harrison Narcotics Tax Act (1914) imposed a much more stringent tax and regulatory structure for opiates and cocaine, and the Eighteenth Amendment to the Constitution (1920) forbade the manufacture, sale, or transportation of "intoxicating liquor."[15] These regulatory regimes arose from the belief that the targeted substances were inherently dangerous and had to be prohibited or strictly regulated to protect the health and safety of the population. As intended, they limited access to psychoactive substances; they also altered patterns of use and changed the demographics of drug users. In the case of narcotics, they shifted drug-taking practices away from medically sanctioned use (where white women once made up the majority of users of many drugs) toward recreational or illicit use, where men, especially those from socially marginal communities and from non-white racial backgrounds, played a larger role and faced more severe sanctions.[16] Moral panics over juvenile delinquency at midcentury, concern over suburban youth in the 1970s, the "war on drugs" of the 1980s, and debates about the legalization of marijuana today show that these issues remain far from settled.[17]

For all the controversy associated with drugs like heroin, alcohol remains the only substance that has merited a constitutional amendment—the Eighteenth, which established national Prohibition in 1920. While concrete data regarding alcohol consumption during Prohibition are scarce and difficult to interpret, Prohibition brought new scrutiny of women's recreational drinking. Many commentators assessed women's consumption as novel and significant, an indication of the success or failure of Prohibition as social policy. Both supporters and opponents of the Eighteenth Amendment claimed that drinking women were newly visible in public spaces such as speakeasies. Men and women drank together, shaping new dating customs and sexual expectations for young people in particular, who claimed cocktails and cigarettes as eroticized symbols of "emancipation."[18] Unlike earlier critiques of lower-class or elite women whose consumption proved their lack of morality and decorum, media attention during the 1920s focused on middle-class women, the very type whose presumed abstinence had ensured their social status in previous decades and animated the temperance campaign. In this way, drinking patterns during the Prohibition era represented a gender convergence, as women acted more like men, and also a collapse of the class-based distinctions that had once marked "respectability."

Yet these changes in drinking patterns were neither as pervasive nor as universally hailed as sophisticated journalists claimed. For one thing, important connections remained between drink and domesticity: Commentators assessed women's consumption in the context of their family roles, insisting that drinking women selfishly put their own pleasure before their maternal obligations and set a bad example for their children. Women who advocated for the repeal of Prohibition used "Home Protection" arguments that evoked the temperance crusade, now emphasizing how the excesses of Prohibition threatened youth and families.[19] Even those Americans who celebrated women's drinking feared that women were especially vulnerable to intoxication, did not know how to manage their intake, and could not be counted on to maintain control.

Journalists and social commentators depicted women's drinking during Prohibition as a search for excitement and enjoyment, eclipsing the earlier view of alcohol as medicine and the corresponding justification for women's drinking anchored in gender difference. Instead, women's consumption now looked like a claim to masculine prerogatives such as pleasure, relaxation, autonomy, and a release from domestic obligations. The very assertion that respectable women desired these privileges could be seen as a threat to family stability and social order. It also meant forfeiting the position women had once held as innocent victims of men's excesses. For those who disapproved of wider changes in women's roles during the 1920s, drinking habits became an obvious target.

The repeal of Prohibition in 1933 both reflected and required a substantial shift in how Americans assessed the substance of alcohol. Constituencies as diverse as scientific researchers and liquor advertisers dismissed the temperance-era depiction of alcohol as an inherently dangerous substance. These efforts, along with narcotics laws that had dissociated alcohol from other drugs, recast alcohol as a legitimate consumer good—even as marijuana, cocaine, and narcotics became increasingly marginalized and their users prosecuted more vigorously.[20] As alcohol became more mainstream, its gendered meanings became more important, rather than less, obscuring other differences of socioeconomic class, ethnicity, and race that had helped define the "inebriate" of the late nineteenth century and that continued to mark the users of illicit drugs in the twentieth century.

As moderate drinking—variously described as recreational, social, or "normal" consumption—became the new code against which pathological drinking would be measured, women's motivation to drink recreationally remained suspect in ways that men's did not, even after Repeal. Middle-class Americans increasingly rejected the notion that abstinence from alcohol and sexual chastity were the only acceptable standards for women, as women, too, partook of a consumer economy oriented toward personal pleasure and self-expression.[21] But how much was too much? Who should decide? How should women balance their own satisfaction with their maternal obligations and with the social expectation that they still modulate men's behavior? As Americans sought to carve out a middle ground of alcohol consumption between abstinence and pathology, women's place in that intermediate zone remained contested.

These debates intensified in the decades after Repeal as researchers reported that women's drinking and associated problems were on the rise. Frequent claims that women were "closing the gap" as their drinking patterns seemed to "catch up" with those of men reinforced the idea of drinking as a masculine prerogative while conveying confusion and disapproval regarding women's behavior.[22] These warnings have proven remarkably persistent, with the most concern aimed at the habits of middle-class women as they joined men in work and leisure and threatened to reject traditionally feminine characteristics such as selflessness, passivity, and restraint. That drinking women faced significantly greater disapproval than men before, during, and after the 1920s suggests that Prohibition and Repeal were not the social and cultural watersheds they are often presumed to be.[23]

Alcohol has thus been many things in American history: a medicine, a toxin, a source of pleasure and recreation. It has had a unique and dramatic legal history, including two constitutional amendments and a patchwork of state and local regulation both before and after Prohibition, even as it has remained embedded in social customs. Alcohol illuminates deeply gendered boundaries between acceptable and unacceptable use, between medicinal and recreational consumption, and between commercialized, public venues and private, domestic space. As legal, medical, and political systems increased the penalties for using other drugs and pushed their users—including smokers[24]—farther to the social margins over the course of the twentieth century, alcohol assumed a larger role as a culturally acceptable psychoactive substance. While other substances such as cocaine, heroin, methamphetamine, and even cigarettes have been categorized as inherently addictive and dangerous by conventional wisdom as well as by legal and medical regulation in the twentieth century, alcohol carries the potential for both "normal" and "pathological" patterns of use; it threatens the health and well-being of some people but not others. Just as temperance rhetoric mirrored and reinforced the ideology of separate spheres, so mid-twentieth-century drinking customs embodied and reflected an emerging gender system that took shape amid World War II and its aftermath. As women's roles looked dangerously unstable, alcohol consumption served as a shorthand to monitor changes in mainstream femininity.

Alcoholism and the Challenge of Medicalization

After Mann was profiled in *Reader's Digest* in 1963, the National Council on Alcoholism received hundreds of letters from individuals who struggled with their drinking, as well as from their concerned family members and friends. These letters provide important clues into American attitudes about alcoholism in the 1960s, about the experiences of those who suffered from problem drinking, and how family circumstances and domestic ideology shaped alcoholic women's lives, including access to treatment. As one woman wrote to Mann: "I've read your article on alcoholism many times and found that the experiences you went through are about the same as I am going through. . . . Can I ask you to help me as you have helped others? *I'm lost*, alone and without a friend in the world, even my folks, sisters and so-called friends and neighbors, just everyone. My husband also hates me and even my four children turned from me. You say alcoholism is a disease!! Can I ever find the cure?"[25] This woman felt a strong sense of connection with Mann's life story, and Mann served as living proof that female alcoholics could stop drinking. But this letter shows the risks, as well as the promise, in calling alcoholism a "disease." Alienated from her family, isolated and scared, this woman's poignant query—"Can I ever find the cure?"—suggests a fear that her condition might be hopeless. At the same time, her wording reflects the expectation that diseases, by definition, could be cured by modern medicine, an optimistic equation of almost mathematical precision and a basic feature of medicalization.

A multifaceted phenomenon, "medicalization" involves the power to define diseases, to diagnose or differentiate between people who manifest illness and those who do not, to provide treatment, and to oversee strategies of prevention.[26] As the just-quoted letter to Mann reveals, medicalization brings with it the presumption that the disorder will be cured and that the sufferer, in exchange for relinquishing control (and privacy) to experts, will find relief. At least in the abstract, medicalization also implies that the person exhibiting sickness should not be blamed for his or her misfortune.

Medicalization is a broad concept that can oversimplify historical developments by suggesting an inevitable forward progress. Scientists, physicians, and the lay public might assume that medicalization reflects a straightforward search for an unchanging biological truth. With a different goal but yielding a similar result of overgeneralizing complex events and motivations, some sociologists and historians used the concept to characterize physicians and other elites as aggressive agents of social control who forced new disease categories on unwitting or unwilling populations in order to strengthen their own status. As recent scholars have shown, however, medicalization is a nuanced, dynamic process, not a fixed end point; accordingly, it need not be an interpretive "blunt instrument."[27]

The concept retains significant utility because it reminds us that naming an aspect of human experience a "real disease" is to make "a historically contingent, political statement."[28] Those who called alcoholism a "disease"—whether they were doctors, scientists, public health advocates, or individuals who struggled with their own drinking—were not simply quibbling over nomenclature but staking a claim to an entire constellation of values and resources in modern America for a category of people frequently dismissed as unworthy and abject. To assert further, as Mann and others did, that drinking women—viewed as a morally compromised, deviant minority even among alcoholics—also deserved sympathy, understanding, and the best that modern medicine could offer was an even more radical declaration.

Many people might assume that characterizing addiction as a medical matter is a recent development, but as early as the eighteenth century, the physician Benjamin Rush called excessive drinking a "disease of the will," a phrase that captured the persistent paradox that still underlies the diagnosis.[29] Following Rush, some nineteenth-century physicians defined "dipsomania" and "inebriety" as distinct conditions that were characterized by chronic drunkenness but not reducible to it. These diagnoses coexisted awkwardly with a popular view that excessive drinking was a sin and that those who did it simply lacked willpower. As we have seen, women were expected to serve as a morally pure counterpoint to drinking men, and it seemed to follow that fewer women than men should drink to excess. Accordingly, most people did not share the sympathetic view of inebriate specialists but instead regarded women with drinking problems as especially debased. And gradually, the temperance argument that alcohol itself should be prohibited because of the widespread danger it posed to health and social stability overshadowed alternative approaches such as individualized medical treatment.

Although it is not generally thought of as such, Prohibition represented a large-scale public health measure—itself a form of medicalization—designed to remove a dangerous toxin from American life. Antiliquor advocates and many physicians and scientists predicted that alcohol-related health and social problems would disappear once Prohibition took effect. Their optimism proved unwarranted, but meanwhile medical attention dwindled, inebriate asylums closed, and aging specialists retired or died, leaving room for new constituencies to step forward after Repeal.

The National Committee for Education on Alcoholism (NCEA), along with research bodies such as the Yale Center for Alcohol Studies and the lay health movement of Alcoholics Anonymous (founded in 1935), have been dubbed in retrospect the "modern alcoholism movement." This wide cast of characters included social workers, psychologists, and psychiatrists; clergy; lawyers and policy makers; and the basic scientists whose findings can inform clinical practice—as well as alcoholics and their family members. The diversity of these groups, and their emergence and interactions in the 1930s and 1940s, illustrate important dynamics of medicalization, a messy process that unfolded unevenly over time and can even be reversed.

This new generation of disease model advocates faced a challenging situation. By this point, the medical landscape had changed in fundamental ways since the days of Benjamin Rush. In the twentieth-century United States, medicalization flowed in part from dramatic therapeutic and public health successes, each adding to the cultural prestige of medicine and raising the expectations of the general public. Clean water, pure milk, and the eradication of some infectious diseases all reinforced the power of scientific medicine, as did "magic bullets" such as vaccines and antibiotics. Each new triumph strengthened a definition of "disease" as something that is caused by a specific germ, verified by a laboratory procedure, and cured by a particular therapeutic agent. Yet alcoholism did not fit this typical medicalization script; it lacked a clear cause, a precise diagnostic test, and a standardized treatment regimen driven by scientific research. Rather than victims of an invisible infectious agent, alcoholics seemed to drink deliberately even when they claimed they wanted to stop.[30]

As they navigated the legacy of Prohibition, Marty Mann and her allies sought to translate alcoholism into a "disease," thereby capturing the enthusiasm and optimism associated with medicine in the middle decades of the twentieth century.[31] They carefully sidestepped the issue of social or recreational drinking lest they be accused of lingering prohibitionist sentiments. "Normal" drinking, they declared, was not their concern; rather, they directed their efforts toward those individuals whose extreme drinking patterns showed they belonged in a special category, that of alcoholic. In this way, disease model advocates articulated a key element of medicalization: drawing a line between the sick and the well, the pathological and the normal.

If some people could drink alcohol occasionally with no ill effects while others could not, the difference must be in the people; it was harder to blame alcohol in the post-Repeal climate. Various experts, along with the AA fellowship, all located the source of alcoholism in the body or mind of the person who became alcoholic, even if they disagreed about the causal mechanism and what should be done about it. Psychiatrists focused on underlying neurosis and recommended psychotherapy and, in some cases, hospitalization. Social workers helped clients cope with life circumstances and family roles. The AA fellowship and the advocates it influenced offered a way to understand alcoholism that was elegant in its simplicity even as it risked circularity: Alcoholics drink the way they do because they are alcoholics. The solution was to stop drinking, which was possible through spiritual reflection, intensive self-scrutiny, and the support of the fellowship.

The mutual construction of a disease model of alcoholism and a "new normal" in drinking customs in the post-Repeal era shows that the medicalization process does not only involve dramatic, life-threatening conditions but also common behavioral norms. In this sense, medicalization brings, not only the authority to care for those judged to be sick, but also the power to create regulations and guidelines for everyone's behavior in the interest of health.[32] Indeed, the more mainstream alcohol became in American life, the more expansive the power of experts to scrutinize it, since "normal" drinking represented the necessary counterpoint to pathology. But that degree of monitoring rests on a presumption that the line between health and illness be clear and consistent, and such was not the case when it came to drinking.

The repeal of Prohibition in 1933 marked alcohol as distinct from other drugs, and organizations like the NCEA and AA contributed to this separation as is evident in their names. Focusing only on alcohol had the potential to lower stigma for alcoholics. After all, their substance was legal, and they were not junkies.[33] Race played a critical role here as well. As illicit drugs became more associated with African Americans and other minority groups in the twentieth century, the stigma grew, for men and women alike, as other scholars have shown.[34] But as alcohol became more normalized, the stigma attached to alcoholic women diverged from that associated with alcoholic men. Exclusive attention to alcohol obscured an earlier model of inebriety in which individuals might become dependent on a substance out of medical need—whether morphine, patent medicines, or alcohol itself. Because that pattern of use had been more common for women and that definition of inebriety more often associated with them, its eclipse meant that addicted women lost the sanction—limited as it might have been—attached to alcohol as a therapeutic drug.[35] Alcohol might no longer be a poison, but it was no longer a legitimate medicine, either—for women or for anyone else. As a result, the recreational meaning attached to alcohol consumption became more important than ever.

Because disease model advocates like Mann tried to avoid detailed discussion of social drinking, they defined "normal" mostly by default, leaving an interpretive vacuum that could easily be filled by the belief that a woman's motivation to drink must be suspect. Even acknowledging that such a double standard persisted—as some psychiatrists did—risked embedding pejorative assessments into the diagnosis, since those experts often resorted to judgmental language when emphasizing the degree to which their patients' drinking violated social custom. The experiences of alcoholic women show that an ostensibly objective, universal standard of identifying diseases and treating patients never fully eclipsed an earlier model in which the sufferer's personal characteristics and behavior were always already implicated in her illness.

The idea that drinking by women was more unusual—and therefore more clinically and socially significant—than the same behavior in men also shaped a concern with numbers, the persistent idea that alcoholic women might be fewer than their male counterparts but that they demonstrated greater pathology. Just as women's recreational drinking took on exaggerated symbolic value, especially during and after Prohibition, so, too, female alcoholics prompted alarm and confusion disproportionate to their numbers. Scientific and popular commentators from the temperance era through the mid-twentieth century concluded that far fewer women became alcoholic than did men, but the number of alcoholic women seemed always to be increasing, converging with the rate among men. Warnings about women's drinking and alcoholism rates thus closely mirrored generalized concern that women were abandoning conventional roles and behavior in many realms.

Statistical and scientific conventions in the twentieth century reinforced the idea that women formed a particularly intractable subset of alcoholics. In tracking alcoholism after the repeal of Prohibition in 1933, many researchers reported their findings in terms of a sex ratio rather than in absolute numbers, partly because it was a more convenient measure as they simply indicated the gendered distribution in their patient population or study sample. But framing the issue in this way also communicated the idea that male alcoholics were always the baseline against which women's changing behavior should be assessed. In the three decades following Repeal, estimates of the sex ratio among alcoholics varied widely but tended to cluster around 6:1 (six male alcoholics to every female alcoholic). While some scientists maintained that this ratio was consistent over time and that any apparent increase resulted from women's greater willingness to seek treatment, other experts insisted that more and more women were drinking to excess.[36] The popular media promoted this latter conclusion; newspaper articles reported that drunk driving, arrests for public intoxication, and hospitalization for alcoholism were all increasing among women.[37]

These assertions were especially alarming since clinicians, including leading psychiatrists, reported that alcoholic women were harder to treat and less likely to recover than their male counterparts. Initially responding to women with resistance or at least ambivalence, the Alcoholics Anonymous fellowship similarly characterized women as a distinct class, even when they were accepted into the group. Because women seemed to be an unusual minority, alcoholism scholars frequently excluded them from field-defining research during these decades. In a vicious cycle, this marginalization of female alcoholics allowed harmful stereotypes to persist and made it more difficult for many alcoholic women to receive appropriate care.

Disease model advocates like Marty Mann believed that only the prestige of science and medicine could counteract the stigma and other challenges alcoholics faced, yet it was not always easy to separate medicalization from criminalization (even with an exclusive focus on alcoholism rather than illicit drugs). Public intoxication and drunk driving remained crimes; some of the individuals who were arrested and prosecuted for these violations may have been alcoholics, while others were not. Moreover, commitment in a hospital for "treatment" could resemble incarceration in some ways.

So even as advocates insisted that medicalization represented a humane alternative to criminalization as well as to neglect, we must recognize that medicalization, too, involves questions of power, sometimes in surprising and indirect ways. Alcoholism shows that disease concepts evolve over time through oblique and overlapping processes in which doctors and scientists do not always play the leading roles.[38] Mann and other advocates tried to convince medical professionals that they should provide care to alcoholics, complicating the view of medicalization as an ever-expanding process in which doctors take an enthusiastic lead. Alcoholism, by contrast, demonstrates that expertise also gives professionals the authority to refuse to bring a condition under the umbrella of medical sanction and care—and the ability to deny attention is also an expression of power.

Lady Lushes focuses primarily on middle-class white women because they were the ones most likely to have access to (or be subjected to) the medicalization process. Patients and family members sometimes welcomed and even sought out medical intervention, as the letter to Mann, cited at the beginning of this section, demonstrates.[39] Others preferred to avoid it. Some members of the general public viewed medicalization as a positive result of scientific progress, while others dismissed it as a troubling and expensive interference in aspects of life that should be "natural," or private, or—in the case of alcoholism—a matter of willpower or sin that was not "medical" at all. Because medicalization includes multiple elements, doctors, patients, or the public could embrace a diagnosis like alcoholism but reject its treatment or policy implications;[40] alternatively, they might covet the funds or opportunities that come when a problem is defined while rejecting the interpretive framework that made those resources possible.

The various forms of authority inherent in medicalization often affected women even more directly than men, for economic, familial, and social reasons. Men were more likely to have the personal autonomy and financial control necessary to seek treatment, if they wished it, or to refuse it. Furthermore, while men's drinking took a toll on their families—as temperance rhetoric had long highlighted—a wife was expected to rally to her husband's support, providing emotional resilience and a commitment to his sobriety and family stability. For women, however, the diagnosis of alcoholism, let alone hospitalization or incarceration, became deeply entwined with dependence in the family, domestic obligations, and opportunities (or lack thereof) in the wider society. As long as motherhood remained central to definitions of womanhood, women's drinking drew particular scrutiny for "the sake of the children," even if not for women's own health. By the middle decades of the twentieth century, alcohol was no longer characterized as a literal poison to the next generation as it had been previously (and would be again). Still, experts warned that the psychological and social implications of drinking, including intoxication, remained incompatible with successful adjustment to, and fulfillment of, the maternal role.

Even as they insisted that alcoholism should be viewed and treated as a disease, researchers, clinicians, and advocates acknowledged that they lacked a cure. As Sarah W. Tracy and Trysh Travis have shown, alcoholism thus raised critical questions about how clinicians, patients, and historians might define "health" in the face of illnesses that are understood to be chronic.[41] In alcoholism, improvement could not be measured by a negative result on a laboratory test, the absence of virus, or the removal of a tumor; it was, instead, a state of being, one to be cultivated and demonstrated, in which abstinence from alcohol was a necessary but not sufficient therapeutic indicator. Recovery could be shown particularly through a return to respectability and productivity, including conformance to conventional gender roles. In this way, alcoholism presaged late twentieth-century "lifestyle" diseases such as hypertension, Type II diabetes, and obesity, where the individual takes on responsibility, understood in both medical and moral terms, for regulating the appetite that created the condition in the first place. Health is not measured simply as a neutral state in which disease is absent; rather, it is a purposeful way of life that recursively articulates ideas about alcoholism, even though recovery itself is not necessarily understood in primarily medical terms. Paradoxically, alcoholics who have arrested their drinking can claim an ongoing, permanent identity as alcoholics (always "recovering") even as they demonstrate, through their current health and normalcy, the mirror image of illness and deviance. As Marty Mann understood very well, the stakes in demonstrating recovery could hardly be higher for those who wanted to prove that alcoholics could stop drinking and deserved help in doing so.

But decades of temperance rhetoric and subsequent criticism of women's consumption as unfeminine had primed Americans to believe that drinking was not something that came naturally to women, and therefore women who did it, especially to excess, were unusual in some way—more sinful, more deviant, more pathological, simply *more* of whatever explanatory model was in vogue. For female alcoholics, this disease begged the question of what kind of women they were, creating ongoing comparisons with alcoholic men, on the one hand, and non-alcoholic women, on the other. That they even had the disease indicated that something was wrong with them as women, and this judgment became built into the diagnosis itself.

In this context, Mann insisted that the disease of alcoholism could strike anyone; gender was secondary at best and generally irrelevant. This posture could assert an equivalence between men and women and thus stake a wider claim for equality. Yet Mann and other prominent alcoholic women in recovery used traditionally feminine symbols to reassure audiences that not only had they stopped drinking, they were back to normal as women. Mann, for example, concealed a decades-long lesbian relationship from the public. Her overall strategy is understandable, since her goal was to use the cultural prestige of scientific medicine to reduce the stigma associated with alcoholism for men and women alike, not to remake gender roles. As a result, her prominence as a female alcoholic expanded Americans' understanding of who could suffer from the condition. But her identity as an alcoholic woman did not similarly transform definitions of womanhood, as disease-model advocacy collided with the unsettled gender-role system of mid-twentieth-century America. Even Mann's efforts were not enough to remake the therapeutic and social landscape for alcoholic women. The story of alcoholism thus demonstrates that medicalization may reinforce harmful, stereotypical judgments and unequal treatment, rather than erasing them.

The "Disease of the Will": Feminism, Biology, and Historical Agency

I have been inspired by pioneering scholars of the 1960s and 1970s who defined women's health as a legitimate topic for historical inquiry. Themselves immersed in the cultural milieu of second-wave feminism, they analyzed nineteenth-century patterns of birth control and abortion, gynecological surgery, and the meaning of illness for women, often scrutinizing power dynamics between women and their doctors. These scholars demonstrated that nineteenth-century women were subjected to unnecessary and even dangerous medical procedures and institutionalization against their will.[42]

While this attention to intersections of expertise, gender, and power yielded critical insights about the effects of medicalization on women, especially in male-dominated systems of care, more recent studies have emphasized the ways in which individual patients and families negotiated with and even manipulated doctors and other health professionals to meet their own needs.[43] For example, twentieth-century women's health advocates demanded more research and aggressive treatment for illnesses, such as breast cancer, that had been overlooked because they disproportionately affect women.[44] In other cases, women fought for interventions that seem troubling in retrospect but represented the most promising strategy at the time. Women in the early decades of the twentieth century wanted to give birth under "Twilight Sleep," a combination of drugs that rendered women unconscious during childbirth and amnesiac afterward but that promised relief from pain.[45] Later generations of women reversed this equation and viewed childbirth without drugs as empowering, but in both cases, birthing women sought to negotiate with medical professionals to get the care they wanted. And as Judith Houck reminds us in her study of menopause, "Feminist scholars cannot claim that women have agency only when they make choices we like."[46]

It is also worth noting that, in all these instances, the health condition reinforced the salience of biological sex differences and the identity of patients as women. Alcoholism, generally considered a man's disease, marked female sufferers as different, unusual, even "unnatural" among those who manifested the condition, and as such, it illustrates the intersection of medical authority with gender-role ideology differently.

Alcoholism poses particular challenges in assessing the intent of historical actors, and I attend to issues of power and voice regardless of the demographic characteristics of the women in question. To that end, this book draws on a range of sources, including medical and social science literature; archival materials of the National Committee for Education on Alcoholism, Alcoholics Anonymous, and the personal papers of Marty Mann; autobiographical writings of alcoholic women; and depictions of alcoholic women in the popular media, such as fiction, film, and press coverage of alcoholic celebrities. In each case these sources need to be read with care, and each comes with its own caveats. When considered in combination, however, they offer a wider perspective on the issues at play. The vast amount of popular culture materials, in particular, could merit a full book of its own. Here, I have drawn on them selectively to illustrate this book's central themes of medicalization and gender-role transformation.

While some female patients have faced medical interventions they never desired, other suffering women have searched in vain for any care at all. These contradictory forces shaped the experiences of women who drank: Such a woman might be pressured into treatment she did not want, on the one hand, or denied professional attention because neither she nor anyone around her viewed excessive drinking as a legitimate medical problem, on the other. Some alcoholic women like Marty Mann conquered their compulsion to drink, created productive lives, and articulated a new sense of self—but many others did not. It may be impossible to reconstruct their experiences. And the drive to drink—whether a "disease" or not—may itself have cost some women their voices.

Tracing the metamorphosis of the "fallen angel" and female inebriate of the late nineteenth century into the "lady lush" of the post–World War II era also raises thorny questions related to feminism and the politics of alcohol consumption. It can be difficult to achieve an appropriate balance regarding autonomy and choice. In the 1990s, two social scientists, Laura Schmidt and Constance Weisner, coined the terms "dry feminism" and "wet feminism."[47] According to their model, dry feminists focused on health and safety, emphasizing the risks associated with alcohol consumption and recommending moderation or abstinence. In contrast, wet feminists interpreted women's access to alcohol, drugs, and other forms of public recreation and pleasure as progressive and emancipatory. These terms emerged to characterize how dry feminists—professionals and activists who worked in alcoholism treatment settings—sought to include more women in alcohol-related research designs, policy and funding priorities, and treatment facilities. Wet feminists celebrated women's right to engage in recreational alcohol use and generally avoided the question of addiction. Dry and wet feminism echoed a division in second-wave feminism between "difference" feminists, who emphasized the distinctive character of the female body and celebrated qualities such as nurturance that seemed to follow from it, and "equality" feminists, who sought to create a society that rendered biological differences between men and women irrelevant.[48]

I argue that these concepts of dry and wet feminism offer analytical utility beyond the chronological period that spawned them.[49] For example, temperance advocates highlighted the danger that alcohol, when consumed by men, posed to women and thus can be seen as part of a dry feminist impulse. Conversely, the "New Woman" of the 1910s and the "flapper" figure of the 1920s came to symbolize wet feminism and the claim that drinking and smoking went along with the right to vote, to drive, and to work for wages. Still, not everyone fits neatly into one category or the other. Marty Mann, for instance, attempted to transcend these divisions as she pushed for a disease model that she hoped would neutralize gender difference even as she conveyed a conventionally feminine persona. Moreover, alcohol consumption does not necessarily confer autonomy and freedom on the drinker—in light of other restrictions women face, drinking might render a woman less powerful and more vulnerable. Even if it has symbolic value in cultural terms, access to alcohol does not guarantee political, economic, or social equality.

In fact, some scholars and critics have depicted drinking by women (and other groups such as American Indians) not as a positive choice to seize the privileges and pleasures of a modern consumer culture but as a desperate attempt to cope with oppression.[50] This insight is important, yet it risks shading into a glorification of resistance. While it is easy to imagine individual cases in which a woman drank as a coping strategy, to opt out of her domestic responsibilities, interpreting women's drinking as a liberating, protofeminist strategy carries its own, significant risks.[51] We must not minimize or overlook the emotional anguish, physical health consequences, and damaged personal relationships that accompanied women's problem drinking, as the dry feminist perspective reminds us.

Historians have shown that it is possible to analyze the evolution of ideas about disease without losing sight of the experiences of real people in the past. I have found the models offered by several other historians of gender and medicine particularly helpful in organizing these themes. In particular, Joan Jacobs Brumberg offers a fascinating and useful conceptual framework in *Fasting Girls*, her study of anorexia nervosa. She maintains that the etiology of anorexia nervosa has three major components: biomedical, psychological, and cultural, and each plays a role, separately and together. Social and cultural cues shape young women's relationships with food and attitudes toward their bodies, yet clearly individual factors are also involved, as not all young women respond to cultural messages in the same way.[52] Similarly, we know that alcohol has exerted a special kind of pull for some individuals, who are attracted to it for a variety of psychological, physiological, and social reasons despite the distress it can cause. Historical context and cultural cues clearly shape the incidence and expression of symptoms in a condition like alcoholism; they help to explain both the changing frequency of the condition over time as well as the different rates of occurrence among men and women.

Scholarship in the history of medicine has been so successful in illuminating the political, cultural, social, and medical meanings of various drugs that it can be easy to overlook pharmacology.[53] This is a mistake. Alcohol is more than a symbol; it is also a biological and psychoactive agent, and only by acknowledging that reality can we fully appreciate how its physiological effects have been highlighted or obscured in cultural terms. Scientific and popular depictions of drinking women suggest an underlying fear that the substance alters them profoundly, that the state of intoxication is especially dangerous for them and those for whom they bear responsibility. Similarly, the scientific and social characterization of alcohol as a poison largely faded after Prohibition—until it was revived and linked to maternal drinking in the last third of the twentieth century.[54]

The history of drinking women shows that, despite major shifts in gender roles, social transformation has foundered on biological sex differences and their implications for human reproduction, family responsibilities, and public comportment. Whatever the health and social consequences of drinking may be, women embody heightened risks and responsibilities. Today, any woman of childbearing age—even if not visibly pregnant—might face a disapproving look or even a refusal of service when she orders a drink. If she is known or presumed to be in the market for motherhood, bystanders may remind her that drinking and pregnancy do not mix. The Eighteenth Amendment is no longer the law of the land, but even today, women can be subjected to de facto prohibition.

Terminology

A few words about terminology. Studying problem drinking over a period of one hundred and twenty-five years requires sensitivity to many shifts in language, which themselves reflect changing ideas about the nature and significance of alcohol use and dependence. During the late nineteenth century, for example, physicians involved in the American Association for the Study and

Cure of Inebriety, a group that wanted to medicalize excessive drinking, used the term "inebriety" to refer to the condition and "inebriate" as a label for the individual drinker. "Dipsomania" was also a term used by medical and popular writers of the period to connote a medicalized view of the condition. Both inebriety and dipsomania were self-consciously used to contrast with the more common terms "drunk" or "drunkard," to emphasize that excessive drinking was neither a sin nor a lack of willpower but a problem to be handled by physicians and others with scientific expertise.

In the early years of the twentieth century, "alcoholic" became an adjective to describe certain types of beverages at the same time that, used as a noun, it referred to individuals addicted to alcohol.[55] "Alcoholism" gradually became the preferred term for the condition within the medical community and for educated laypeople alike, although older terms such as "drunk" have persisted. Other pejorative terms, such as "lush," came in and out of style. The concept of "addiction" has been greatly broadened in our own day, but the underlying notion (and the label "addict") was used in earlier eras as well, often interchangeably with "habit" and "habitual drinker." Similarly, while scientists and physicians debate the precise clinical meaning of "dependence" on alcohol and other drugs, the concept has a commonsense quality that makes it a useful term for most laypeople. Both medical and lay writers frequently felt the need for a modifier when a woman was the subject of any of these: female alcoholics, for example, or lady lushes. I have tried to avoid anachronistic usages of all these terms by following the conventions of the period under discussion; in some cases, however, I do default to "alcoholism" or "alcoholic," as those are the terms most familiar to readers today.

Finally, I use "alcohol" to refer to any intoxicating beverage, occasionally alternating with "liquor" as another generic term. As appropriate, I use "beer," "wine," or "spirits" for specific references to those beverages.

Plan of the Book

Chapter 1: "The Female Inebriate in the Temperance Paradigm." The book begins with the "inebriety movement" of the late nineteenth century, when some physicians argued that respectable women drank in order to cope with the pain and discomfort of being female. These doctors created a relatively sympathetic model of women's excessive drinking, centered on the idea of gender difference. Although these women were not necessarily blamed for their habit, concern with the reproductive implications of women's alcohol use served to justify a lasting double standard in the treatment of inebriate women.

This chapter also analyzes fictional accounts and a nineteenth-century recovery narrative to show that these sources, like medical literature, emphasized connections between women's drinking and the biological and social dimensions of motherhood.

Chapter 2: "'Lit Ladies': Women's Drinking during the Progressive Era and Prohibition." This chapter addresses debates about women's public drinking during the late nineteenth and early twentieth centuries, culminating in the Prohibition period. These drinking customs—in public places and in mixed-gender company—served as a dramatic counterpoint to the hidden drinking of delicate female inebriates. Changes in women's comportment accelerated in the 1920s when the flapper—a young woman with bobbed hair, short skirt, and a cocktail in hand—became an emblematic figure. Even more disturbing were "lit ladies," adult women who tried, often unsuccessfully, to learn to drink and whose intoxication threatened conventional roles and respectability. These images contributed to the persistent belief that alcohol consumption, especially among women, increased during Prohibition—despite evidence to the contrary. In fact, women's overt alcohol use remained a powerful symbol of rebellion or modernity precisely because many Americans remained ambivalent about women's new behaviors. Yet one thing had changed: Women forfeited the position they had once held as innocent victims of men's excessive use of alcohol.

Chapter 3: "'More to Overcome than the Men': Women in Alcoholics Anonymous." A mutual-help organization, established by alcoholics soon after the repeal of Prohibition, Alcoholics Anonymous was originally structured around alcoholic men and their nonalcoholic wives, reflecting both a demographic reality and a persistent cultural echo from the temperance era. As a result, the fellowship perpetuated a stereotypical distinction between "good" and "bad" women, and alcoholic women who approached the group often confronted exclusion and discrimination that stemmed from the belief that they were especially degraded. Despite these challenges, pioneering women such as Marty Mann achieved sobriety through the fellowship, sometimes by creating women-only groups. This strategy highlighted a tension between their identity as women and the emerging, ostensibly gender-neutral, category of "alcoholic." The belief that women formed a separate category of alcoholics persisted for decades, as evident in the 1962 film *The Days of Wine and Roses*, analyzed here, as well as in the retrospective competition for the title of "First Woman in AA."

Chapter 4: "Defining a Disease: Gender, Stigma, and the Modern Alcoholism Movement." Along with Alcoholics Anonymous, research scientists, clinicians, and advocates sought to define and explain alcoholism and to facilitate treatment in the post-Repeal period, and their collective efforts have been dubbed the "modern alcoholism movement." Marty Mann emerged as the movement's charismatic spokesperson, energetically spreading the news that alcoholism was properly understood as a disease and that recovery was possible. This chapter finds ironies in the complex process of medicalization, analyzing the gendered implications of Mann's public health campaign. As she carefully negotiated the legacy of the temperance movement, Mann offered herself as living proof that alcoholism could afflict anyone. Yet despite claims that women's drinking was on the rise in the World War II era, research methods in the social and natural sciences tended to exclude women's experiences—just as important new models were taking shape. This pattern was especially unfortunate as biases about alcoholic women became embedded into the diagnosis of alcoholism, with the growing prestige of scientific medicine making them that much harder to dislodge.

Chapter 5: "'A Special Masculine Neurosis': Psychiatrists Look at Alcoholism." Psychiatrists and other mental health experts asserted themselves as another influential constituency shaping post-Prohibition understandings of alcoholism. While the Alcoholics Anonymous fellowship and advocates in the modern alcoholism movement often sidestepped issues of sexuality and related matters, psychiatrists highlighted them. Psychiatrists understood alcoholism as the result of a failure to "adjust" to conventional roles because of underlying psychological conflicts and weaknesses. Recognizing that American society retained a double standard regarding even casual drinking, psychiatrists insisted that those women who turned to alcohol despite social sanction must be especially disturbed. Psychiatric discussion of alcoholism during the middle decades of the twentieth century reinforced ideas about masculinity and femininity as Americans grew concerned about the effects of economic crisis and war on family stability.

Chapter 6: "'The Doctor Didn't Want to Take an Alcoholic': The Challenge of Medicalization at Midcentury." The modern alcoholism movement achieved important successes by the late 1950s and early 1960s, when various professional groups—including the American Medical Association—declared that alcoholism should be considered a disease. But simply articulating this view did not lead automatically to a standard treatment regimen or even an agreed-upon diagnosis or definition of cure. This chapter assesses treatment protocols to explore how women's experiences differed from men's in terms of diagnosis, access to care, and hospital commitment. Even in the most cutting-edge and ostensibly objective forms of medical care, social perceptions of women and women's roles continued to inform treatment approaches and patient evaluation. Doctors consistently reported that women did not respond well to treatment. Although this finding might have thrown the entire disease model into question, it instead reinforced the idea that women were a particularly intractable subset of alcoholics. In contrast to specialized medical regimens overseen by physicians, social workers who ran programs in jails and hospitals that focused on women provided a wider range of support services tailored to women's particular needs—even as they drew on the prestige of medicine to do so.

Epilogue: The early 1960s represent a capstone moment, as demonstrated by the juxtaposition of Mann's confessional profile in *Reader's Digest* with the 1962 film *The Days of Wine and Roses*, in which a young woman was depicted as an irredeemable alcoholic even as her husband recovers from the same disease. This book's epilogue touches on several post-1960s developments to underscore how some ideas about gender and alcohol have remained remarkably persistent, continuing to shape medical and scientific knowledge about problem drinking and its effects. I explore the late twentieth-century phenomena of Fetal Alcohol Syndrome, which demonized alcoholic women, and Mothers Against Drunk Drivers, an organization that echoed temperance discourse in identifying women and children as innocent victims of male drunken excess. The cultural power of these contemporaneous movements demonstrates the staying power of alcohol as a force that in important ways still channels, and sometimes challenges, gender roles in modern America.

Chapter 1

The Female Inebriate in the Temperance Paradigm

In 1888, twenty-five-year-old Mrs. C. of Davenport, Iowa, once a "most exemplary wife and devoted mother," became transformed almost beyond recognition when she drank.[1] Mrs. C.'s dependence on alcohol stemmed from chronic health problems associated with the birth of her second child. A lengthy labor, the use of forceps during the delivery, and extensive maternal bleeding had all resulted in "general debility and nervousness which persisted for weeks." Ongoing problems with her uterus and a severe backache made Mrs. C. "faint and dizzy" when she tried to get out of bed. To help her cope, her doctor had recommended wine, which "promptly relieved the horrible sinking feeling" she experienced. Unfortunately for herself and her family, Mrs. C. turned to wine "with increasing frequency" and built up a considerable tolerance. Finding that "something stronger was necessary to satisfy the uncontrollable craving" she had acquired, she switched to whiskey and then brandy. As her drinking increased, she developed other health problems, including neuralgia, a disordered appetite, and constipation. Most troubling of all, she was no longer the kind and dedicated mother she had been but was instead "entirely indifferent to her children, irritable and abusive." Despite her husband's pleas that she abstain, she could not resist the "insatiable craving" at each menstrual period, when she "drank to stupefaction."

Mrs. C. fell victim to what is known as an "iatrogenic addiction," where sanctioned medical use of a substance evolves into dependence. According to the doctor reporting her case (who was not the physician who had originally prescribed the wine), female physiological and reproductive events had sparked Mrs. C.'s drinking problem. Accordingly, alleviating her uterine condition represented the first step in addressing her reliance on alcohol. With a combination of the "most strict surveillance which kept temptation out her way" and "the exercise of strong will-power," she refrained from drinking for one year. At that point, she suffered a miscarriage with severe hemorrhaging, a situation which "brought to light the smothered propensity." The urge to drink made it impossible for her to fulfill her domestic responsibilities; as the reporting doctor explained somberly, "the morbid craving proved stronger than maternal love or family pride." As before, the doctor's first step was to restore her physical health, then she "more gradually regained her self-control." Although she apparently abstained from then on, she still felt the "impulse" to consume alcohol at "every menstrual period."

Mrs. C.'s story appeared in the *Quarterly Journal of Inebriety*. Beginning in 1879, this journal was published by the American Association for the Study and Cure of Inebriety, a group of physicians and asylum superintendents who challenged the widely held view that drinking to excess was a sin and that those who did so simply lacked willpower. These doctors argued instead that such a compulsion should be understood as a medical problem, one that could be cured through treatment by professionals, often in specialized institutions.[2] Their efforts can be seen as part of a wider professionalizing impulse during the late nineteenth century, a period when Americans increasingly believed that science could resolve many of the social and economic problems that seemed to threaten the country. This chapter explores how doctors involved in this "inebriety movement" made sense of women's drinking in the context of wider ideas about women's health and women's roles. Medical literature and treatment protocols, patent medicine advertisements, and even popular fiction all rested on the belief that men and women were fundamentally different, and all reinforced a connection between women's drinking and the biological and social dimensions of motherhood.

Temperance, "Female Complaints," and Drinking in the Post–Civil War Era

Although many Americans considered alcohol a central part of dietary and social customs during the colonial era and the early years of the republic, mid-nineteenth-century reformers channeled their increasing concern about the health and social consequences of liquor consumption into a political movement. Like other nineteenth-century movements, including abolitionism and woman's rights, the temperance campaign included individuals and constituencies who did not always agree on priorities or strategies. Temperance advocates gradually shifted from a tactic of moral suasion—convincing people that alcohol was so dangerous they should moderate its use or give it up voluntarily—to that of prohibition through legislation, using the law to rid society of liquor. Stretching from antebellum initiatives to national Prohibition, the temperance campaign was one of the longest-lasting and most influential social reform movements in American history.

During the nineteenth century, most Americans believed that social roles followed automatically from biological differences between males and females. Reproduction was women's central function; family and social organization built upon the physiological reality that women, not men, became pregnant, gave birth, and fed infants. Many Americans subscribed to the doctrine of "separate spheres," distinct but complementary realms, one for men in the public world of paid work and the other for women (and children) in the private domain of the home. Drinking customs reinforced separate spheres: Men might venture into saloons, but women should stay home. As representatives of a pure and moral domestic space that served as the counterweight to the masculine excess of saloons, respectable women—whose abstinence from alcohol marked them as decent and upright—converted their moral authority into temperance advocacy under the slogan "Home Protection." The Woman's Christian Temperance Union became the largest women's organization in late nineteenth-century America and exemplified "dry feminism." Calling on men to honor their commitments to their families and emphasizing women's purity and vulnerability, temperance advocates offered a way to achieve respectability—a key component of middle-class status in America—through behavior.[3]

While early scholarship focused on the political and social dimensions of the temperance movement, more recent work has explored the ways in which literary, legal, and medical debates about drinking and temperance shaped the meaning of the family; concepts of masculinity as well as femininity; and nineteenth-century notions of the self. Although drinking was a masculine act, the state of drunkenness and a reliance on alcohol threatened a man's self-control, a fundamental trait for Americans in this era. Too much drinking might render him dependent and undermine his position in his family as well as his status as a citizen. Men and women involved in the temperance movement crafted narratives in which they reflected on how drinking—their own or, in the case of women, usually that of a family member—had influenced their lives. The authors of these narratives articulated both a renewed sense of self and a new vision for society, and this narrative genre—which built on religious conversion stories—became a permanent part of American literary and popular culture.[4]

Temperance tactics and priorities changed over time, but two central premises remained remarkably consistent. The first emphasized the destructive potential of alcohol itself; in this view, alcohol was a toxin or poison not just to the individual drinker but also to family stability and social order. The second principle held that women embodied innocent victims of male drunkenness; they should not drink themselves. Indeed, if women imbibed, the whole system might unravel. As one scholar has explained about the antebellum period, "women's alcohol abuse threatened not just domestic ideology but the bedrock binary gender assumptions on which it was based."[5] Activists tried various explanations to make sense of this paradoxical behavior, which contradicted everything they thought they knew about the complementary roles of men and women. Since most women in the temperance movement were native-born Protestants, perhaps only immigrant women—especially Irish—drank. An even more satisfying rationale blamed alcohol itself for these "fallen angels." If even women could succumb, that only showed how dangerous alcohol could be and how much temperance—or even outright prohibition—was urgently needed.[6]

By the time Mrs. C. was drinking her wine in 1888, the temperance campaign had accelerated, and so had the efforts of doctors to assert their authority over women's health habits. Increasing standardization characterized many aspects of American life during the late nineteenth century. In medicine, the professionalizing process brought a shift away from informal practices in which women played key roles, such as midwifery, to male-dominated systems of care with formally trained physicians—disproportionately men—at the top of a hierarchy. Influential doctors buttressed the doctrine of separate spheres by insisting that women's health—especially the turning points of the female life cycle—must be carefully managed to assure the future of the "race." By "race," they did not mean the human race, but native-born whites of the respectable classes—the same sorts of people who tended to join the temperance movement. Concerned at falling birthrates among this demographic group, they insisted that activities outside the home, especially higher education, risked damaging women's reproductive organs. For their own health and for the well-being of society, women should focus their energies on motherhood and domesticity. If not quite inherently pathological, the female body seemed always at risk of becoming so, which called for extensive medical management.[7] And in fact, repeated pregnancies and deliveries could bring long-lasting health complications, even when mother and baby survived—as in the case of Mrs. C.[8] For doctors, and perhaps for many women, "separate spheres" was not only a behavioral prescription but an assertion that a male or female essence was located in the body, with implications for health and disease.

In contrast to those temperance activists and members of the general public who regarded drinking women with horror, inebriate specialists insisted that Mrs. C. deserved care and understanding. Rather than viewing her as especially debased, they believed she proved their point that women's dependence on alcohol represented a disease state, not a vice or sin. Such an understanding was based on two fundamental principles: that women, especially middle-class women, were frail and vulnerable to the vagaries of their reproductive systems; and that alcohol could be grouped with other drugs as a form of medicine rather then a recreational substance. Even nineteenth-century temperance advocates granted women some leeway to use opiates or other drugs to address ill health.[9] Classifying alcohol as part of a spectrum of substances, including patent medicines and commercial nostrums, narcotics, and even tea, which women used for medical reasons, inebriate specialists avoided thorny questions raised by women's recreational liquor consumption. Doctors could assert their expertise without threatening conventional standards for how women should behave, in fact offering reassurance that inebriate women had not forfeited their femininity and could be restored to sobriety and health.[10] What's more, such a cure did not require these women to engage in the soul searching of temperance narratives; instead, physicians simply repaired whatever underlying physical problems caused the desire for drink in the first place.

Depending on the circumstances in which they imbibed, then, drinking women occupied one extreme or the other: Those who consumed alcohol in public settings for recreational purposes could be dismissed as "fallen angels," especially degraded and unlikely to reform.[11] But those who drank for pain relief rather than pleasure represented the best evidence that victims of inebriety deserved sympathetic professional care. Although the doctors of the American Association for the Study and Cure of Inebriety were not the only voice on alcohol-related problems in the late nineteenth-century United States, they illustrate critical aspects of the ongoing relationship between medicalization and gender-role ideology. If some women became dependent on alcohol because of inherent frailty and weakness exacerbated when they carried out their prescribed roles, they could hardly be blamed. Yet this biologically reductionist view of womanhood was both limited and limiting, as it was restricted to those women—usually white, middle-class, married, and bearing children—who followed a conventional social script. This worldview also led medical experts to regard the biological implications of alcohol use very seriously indeed, categorizing alcohol as a potent substance, even a toxin, that altered the body as well as the mind and could damage the offspring of the drinker. According to these experts, women's reproductive roles might help explain their drinking but simultaneously made it a pressing problem that required professional intervention.

Mrs. C.'s case also reinforced the common belief that all aspects of a woman's health, not just her childbearing capacity, followed from her reproductive organs. As a result, many treatment regimens, including surgical removal of these organs, focused on that region of the body even for symptoms that might seem unrelated. Doctors insisted that their expertise allowed them to identify underlying connections and take appropriate action, maintaining that they, not mothers or sisters, had the knowledge and skills to be caretakers of women's health.[12] As patients, women both welcomed and feared medical attention; although the scrutiny of male doctors might be discomfiting and surgical procedures frightening, the most up-to-date scientific methods promised relief from pain and ill health.

Doctors and laypeople considered all of the physiological turning points in a woman's life cycle to be danger zones, making her especially vulnerable to ill health.[13] According to inebriate specialists, the risk of female inebriety could begin at menarche. One inebriate woman, for example, had followed the recommendation of a neighbor and started drinking gin in her teenage years to cope with painful menstruation.[14] General "pelvic pain" or "uterine troubles" also made women use alcohol or drugs. The prominent neurologist George M. Beard described a case in which a woman who suffered from neurasthenia with uterine complications could only sleep "after taking a large quantity of beer at night."[15] Like Mrs. C., women who experienced painful childbirth sometimes drank alcohol during their recovery.[16] Many women resorted to "stimulants" (which alcohol was believed to be at this time) while they breastfed their babies. Some doctors prescribed spirits after women suffered miscarriages.[17] Finally, even menopause—the "sufferings due to the change of life," according to one doctor in 1898—could trigger inebriety in women.[18] In short, women had a "peculiar susceptibility . . . to contract habits of intemperance at the times of pregnancy, lactation, and middle age."[19] These episodes were doubly dangerous: The pain, discomfort, and fatigue that some women experienced encouraged them to try tonics or alcohol for relief, but doctors also concluded that the particular stresses that women's bodies were under during these periods made them more vulnerable to developing dependence than they might have been at other times.

Medical authorities believed as well that women were at risk owing to a generalized frailty, exacerbated by environmental circumstances. Women often explained their drinking this way, noting that they used alcohol and highly alcoholic tonics as "pick-me-ups." One thirty-two-year-old Iowa milliner, for instance, drank strong tea to stay awake when she had to work long hours, then switched to alcohol when she had to complete a particularly large order.[20] As this example suggests, women alternated among different substances, understanding their use in medical, or at least health-related, terms. "Caffeinism" itself could be a diagnosis, leading to reliance on other substances as well, as one doctor warned: "[Such] cases, after beginning on tea, take other drugs, and become alcohol, opium, or chloral takers."[21]

Entire industries, most notably the patent medicine business, capitalized on women's perceived ill health.[22] Women often turned to these nostrums, many of which were highly alcoholic, as an alternative to other kinds of medical treatment; at times, these medicines were even used to treat addiction to other "stimulants." Lydia E. Pinkham's Vegetable Compound, probably the best known of these products, even advertised to healthy women, too, expanding their market while also reinforcing the idea that women were inherently fragile. It is impossible to know today how many women who consumed these products knew they were imbibing alcohol or other drugs that they otherwise might have shunned, since these potions were unregulated and unlabeled until the first decade of the twentieth century. Ironically, even the Pinkham family supported temperance efforts, insisting that the alcohol in their product was essential as a preservative and medicine.[23] Regardless of individual women's awareness or motivation, the patent-medicine industry created an alternative means for women to acquire mind-altering substances in a much more socially acceptable manner than public drinking in commercial venues. This industry also fostered a medicinal rather than recreational understanding of why women used alcoholic products.

Narcotics offered another substitute for alcohol and its association with the saloon. Some doctors argued that narcotic abuse was more of a problem among women than alcohol.[24] T. D. Crothers, a leading inebriety specialist, maintained that among children with a "nervous" or "alcoholic" heredity, boys would grow up to drink liquor while girls would choose narcotics.[25] Doctors reported that some women alternated between liquor and narcotics or simply used both, and they noted cases in which the combination could be especially dangerous.[26]

Recognizing that social sanction shaped women's selection of substances, doctors insisted that the common denominator in women's use was biological and therefore medical. It followed that the legal status of any particular drug including alcohol was not primarily a political question but rather a scientific one. In adopting this position, doctors could and did hold themselves apart from the temperance debate or, on occasion, engage directly with it from a position of authority by critiquing the use of alcohol for female complaints as an outmoded and dangerous folk practice.

This view contrasted so sharply with wider ideas about chronic drunkenness that some doctors insisted that women's dependence on alcohol represented a fundamentally different condition from the same behavior among men. According to Dr. Agnes Sparks, one of the first female physicians in the field, "Inebriety from a fondness of alcohol *per se*—vicious indulgence—obtains less often in women." The reason for this difference, she insisted, "goes without saying." The occurrence of inebriety in women, Sparks maintained, "presents the strongest possible proof that its origin lies in perturbed *physical* conditions."[27] For Sparks, female inebriates were not especially degraded creatures unworthy of help; they proved that inebriety should not be viewed as a "mere moral obliquity" but instead as a condition that called for medical attention. Her assumption that she need not elaborate on why women did not engage in drinking as "vicious indulgence" showed the pervasiveness of traditional standards for female behavior. In her view, the social conditions and domestic expectations that led to exhaustion were no more amenable to change than the biological dimensions of womanhood. Both were immutable characteristics of being female. Invoking medical expertise to manage both these realms, doctors such as Sparks simultaneously defined a disease and monitored appropriate femininity. Understood in this way, female inebriety did not violate expectations for how women should behave but instead reinforced them.

"Handed Down for Four Generations": Alcohol and Reproduction

Inebriety specialists offered a relatively sympathetic interpretation of the *causes* of women's excessive drinking, but they could not be cavalier about its *consequences*, which they believed extended well beyond any individual woman's consumption. Medical and popular writers during this era devoted significant attention to the ramifications of alcohol use on future generations: In the language of the time, physicians maintained that alcohol was a factor in "race degeneracy." Just as temperance campaigners linked the saloon with a range of social problems, many doctors and scientists who studied inebriety viewed it much more broadly than a simple clinical diagnosis for the afflicted individual. Reflecting the scientific and popular view that heredity shaped human traits and behaviors, doctors were practically unanimous that inebriety—as well as a host of medical and social problems of which inebriety could be both cause and effect—could be transmitted to offspring.[28] This emphasis on the hereditary nature of drinking aligned with the social Darwinism of the period, in which scientists and other commentators used the theory of evolution to make judgments about the health and worthiness of people, buttressing racial and class divisions through a language of science.[29]

Temperance rhetoric grouped women and children together as victims of men's alcohol consumption; women's drinking raised troubling questions in this context. Focusing on the reproductive consequences of women's drinking complicated the depiction of female inebriates as innocents who suffered from their own frailty, while the temperance-inflected belief that alcohol itself was a toxin raised the stakes for any drinking by women.[30]

Physicians identified many ways that a parent's drinking could adversely affect children, including biological mechanisms such as prenatal influences and breast feeding as well as psychological and social aspects of parenting, such as example and neglect. It seemed self-evident to doctors and laypeople alike that the mother's impact on offspring was much greater than the father's in all these realms. A number of writers recalled the declaration attributed to Aristotle that "a drunken mother would produce drunken offspring," and they emphasized that it had been "known since antiquity" that a mother's use of alcohol could damage her child.[31] Restating this observation as a truism allowed commentators to attach themselves to timeless authority while offering updated scientific findings. Their analysis, which enumerated health and reproductive risks associated with women's alcohol use, thus served as a counterpoint to wider temperance discourse, which generally addressed problems linked with men's drinking.[32]

One major source of concern was the transmission of inebriety itself. A minority of doctors held to a Lamarckian view, arguing that the "acquired habit" of intemperance could be transmitted to offspring, but most maintained that some sort of "constitutional predisposition" that led to problem drinking—not the drinking pattern itself—could be inherited.[33] This "taint," sometimes described as an "inherent fondness for liquor" or a "thirst" that was "engrafted" onto the offspring, might be invisible while the child was young, but once it surfaced—and it could "break out in full blow at any period"—it was "almost irresistible," according to many physicians.[34] Observations showed that even when the children of inebriates were taken away from their parents and "reared in changed and favorable surroundings," these children nevertheless "developed the desire for drink in later life."[35] Physicians' estimates of the percentage of cases of inebriety and related problems in which heredity was the main cause ranged widely, from one-third to more than three-quarters, while numerous studies calculated the number of an inebriate patient's relatives who were also inebriates, tallying parents, siblings, grandparents, and cousins.[36] Women with drinking problems were aware of this interpretation and used it to explain their condition, like the actress who justified her reliance on absinthe this way: "My father was never sober, and my mother a morphine eater. Conceived under such circumstances what can you expect of me?"[37]

Such concerns were not limited to medical literature but appeared in fiction as well. The possible transmission of a drinking habit across the generations drives the entire plot of *Daughter of the Vine*, an 1899 novel by the well-known writer Gertrude Atherton. The story focuses on a well-to-do family in late nineteenth-century San Francisco. Dudley Thorpe, a visitor from the East, is smitten with the attractive daughter Nina. As he courts her, Thorpe senses a family secret, which he tries to discern with a litany of questions that provide insight into the sorts of problems that would disqualify her as a potential wife: Has she had a lover or a child, or is there insanity in the family? She denies it all, but still will not tell him the real reason, nor will her father when Thorpe asks for Nina's hand in marriage. Then, Thorpe sees Nina's mother experiencing some sort of fit, and Nina finally explains that her mother had been a British barmaid with an "insatiable appetite for drink," who even gave liquor to Nina when she was a child. As a result, Nina explains to Thorpe, "the cry was in my blood." Nina is convinced that she must conquer the habit in herself before she can consent to marry Thorpe, and after an intense scene together, Thorpe agrees to return to the East while Nina attempts to master her craving.[38]

While the spread of inebriety to future generations was bad enough, experts warned that other medical and social problems associated with it could also be inherited. Doctors offered a litany of diseases that they believed were the result of inebriety in parents, including epilepsy, lunacy, imbecility, tainted blood, consumption, hysteria, paralysis, crooked eyes, deafness, and hydroencephalus.[39] Other conditions that were less clearly defined but no less troubling also appeared in children of inebriates, including a weakened constitution; an irritable, unstable, "vicious moral disposition"; and high rates of miscarriage, stillbirth, and infant mortality.[40] Remarking that the "children of alcoholics are not all of necessity idiots, lunatics, or epileptics," one physician nevertheless warned, "There are few that present nothing abnormal."[41] Reflecting the attitudes of many of his colleagues, another doctor concluded, "One thing is certain—the whole tendency is downward, physically, mentally, and morally."[42] The results of such a trajectory could be seen in institutionalized populations, and doctors and others who worked in jails, asylums, and poorhouses asserted that parental alcohol use led to crime, prostitution, and poverty.[43]

Searching for explanations, doctors drew parallels with congenital syphilis, concluding that, while the father's role might be important, the mother's was much more so because her body was the environment in which the fetus developed.[44] Physicians speculated that liquor consumed by a pregnant woman could damage the fetus in fundamental biological ways. The alcohol might "[carry] into the fecundating material certain unknown modifications" that could lead to "malnutrition of the embryo."[45] In short, the offspring of inebriates were "hopelessly tainted" in their cells, according to Lucy M. Hall, an American physician who worked extensively with inebriate women in prison.[46] Although the language might seem imprecise by our standards, these descriptions reinforced the notion of alcohol itself as a dangerous substance that could hurt anyone, even among the "better" classes.

The risk posed by the mother's use of alcohol or drugs did not end when the child was born. Analyzing the health problems, habits, and death rates of children who were nursed by women who drank or used narcotics, doctors became convinced that these substances could be transmitted through breast milk.[47] In many cases, doctors were puzzled by an infant's symptoms—convulsions, nervousness, stupor, diarrhea, indigestion, anemia, and even death—for which they could find no cause. Eventually the physician discovered that the mother—or, in most European examples cited in the *Quarterly Journal of Inebriety*, the wet nurse—used alcohol, opium, or morphine.[48] Here, too, the danger crossed class lines; not just poor women but elite women as well might endanger their children. In addition to these immediate health risks during the breast-feeding period, doctors believed that ingestion of drugs through breast milk, like exposure to drugs in the uterus, made offspring more likely to become inebriates themselves—even in cases where the mother was not an inebriate but was using the substance for medicinal purposes.[49]

Doctors criticized mothers who gave alcohol to their children, whether allowing them a sip of wine or beer at dinner or "dosing" them with whiskey and soothing syrups to treat illness or simply to quiet them. These critiques of women's behavior emphasized the risks of using alcohol as a medicine, and physicians also warned of the dangers of prescribing opium and morphine, to which patients often became habituated. Doctors blamed folk practices in which liquor was used to treat a variety of ailments (thereby highlighting their own authority as professionals) and also chastised their colleagues who continued to prescribe these substances.[50] As well as complicating the child's health status, the use of any drug during childhood could set the stage for inebriety later. For example, Crothers was puzzled when a "very highly cultivated woman" began to use morphia "without any apparent cause in pain or sickness" and was thus inconsistent with the model of female inebriety. The mystery was solved when "the remarkable fact appeared that opium was used very freely in the first two years of her life."[51] Doctors noted with concern that some mothers even allowed their children liquor that was not intended medicinally. The sight of a four-year-old child sipping wine in a Chicago restaurant in 1898 prompted one doctor to insist that mothers should be taught that children could become inebriates, too.[52] Secret drinking at home could exacerbate this; in some instances, a child would find and sample the mother's hidden stash of liquor, while in others the mother would reward the child with a drink for bringing her more alcohol.[53]

Children faced additional dangers in an "alcoholic milieu"—a home environment characterized by neglect and accidents because of parental drinking. Doctors told of children of inebriate mothers who died in violent circumstances, by scalding, burning, suffocation, cold, and deprivation.[54] Children in poor families often faced the worst risks. The chaplain of a British prison described how babies died from being "overlain," suffocated by the mother's body, often on Saturday night "when the alcoholized mother is unable to hear or feel the cry or the struggle of the infant, if that be not already narcotized by the alcoholized milk from her breast."[55] In other cases, drinking mothers were unwilling or unable to care for a sick child. Checking on a child who had been treated for fever, a doctor's assistant found the parents and friends enjoying a "Bacchanalian orgy" while the child lay "helpless and unnoticed" in the next room of the family's tenement apartment. Reflecting a belief that mothers should be more responsible for children, the supervising physician in this case remarked that it was "bad enough that the father is a drinking man, but when it is the mother, or both parents, the poor little ones appeal most urgently to the doctor who has a thread of sympathy in his composition."[56]

Fictional accounts played on many of the same themes, underscoring their resonance beyond medical literature. Stephen Crane's novella *Maggie: A Girl of the Streets* (1893) is today hailed as a pioneering work of literary naturalism, providing a glimpse into the complex social and economic customs surrounding saloons and their implications for family life in the late nineteenth-century city. Crane's portrait of Mary, the drunken mother, represents a horrific inversion of conventional ideas about drinkers and their victims. Mary is nothing like the pure and subdued wife and mother portrayed in temperance rhetoric, nor does she resemble the frail female inebriate in medical reports. Instead, Mary embodies the ways in which women's excessive alcohol use seemed unnatural. Crane frequently describes her immense physical size and strength: "Her massive shoulders heaved with anger" as she cleans up her young son Jimmie after he has been in a fight, and she engages in physical battles with her husband when she has been drinking. Moreover, she is portrayed as violent and cruel to her children. When daughter Maggie breaks a dish, the mother erupts in fury: "Her eyes glittered on her child in sudden hatred. The fervent red of her face turned almost to purple."[57] Her physical and verbal abuse and her inability to protect her daughter from the dangers of the streets illustrate the alcoholic milieu.

The family Crane describes in *Maggie* resembles the tenement dwellers and prison inmates who often appeared in medical and social reform literature. But other accounts show that the risks of maternal drinking to children crossed class and regional boundaries; even Mrs. C. from Iowa became "indifferent" and "abusive" to her children when she drank. Similarly, "The Victim of Excitement," a short story published in 1870, relays the story of Anne Weston, an otherwise respectable wife and mother whose drinking habits bring tragedy to her family.[58] When her father dies "of a broken heart" upon learning about Anne's drinking, she abstains and focuses on domestic matters. Her resolve is undone when her cook asks her to sample the brandy required for a cake recipe and the first sip launches her on a binge. Passed out in her bed, she fails to protect her young child who falls and hits her head, ultimately dying from the injury. Anne's drinking has caused death in multiple generations of her family and disrupted her husband's masculinity as well, causing him to faint in grief. He recovers his authority to send their surviving child to live with a family friend. Even with the loss of her children, Anne does not stop drinking and her condition deteriorates. Although the reader is reassured in a deathbed scene that Anne has hope of going to heaven, the story is intended as a cautionary tale that women of any background can fall victim to the corrupting power of alcohol.

Concern with familial consequences thus animated much of the discussion of women's use of alcohol and other drugs in medical and popular literature, just as temperance advocates emphasized how much men's drinking harmed families. This focus is hardly surprising, given the central role of nurturing in nineteenth-century definitions of womanhood,[59] but it put inebriety experts in a difficult position as they sought to finesse issues of disease, motivation, and blame. If any alcohol use by women posed a threat, then defining inebriety as a specific diagnostic category became more challenging. And even if drinking women were victims of their own ill health or social circumstances, their actions endangered others and demanded a response.

Individual Treatment and Medicalization

While temperance advocates focused on the elimination of alcohol from American life through legislation and other reformers took aim at the patent medicine industry, inebriety specialists—as well as people who wanted to stop drinking—experimented with strategies that did not hinge on the legal status of beverage alcohol. This wide range of approaches shows that Americans understood problem drinking as a multifaceted phenomenon, and various constituencies developed methods in keeping with their own expertise and perspective. Yet they shared a focus on abstinence and the cultivation of regular habits. While physicians insisted that they could cure the condition, social reformers as well as fiction writers were relatively pessimistic about the prognosis for women who drank to excess.

One early and innovative approach came from the Washingtonians, a "mutual-help" group of reformed drinkers who began meeting in Baltimore in the 1840s. Unlike previous temperance groups whose efforts were aimed at the drinking customs of others, the Washingtonian movement was made up of individuals who wanted to achieve abstinence themselves. To do so, they talked about their experiences, offering emotionally charged accounts of drinking and sobriety and creating a genre called "temperance narratives."[60] Other scholars have written in depth on the wider movement, its significance in antebellum reform, and its legacy for alcoholism treatment, particularly in foreshadowing Alcoholics Anonymous decades later.[61] Its different implications for women and men also deserve attention. Although women could sign the Washingtonian pledge to abstain from drinking, they were forbidden to speak at meetings.[62] Following nineteenth-century conventions of gender segregation, wives and sisters of male participants did not join the men's group but instead founded Martha Washington societies, which initially sought to rescue female inebriates as well as support men in sustaining sobriety. But these efforts did not last long, and soon the working-class, nondrinking women who were active in the Martha Washingtonians came to exclude, even ostracize, inebriate women. These "good women" played critical supporting roles to inebriate men, but such a constellation left no room for inebriate women, who occupied an awkward position in reform and treatment efforts.[63]

At least one temperance narrative purportedly written by a woman in the Washingtonian movement has survived. "Confessions of a Female Inebriate" relays the story of "Mrs. L.," a young married mother of two small children, who starts drinking wine when a well-regarded physician prescribes it for her (just like Mrs. C. at the beginning of this chapter). The author provides no specific reason for the deterioration of Mrs. L.'s health, suggesting that readers shared the belief that women were often sickly, especially during their childbearing years. As Mrs. L.'s tolerance and dependence grow, she finds it "impossible to relinquish my wine." The pressures of caring for ill children accelerate her drinking, and she experiences a loss of control: "With the first stimulant, my resolutions were gone."[64] Tragically, in her incapacity she gives her daughter the wrong medicine, and the girl dies. Although her inebriety originated in a doctor's prescription, she does not seek medical advice to help her *stop* drinking. Instead, her guilt at her daughter's death is sufficient shock that she resists the urge to drink until she is overcome by nervousness while planning a party at her husband's request and yields to her craving to assuage her fears. At the event she is "far too loudly talkative for a lady hostess," ultimately falling down intoxicated in front of her guests. Announcing that he will return if she remains sober for one year, Mr. L. departs. The narrator notes in an aside to the reader that wives tend to remain devoted to husbands even when they imbibe excessively, whereas husbands are more likely to leave their drinking wives for fear of disgrace. Although Mrs. L. does abstain given this ultimatum, she does not earn a happy ending, receiving word eight months later that her husband has died in England.[65]

"Confessions" is a puzzling document: The fact that it was written at all, even if by a man (as scholars believe likely),[66] shows that some Washingtonians thought that women's drinking merited attention. This narrative illuminates fundamental elements in female inebriety: the medicinal use of alcohol to cope with female complaints; the sanctioning or denial of such use by male authorities as an element of their control over women's bodies and lives; the troubling, even tragic, consequences of maternal drinking; women's less-powerful position within marriage and a double standard in the behavior of nonalcoholic spouses; and a warning that inebriety does exist among women, including those of higher-class status. Even though Mrs. L. does not receive the promised reward of her husband's return despite her sobriety, the narrative suggests that she refrained from drink thereafter, conveying the wider Washingtonian message that inebriates can change.

In contrast, female inebriates in fiction are usually left to rely on individual willpower, not the mutual support of the Washingtonians or the expertise of the medical profession, and they do not always survive. In *Daughter of the Vine*, Nina discovers she is pregnant after Thorpe leaves California. When the baby dies soon after birth, Nina can no longer resist the urge to drink and declines rapidly. She then agrees to marry a manipulative suitor so that she will not ruin Thorpe's life now that she has resumed drinking. Several years later, Thorpe returns to California to settle some family business and encounters Nina, now "an ugly old sot" and much changed. Through all this, Nina never consults a doctor regarding her drinking, even though her family is sophisticated and financially comfortable and her father had previously threatened to send her mother, whom he kept a virtual prisoner, to the "inebriate home." Inspired by seeing Thorpe once again, Nina stops drinking abruptly, explaining that the withdrawal is killing her, but she is "glad."[67]

Within the genres of Washingtonian temperance narrative and fiction, readers did not have any reason to doubt that Mrs. L. and Nina suffered from inebriety. In real life, however, even diagnosing women who drank to excess could be challenging for doctors, a dilemma they debated at some length given that the authority to create categories of disease and to identify those patients who manifested them was a critical part of medicalization. Doctors insisted that women were even more determined than their male counterparts to deceive others regarding their drinking habits.[68] Physicians repeatedly reminded one another that female patients' duplicity required sensitive diagnostic skills honed through experience. One physician explained, "Happily it is still regarded as a great disgrace for a woman to be intemperate; and so she is bent upon deceiving us. We need expect no help from her in arriving at the real cause of her ailments, and it is very probable that the young and inexperienced practitioner will be unable of himself to arrive at a correct diagnosis or appropriate treatment."[69] Similarly, doctors, nurses, and other attendants described elaborate schemes women used to obtain and hide liquor, failing to note that the typical male inebriate had more social and financial freedom to drink as he chose. One nurse who cared for a young inebriate woman recounted how the patient gave her jewelry to the gardener, which he pawned in order to procure liquor for her. He then piped the alcohol into a false flowerpot on her windowsill.[70] Stymied by the patient herself, many doctors had no qualms about acquiring information from her husband or other family members or friends, noting that such "confessions" (by others) made a case much easier.[71] Indeed, it is striking that it was a woman physician, who may have had a better rapport with her female patients, who maintained that doctors should simply ask their patients directly about their drinking habits.[72]

Doctors also noted that inebriate women, fearing "exposure and publicity" for their drinking habits, showed a "disposition to retreat behind the mask of various nervous diseases," as T. D. Crothers explained.[73] Using alcohol and other drugs for "female complaints" allowed women to claim a more conventionally feminine diagnosis, but this overlap illuminated a central dilemma of medical treatment. If the underlying cause of inebriety was physical pain or discomfort associated with female reproductive functions, many doctors maintained their first task was to cure or otherwise relieve this underlying condition. Once that was done, some argued, the woman's inebriety would disappear.[74] While excessive pain could be understood as pathological and thus within doctors' purview, it was difficult to see how they might "cure" conditions fundamental to womanhood. In other words, the notion that all women passed through physiological danger zones as an inevitable part of life, and the corollary that many women—especially the "better sort"—were inherently frail and vulnerable to ill health, made it that much harder to demarcate inebriety as a specific condition in women.

Nevertheless, inebriate specialists insisted that they could offer systematic treatment to women as well as men. Although a few physicians noted that female patients could be more difficult to treat, most doctors, responding to the popular view of all inebriates, but especially women, as degraded and hopeless, insisted that women could be cured just as men could. Some even argued that women were easier to care for because they were more "tractable" and therefore offered a better prognosis than male inebriates.[75] While Mrs. C.'s doctor had cared for her at home, inebriate specialists also established asylums where patients could be admitted for intensive, long-term treatment. These doctors contrasted the care they could provide with the methods—or lack of same—currently in use. They condemned the use of prison for inebriates, criticized family members for their clumsy, ineffective, and even dangerous attempts at home cures, and recommended asylum treatment.[76] This advocacy was not only altruistic or the result of scientific advances; institution building, like publishing a journal, helped established this field as a legitimate medical specialty. These inebriate asylums could be public or private, Christian or secular, but they shared a basic orientation, incorporating a "holistic approach to reforming the inebriate."[77] Often located in rural settings, asylums were intended to provide "nerve and brain rest," away from the "exciting causes" that contributed to inebriety. Therapy included baths, nutritious food, rest, exercise, tonics, and sometimes even hypnosis and electricity.[78] Patients often worked at gender-specific tasks, both because their labor was essential to the maintenance of the institution and because doctors believed it aided their recovery.

Despite rhetorical attention to women's drinking and optimistic and inclusive attitudes among some inebriety specialists, resources to treat women did not necessarily follow. Most Americans believed that inebriety was a much greater problem among men than among women, and institutional data from the period yield a sex ratio of men to women between 3:1 and 9:1.[79] As a result, facilities for male inebriates were viewed as a higher priority. For example, the General Court of Massachusetts voted in 1889 to establish an inebriate hospital to serve both men and women. But a funding shortfall and concern that mixing men and women would have a detrimental effect on inmates' morals meant that women were ultimately excluded.[80] Without access to a hospital, women who were arrested for drunkenness were thus relegated to other kinds of institutions, such as jails and insane asylums, where they were denied the care that inebriate specialists considered essential.[81] Nationwide, while some inebriate asylums accepted women, and a few were established exclusively for them, the majority did not accept female patients.[82] Additionally, middle- and upper-class women who could afford care might have feared social sanction too much to do so, while working-class women, who may have faced less stigma for their drinking, lacked the resources to pay for care, and the limited number of public facilities that existed rarely accepted women.[83]

Even facilities that accepted women, such as the Keeley Institute, stumbled over how to provide equivalent care. The Keeley Cure combined a specific, proprietary formula—the "bichloride of gold"—with a carefully structured environment at its institute in Dwight, Illinois. By the 1890s, the Keeley Cure had become immensely popular: The inventor of the formula even hosted a booth at the Chicago World's Fair of 1893. The Keeley Institute accepted female patients, many of whom sought treatment for their use of morphine and other narcotics as well as alcohol. Sensitive to the additional stigma faced by female inebriates who were greatly outnumbered by the men, Keeley doctors sought to protect women's identity by housing them in a separate building and providing their injections in private. Structuring the program in this way represented a laudable attempt to neutralize the particular disgrace that female addicts faced, yet it implied that they had more to hide and risked reinforcing the very double standard that these doctors hoped to avoid. Looking back at the Keeley program, it may be that the real innovation was not the secret formula but rather the "therapeutic community" of Dwight itself.[84] If so, then the segregation of women, however well intentioned, denied them the central benefit of this treatment program. Gender division also continued in the Keeley Leagues, local associations of former patients who continued to meet after leaving Dwight. League meetings grouped female veterans of the program with female relatives of the men who had taken the cure, rather than with the male patients.[85]

As these examples suggest, the spatial arrangements of nineteenth-century treatment facilities and the ways in which problem drinking was understood reinforced the notion of gender difference. The implicit goal of many treatment efforts was a return to conventional roles, for men and women alike. Although they believed the stresses of the maternal role often served as catalysts for women's drinking, many observers held that female responsibilities should also be incentives to abstain. At the New England Home for Intemperate Women, for example, inmates worked at domestic tasks such as sewing, cooking, and washing, both to inculcate good habits and a sense of self-worth and to prepare the women to support themselves or manage their own homes.[86] Making a "best dress" was part of the regimen at another facility, while female inebriates ran a nursery for poor children at yet another. Some doctors went even further, with at least one maintaining that marriage and lactation cured some cases of female inebriety.[87] This belief shaped fictional plots, too—for example, in *Daughter of the Vine*, Nina resists the urge to drink during pregnancy and while caring for her newborn but abandons herself to her craving after the infant's death.

Although many of them maintained a dogged optimism in their publications, doctors recognized that some women simply did not improve, and they debated what to do about the reproductive consequences. Some physicians recommended that inebriates, whether male or female, should not marry,[88] but most such prophylactic measures were aimed at women. Although he did not advocate it as a standard procedure for inebriate women who became pregnant, one doctor observed that when female inebriates were imprisoned during pregnancy, their children were healthier.[89] Finally, some physicians recommended that female inebriates who did not respond to other treatment should be sterilized. Even Dr. Agnes Sparks, who expressed considerable sympathy toward inebriate women, endorsed this view: "One remedy, radical and a *dernier resort*, remains to be noted. Granting that the woman has been given treatment, proper, persistent, and prolonged, without avail, she should be [de]sexualized. This whether maid or matron. . . . It might be curative: it surely would be preventive, and better, by far, to unsex the woman, than have her beget a brood tainted with this curse of the world."[90] Sparks and doctors like her understood female inebriety in fundamentally biological terms: Removing the ovaries might actually cure the desire for drink. And if not, the consequences were dire enough that "unsexing" seemed the only solution. While this form of treatment might seem extreme to readers today, it was not unique to inebriety but was used in response to a variety of complaints and symptoms. In this way, inebriate specialists aligned themselves with advanced surgical techniques and medical progress. It is ironic and unfortunate that some women may have begun their use of patent medicines and related substances in an attempt to avoid gynecological surgery, only to develop inebriety and face such a procedure after all.

Gendering Policy: Temperance and Drug Control

Beginning in 1904, the *Ladies' Home Journal* printed a series of articles that exposed various practices of the patent medicine industry, including the use of potentially addictive ingredients in nostrums aimed at children (soothing syrups) and at women. This crusade was part of a wider Progressive Era impulse to use investigative journalism to reveal and correct harmful and corrupt practices. It soon spread to *Collier's* and other publications, with additional charges of collusion between patent medicine manufacturers and newspapers that profited from the industry's extensive advertising. One prominent muckraker declared that women—even those in the Woman's Christian Temperance Union!—got drunk from alcoholic tonics. This campaign, along with publication of *The Jungle* by Upton Sinclair in 1906, which detailed horrific conditions in Chicago's meat-packing industry, helped lead to the Pure Food and Drug Act of 1906, which established standards of purity and labeling for proprietary medicines in interstate trade. As a result, remedies like Lydia E. Pinkham's Vegetable Compound had to be more forthcoming about the inclusion of certain ingredients and soften the claims they made about the effectiveness and versatility of their products.[91] Less than a decade later, the Harrison Narcotics Tax Act (1914) sharply restricted the use of opiates and cocaine.[92]

Both of these laws demonstrated Progressive Era desires for social order through regulation, and they reflected a concern with alcohol and drugs as dangerous substances that harmed families and society as well as individual drinkers and users. Warnings about patent medicines, like case reports of drinking women such as Mrs. C., reinforced nineteenth-century ideas about alcohol *as* a drug—consistent with the view of many inebriate specialists. These warnings also reflected a common view of women as a particularly vulnerable class whose health and behavior followed directly from their biology.

Against the backdrop of the temperance campaign, the inebriety movement propounded a disease model that incorporated medicinal drinking by otherwise respectable women. Rather than contradicting the "True Woman" standard, this type of drinking instead appeared to be a logical extension of women's nature, which was itself understood as a reflection of women's reproductive functions. Fictional accounts of women who drank to excess largely echoed these themes, showing how widespread they were in nineteenth-century America. Importantly, this depiction of women's drinking stood in marked contrast to the vice of consumption by men in saloons, just as women's social role should complement, not mimic, that of men. In fact, both of these drinking patterns reinforced the doctrine of separate spheres.

This episode in the history of women and alcohol shows that the promise of medicalization to provide care and reduce disgrace often brings other costs. The focus by inebriety specialists on women's medicinal drinking as a consequence of biology could pull in a universalizing direction—to the idea that all women might be at risk and that the actions of drinking women were comprehensible and even forgivable if the cause was simply being female. But not all drinking styles aligned with this logic, and medical authority applied unevenly. Doctors and other experts reinforced distinctions among women even as they underscored differences between women and men. And even those women who were included in this model could only belong if they matched a preferred demographic profile and followed a conventional gendered script.

Chapter 2

"Lit Ladies"

Women's Drinking during the Progressive Era and Prohibition

In the summer of 1909, newspaper headlines across the United States screamed "Mrs. Gould's Life at Home, Drunken Orgy: Coachman, Carpenter, Footman, Maid, Florist and Clerk All Relate Instances When Mistress Was Intoxicated and Profane."[1] Sensational stories covered the divorce proceedings of Howard Gould, son of railroad magnate Jay Gould, and Katherine Clemmons, an actress. Howard and Katherine had been married in 1898 after a long courtship, and the marriage lasted less than a decade.[2] Katherine's drinking had led Howard to impose "stipulations . . . to govern his wife's conduct," including the requirement that she "abstain wholly from the use of intoxicants," but Katherine refused to accede to this, and the couple separated.[3] The question of Katherine's alimony hinged on whether Gould was justified in leaving her owing to her "habits." Testimony came from acquaintances who had observed Katherine's alcohol consumption at parties and other events, as well as from servants who provided tantalizing details about the amount she drank and under what circumstances. A traveling companion insisted that Katherine only had one cocktail before dinner and never touched brandy and soda.[4] In contrast, a valet recalled that he "at one time he served his mistress with two quarts of Manhattan cocktails in as many days, besides the wines and liqueurs which . . . she drank at the table." Despite such attention to quantity, commentators did not focus on whether she was an inebriate, nor did they seem to expect total abstinence, but they marveled at how she seemed altered by alcohol. Servants claimed that they had repeatedly seen her intoxicated, where "she changed from a charming, affable woman to a woman of whims and caprices, ill-tempered, not nice in her choice of language, overbearing, and quarrelsome."[5]

Katherine's drunken behavior thus underscored the transformative power of alcohol to which women, as novice drinkers, seemed especially vulnerable.

Katherine Gould's divorce hit the papers two decades after Mrs. C. began drinking.[6] The two women led very different lives, and their drinking patterns differed as well. The alcohol that Katherine Gould consumed during the early twentieth century was not understood as medicine but as a consumer or luxury good. If medicinal use had reinforced prevalent ideas about women's health and abstinence continued to define middle-class respectability, Gould's consumption demonstrated that women's drinking could be incorporated into a sophisticated lifestyle, provided that women (and men) maintained appropriate limits. But when Gould crossed the line into excess, she was harshly condemned because there was no medical rationale for her behavior, and her intoxication served as proxy for a wider unraveling of social standards.

This chapter explores how women's recreational drinking during the first three decades of the twentieth century became a testing ground for widespread debates about women's proper roles. During these years, the temperance movement gathered momentum, culminating in national Prohibition when the Eighteenth Amendment to the Constitution and its enabling legislation, the Volstead Act, forbade the manufacture, sale, and transportation of intoxicating liquor. While inebriate specialists could explain alcohol use as consistent with conventional femininity, recreational drinking seemed a gender transgression. And while medical authorities focused on the reproductive implications of women's consumption, other commentators emphasized connections between women's social drinking and "promiscuous" sexual behavior, including prostitution.

Katherine Gould's story reminds us that many of the changes in women's comportment that have often been attributed to the flapper of the "Roaring Twenties" were well under way before that decade. Young middle-class women increasingly flouted convention, claiming privileges once reserved for men as well as behaviors and attitudes previously associated with disreputable women on either end of the class spectrum. These shifts in standards, which accelerated during the 1920s as women's drinking took on particular significance as a test of Prohibition policy, raised important questions about women's autonomy and the effects of alcohol on women's conduct as wives and mothers. As medical authority on alcohol-related matters receded during Prohibition, notions of alcoholic excess became ever more embedded with anxieties about rapid changes in women's lives and behaviors.

Saloons and the "New Woman"

Neither Mrs. C., the Iowa farm wife, nor Katherine Gould drank in saloons—and for good reason. For many Americans, the saloon epitomized an unsavory, even violent, subculture where men, often recent immigrants, congregated to squander their wages on liquor and their votes on corrupt machine politicians. There, too, they might cavort with syphilis-laden prostitutes, leading them to infect their wives with venereal diseases. At the very least, a man who frequented saloons might return home drunk and verbally or even physically abuse his wife when she asked for funds for household expenses. In all these ways, saloons polluted the domestic sanctuary that should have been the counterpoint to such commercialized vice. While overly dramatic, this depiction reflected social realities and concerns, particularly the legal and economic powerlessness of most wives in nineteenth- and early twentieth-century America. This view of the saloon as the source of all that threatened the American home had led many women to join the temperance movement which embraced the slogan of "Home Protection."[7]

Still, saloons were not all alike, and historians have shown that they served important social functions in many working-class communities. Moreover, saloons did not always conform to the highly gendered divisions of temperance rhetoric that typically depicted the saloon as a space inhabited only by disreputable men while women and children always remained outside. In fact, many women worked in the liquor industry: Irish widows operated saloons in some communities,[8] for example, while high fees and licensing difficulties in Boston created a thriving "kitchen barroom trade" in which women played a significant part.[9]

Yet working in a saloon or hotel that was owned by one's family was one thing; going there as a consumer could be quite another. Women's position as customers in saloons or any public drinking establishments remained controversial, well into the twentieth century in some places. As a result, much of women's alcohol consumption occurred outside the saloon: Working-class and immigrant women who wanted to drink frequently "rushed the growler," that is, they bought their alcohol to carry out and consume at home. In Chicago, for example, Italian wives would socialize whenever anyone brought a bucket of beer back from the saloon.[10] In Stephen Crane's novella *Maggie*, women consume alcohol but are not necessarily welcome in saloons. When Maggie's mother, a known spree drinker, enters a saloon, she is thrown out. Similarly, when Maggie seeks the lover who has rejected her by going to the saloon where he works, the young man reacts angrily, telling her to leave before the boss sees her or he will lose his job.[11] Women's participation in public drinking customs remained limited, with access shaped by age, time of day, and the presence of a male escort.[12] These practices reinforced complex social codes and gradations of respectability, closely observed but usually incomprehensible to outsiders, including reformers.

In those saloons that allowed women as customers, the typical spatial arrangement marked them as a separate class even as it may have offered some protection. Women could enter by the "Ladies' Entrance"[13] and could partake of the infamous "free lunch" in a segregated back room.[14] But the fear and animosity many reformers felt regarding women's presence in saloons is reflected in a poem from 1910 that warns of the dangers of alcohol through the figure of the "fallen angel."[15] This is no delicate female inebriate but a young woman embarked on a downward path with no turning back: "Corrupt" in her morals and "deep in disgrace," she "sank," drowning in a "river of vice." Once she was inside, there was "no exit for purity." Just as many temperance advocates lumped together all problems caused by alcohol consumption, the quick journey represented in this poem—"through wild pleasure right into despair"—suggests that for women in particular there was no moderation, no chance for a middle ground.

As the phrase "river of vice" suggests, women's public drinking was only one element in a cluster of antisocial activities that frequently included premarital sex and prostitution, another Progressive Era flashpoint. In this era of rapid urbanization, many Americans feared that cities corrupted young people, especially women who moved there from rural areas. Such concerns came to a crescendo in the first decades of the twentieth century as part of the accelerating attack on the saloon. Young women who drank embodied vulnerability: They faced sexual peril but could, in turn, become threats themselves. The naïveté of these young women, coupled with the unscrupulous motives of urban businessmen, proved a dangerous combination. Reformers worried that single women who lived in boarding houses, for example, had few opportunities for respectable recreation.[16] While dancing, attending the movies, or gathering with peers for ice cream might seem innocent, reformers argued that a ruthless "vice complex" lay behind apparently benign establishments in this unregulated environment. As if that were not bad enough, young women, who earned much less than their male peers even when they had jobs, had to rely on men to cover the expenses of urban leisure. In exchange, these "charity girls," as they became known, offered the pleasure of their company, which might include sexual favors. The Juvenile Protective Association of Chicago insisted in 1911 that "the recreation of thousands of young people has been commercialized, and as a result hundreds of young girls are annually started on the road to ruin, for the saloon keepers and dance hall owners have only one end in view, and that is profit."[17]

While reformers' language may sound judgmental and condescending to us today, they recognized that alcohol contributed to the volatility of urban recreation, which made young women especially vulnerable. The differential fates of Maggie and her brother Jimmie in Crane's novella demonstrate the greater risks girls faced, and Maggie's trajectory is exactly what reformers feared for young women in her situation. Living at home with their widowed mother, both Maggie and Jimmie take jobs as teenagers. But Jimmie enjoys relative independence; he goes out to drink at night and returns late. Maggie only gains access to this social world when she is courted by Jimmie's acquaintance Pete, who seems sophisticated and charming to the naïve Maggie.[18] But when Pete abandons her and her family rejects her as "ruined," Maggie has no choice but to become a prostitute, and she ultimately dies.[19]

Liquor could become the first step on a downward path, contributing to the "development of promiscuity"; according to one social worker, "The prelude to her first sex adventure is, very frequently, the partial intoxication of the girl. Taken when off her guard, possibly scarcely remembering what took place, she passes through the experience which may lead to her adoption of prostitution."[20] Then, reformers warned, alcohol could become the attraction, with one even suggesting that women who became prostitutes were nascent alcoholics in the first place: "Desire for drink has long been recognized as playing an important part in the drift toward prostitution."[21] These observers insisted that the association was clear, even if the direction of causation was not. As one reformer explained in 1910, "The habit of intoxication in woman, if not an indication of the existence of actual depravity or vice, is a sure precursor of it, for drunkenness and debauchery are inseparable companions, one almost invariably following the other."[22]

Young women who drank in dance halls and other venues became caught in regulatory systems that attempted to categorize, rescue, or punish them. Although women differentiated among themselves—while she is relatively secure with Pete, for example, Maggie draws back her skirts when passing women in the bar she believes to be prostitutes—reformers, like many casual observers, often assumed that unescorted women in saloons were prostitutes.[23] Reformers' language and the policies they advocated contained a mixture of pity and blame. Saloons commercialized both drinking and sex: Alcohol attracted clientele, provided a source of profit to the madam, "incited" the men, and served as a "stimulant" to the prostitutes.[24] It followed, then, that prohibiting alcohol would curtail illicit sexual behavior as well.[25] Women's public drinking, segregated as it often was, made an obvious target for regulation, an entering wedge for prohibition just as protective legislation aimed at wage-earning women could, some advocates hoped, ultimately improve labor conditions overall. In 1907, for example, the state of Montana sought to eliminate women's drinking in saloons, banning women from them and outlawing any accommodations that had provided space for women to drink, including wine rooms, private apartments, screened areas, and even signs that had advertised ladies' entrances.[26]

Alongside these wider policy initiatives, individual women who drank in public, especially to the point of intoxication, faced sanctions as well, ranging from social disapproval to arrest and incarceration. In Boston during the 1910s, for example, drunkenness was one of the "commonest charges against women offenders in court," and these women exemplified the "river of vice." Of one hundred women so arrested, three-quarters had "become habitually accustomed to [liquor's] use." At least two of the women used drugs as well, and there were also twenty-nine arrests in the group for "offenses against chastity."[27] Similarly, among women imprisoned on Blackwell's Island in New York City in the early 1900s, almost 25 percent had been arrested for intoxication, with almost three times that many arrested for being "disorderly," a category that probably included drinking in many cases.[28] Many of the women were poor, and they seemed very unladylike according to those who evaluated their conduct: "The workhouse class have the greatest number of bad habits and are more unreserved in discussing them. Of 30 women measured, I found 27 used alcohol, 7 chewed tobacco, 8 smoked, 13 swore, 15 used snuff, and fully seven-eighths were immoral."[29] These women violated feminine standards not just by their habits but by their willingness to display and discuss them. In this way, they evoke Katherine Gould, who faced accusations of profanity, careless spending, and sexual dalliances as well as intoxication. But while Gould faced embarrassment, poor women who were arrested could be incarcerated in reform facilities. Doctors were pessimistic about changing their drinking behavior,[30] although it is important to note that physicians and prison officials did not differentiate between women with a true dependence on alcohol and those who drank only occasionally.

Because of who they were and the circumstances surrounding their drinking habits, these women did not appear to be delicate female inebriates, and the experts who dealt with them explained their drinking very differently. Instead of treating them as fragile females who needed sympathetic care, prison officials and even physicians attributed their difficulties to "mental defect," a catch-all term popular in the early twentieth century that encompassed cognitive ability, psychological maturity, and moral values. Other observers blamed environmental factors, including social and economic variables, especially the "low moral standards" that allegedly characterized the families and communities in which these young women had lived. In a passage that could have been written to describe the life story of Maggie, one crusading journalist explained that a large number of prostitutes came from families

> in which the father or mother, or both, used alcoholic liquors habitually.... Many such girls have become accustomed to drink at an early age. Many have so often seen their parents and friends in a state of intoxication that there is no longer, if there ever were, any revulsion at the spectacle of drunkenness. For many such girls the step from casual immorality to which they have almost unconsciously, in many cases, accustomed themselves, to commercialized immorality, is but a short one.[31]

In Maggie's fictional case, her family described her as "ruined" and "bad." By the early twentieth century, many social workers and journalists no longer used that language, seeking, like physicians, to substitute terms that seemed scientific and up-to-date for a language of sin. Yet even these formulations continued to posit an inevitable downward path for girls who transgressed traditional feminine standards.[32]

Middle-class parents and reformers feared that young women from the respectable classes might compromise themselves, too. New drinking customs in which men and women participated together signaled the arrival of the "New Woman." This figure emerged during the 1890s, when the number of women attending college and entering the professions—though still small—gained new attention. Women adopted new clothing styles, too, shifting from heavy dresses and layers of petticoats to blouses and skirts allowing a greater freedom of movement and participation in activities such as badminton and cycling. More women worked for wages, including married women, and the suffrage campaign brought more women into the public realm. This is not to say that all women's lives were suddenly transformed; traditional values and expectations remained strong for many groups, and these changes had significant limitations. Women who worked earned less than men and many regarded their jobs as only a temporary stage before marriage and motherhood. Still, the experiences of men and women overlapped more than they had previously, especially among middle-class Americans, and many observers considered the New Woman to be a symbol of modernity itself.[33]

Because she stood at a particular juncture of gender, class status, and youth, the New Woman's drinking habits looked very different from those of nineteenth-century matrons who turned to alcohol for medicinal reasons. The New Woman entered into new forms of commercialized leisure that reshaped gendered norms of consumption even as they regulated them. For example, cabarets reorganized their interiors, allowing couples to be served at tables, rather than having to stand at a male-only bar. The Cafe des Beaux Arts in New York even created a "ladies' bar" in 1913, where men could not be served without a female escort. Newspapers reported that "society women, actresses, and social climbers" came to the bar, but the very publicity the establishment attracted suggests that women's public drinking retained shock value.[34]

Unlike working-class girls, middle- and upper-class women had the space to entertain at home, but even here they did not escape scrutiny. Inviting guests into her home, the hostess put herself on display, if only to a handpicked audience. Women's drinking in this setting could be acceptable—even obligatory among certain social groups—and serve as an alternative to the saloon.[35] Yet husbands or other acquaintances—or, in Katherine Gould's case, servants—monitored women's consumption carefully. For example, alcohol is served as part of the social milieu described in the 1899 novel *Daughter of the Vine* by Gertrude Atherton.[36] Dudley Thorpe feels justified in commenting on Nina's consumption even before he learns the family secret: "I don't like to see a woman drink when it affects her as it does you," he tells her.[37] While the majority of society women did not drink to the point of drunkenness, one reporter explained, even apparently moderate consumption came at a cost. Drinking brought to these women a quality "quite foreign to their real nature."[38] Here too, we see concern that women were especially affected by alcohol, regardless of their reasons for drinking or the context in which they did so.

The New Woman's class privilege generally insulated her from the legal and social sanctions, not to mention the physical danger, faced by poor women who drank. But even occasional, recreational drinking by New Women carried some risk, if only of social disapproval. Indeed, the excitement of breaking with convention was part of the point for many who indulged and those who wrote about it. Yet as they documented, even celebrated, more social drinking by women, accounts in the popular press and in fiction simultaneously reminded readers of the potential costs involved—lost love, social embarrassment, and a continued reliance on men for access to these new privileges.

Speakeasies and Flappers

Debate over the New Woman's drinking habits played out against the backdrop of a massive temperance campaign. Although it can be hard to appreciate this today, prohibition sentiment represented mainstream views in the early twentieth century. To be sure, many immigrant groups opposed restrictions on drinking, but most native-born Americans and more than a few immigrants believed that eliminating the liquor trade would solve a host of social problems such as poverty and domestic violence, as well as municipal corruption. The decades-long campaign of the Woman's Christian Temperance Union, combined with the brilliant lobbying techniques of Wayne B. Wheeler and the Anti-Saloon League, gained momentum in the early twentieth century, and by 1903 some kind of prohibitory law (state or local) affected more than one-third of Americans, with more than half similarly affected a decade later. In addition, concern with food shortages during World War I brought wartime prohibition, which restricted the brewing and distilling industries. Following these measures, the Eighteenth Amendment was ratified in January 1919. The amendment and its enabling legislation, the Volstead Act, targeted the liquor industry and the saloon, not private consumption. Nevertheless, the Prohibition era is often understood as if drinking itself had been rendered illegal.[39]

Clearly, not all women abstained from alcohol in the years leading up to national Prohibition, which took effect in 1920. Still, alcohol consumption took on new meaning in the context of Prohibition, and the New Woman figure became more familiar as she was transformed into the flapper. Many commentators asserted that women—especially middle-class women who may have shunned alcohol previously—now experimented with it in new ways, by making it, selling it, buying it, and drinking it.

Although women had been involved in alcohol production since the colonial era, Prohibition created new patterns of alcohol manufacture and distribution, and women's participation attracted particular attention. According to one former Prohibition officer, an increasing number of "ladyleggers" plied their trade by the mid- to late 1920s. As liquor runners, women supposedly enjoyed a number of advantages: Police were less likely to stop them, especially since some brought a child along in the car. If stopped, they could more easily talk their way out of an arrest, and if arrested, juries were less likely to convict. While press coverage often depicted such cases in sensationalistic terms that emphasized their novelty, many women who became bootleggers described it matter-of-factly as simply another business. One law enforcement officer explained that "bootlegging is a recognized trade for women, so frequently are they met with by our agents—the same types which furnish the women proprietors of tea rooms and millinery shops—the economically independent-minded, modern young woman who prefers to make her own way." These women could not be dismissed as deviants or criminals; one policeman noted that the women he arrested were "respectable" in everything except a "Volsteadian" sense.[40]

Media coverage of women's consumption featured similar tensions between sensationalization and normalization as commentators sought to make sense of bewildering new standards. As before, Americans assessed women's drinking differently depending on the location of consumption—commercial establishments versus the home—and the age and life circumstances of women who imbibed. Reconstructing actual drinking practices of the Prohibition era is notoriously difficult. Important regional variations existed, with New York City, where drinking was more common than in much of the rest of the country, exerting an outsized influence as a media center. What is clear is that young women especially viewed drinking as an act of rebellion, of a piece with other behaviors like smoking and petting, just as Progressive Era reformers understood alcohol consumption as part of the "river of vice." Press coverage of celebrity flappers such as Zelda Fitzgerald and Lois Long reinforced these associations.[41] The behavior of these young women, and the ways in which Americans understood it, reinforced a narrative of "wet" feminism—that women's drinking represented emancipation from tradition and a move toward social equality.

The saloon had been a primary target of the temperance campaign, representing a male-dominated, uncouth counterpoint to genteel domesticity. Many temperance advocates had hoped that Prohibition would create a single standard in which men acted more like women by abstaining from alcohol.[42] Instead, the rise—and glamorization—of heterosocial drinking establishments in which men and women mingled seemed to represent a substantial break with the customs of the past as well as an ironic inversion of the goals of prohibitionists. As one journalist reported, "It is nothing to write to the papers about these days when you see women—with or without escort—leaning on the bar of a Manhattan speakeasy ordering 'another scotch and ginger, Tony.' In the days of the saloon, such women as frequented them were segregated in a back room and even had an entrance of their own to slink in unnoticed. The speakeasy has changed all that."[43] This movement into spaces previously denied to them and the participation of middle-class women made women's alcohol use seem all the more significant. Not only were women drinking alcohol, but the location and manner of their consumption threatened to unravel the wider gender role and class conventions that previous drinking customs had helped to maintain.

For Marty Mann, who was a young woman during the 1920s, alcohol consumption was a fundamental part of social life. Mann explained, "Every boy in our crowd carried a flask and every girl drank from it. Drinking was a matter of pride with us."[44] She recalled also how exciting it could be to venture into new and slightly risky drinking establishments. The young men in her group, she explained, "would take the girls to little places where they must be recognized through a peep hole before being allowed to enter. I was young and happy and gay and I thought it great fun to take a drink."[45] Mann's memories show how drinking customs mapped onto existing rules of heterosocial courtship and power relations: Girls did not carry their own flasks or go out drinking on their own because boys took the lead.[46]

As they observed women's comportment in the 1920s, many journalists and social commentators pointed to drinking habits as marking a rupture with the past. While the "Victorian woman delighted in martyrdom," one reporter explained, "the modern woman tends toward hedonism."[47] Many journalists argued that the freedom to drink was simply one element of a wider transformation in women's behavior. These writers also welcomed expanded employment opportunities during World War I, equal suffrage, and even the new conveniences of the "machine age." One journalist maintained that women had a right to seek "men's playthings as well as his work." Liquor joined "cigarettes, the vote, golf, motors, and sex 'expression'" as privileges that women now demanded.[48]

At least some young women beyond New York and Chicago, where Mann lived, followed suit. In Butte, Montana, for example, unmarried women of the working and middle classes made, distributed, and consumed alcohol on a bigger scale *after* the adoption of Prohibition. For many, the appeal was not necessarily liquor but, rather, the adventurous behavior that public drinking required.[49] Young women in Butte smoked and bobbed their hair, deliberately violating adult conventions but ironically reflecting peer pressure, as rebellion came to be expected among youth. Similarly, college newspapers explained drinking by both men and women as a way of demonstrating disregard for traditional rules and standards.[50] These behaviors were not, however, as novel as participants and commentators claimed. What was different was that increasing numbers of middle-class women were now drinking publicly, and the same acts that might have brought severe social sanction or even arrest only a few years earlier were celebrated, at least in some circles.

While some young women hoped that a short hairstyle, the ability to drive a car, and a cigarette signaled emancipation and equality, they found that a double standard, rooted in differential power relations between men and women, persisted in courtship and sexual matters. The psychoactive effects of alcohol could amplify rather than erase that disparity, especially as young people created new dating practices and expectations. One Chicago woman described in her diary an encounter with her boyfriend in the summer of 1930, when she was nineteen. Taking advantage of the privacy of an automobile, the couple shared several drinks, making her "just tight [intoxicated] enough" to get "awfully worked up." Confessing that she was "frightfully ashamed of myself the next morning for letting him go so far," she nevertheless recorded, "I enjoyed myself."[51] It is impossible for us to know today whether her boyfriend took advantage of her in this situation. Her language suggests that he took the lead, yet she held herself responsible for the outcome even as she acknowledged the disinhibiting effects of alcohol.

The concern of an upper-middle-class father about his daughter's upcoming European trip because of "loose" mingling on the ship exposes similar tensions. Using a language of contagion, he feared for his daughter in a setting where "more hardened girls . . . sat in the bar hour after hour, day after day, singing barroom ballads with the regular fellows and taking part in the drinking races." The girls might believe they participated as equals, but the father emphasized their vulnerability. "Girls not quite 'themselves' visited boys' staterooms late at night and barely escaped seduction," he explained.[52] Although the term "seduction" could sound like an old-fashioned depiction of girls as innocent victims, he nevertheless seemed to suggest that these girls drank enough to cloud their judgment and would have only themselves to blame if something went wrong. The combination of concern and censure here recalls reformers' depictions of charity girls and prostitutes during the Progressive Era. Yet by denying that they needed rescue, young women of the 1920s contributed to the belief that they did not deserve protection.[53]

Although flappers self-consciously violated many traditional standards, their young age circumscribed the challenge they represented to middle-class womanhood. Their behavior could be understood as a rebellious phase, even a necessary part of development. This latitude for a short episode constituted a new privilege, but it did not ultimately threaten the goal of marriage and motherhood.[54] Even so, the flapper phenomenon could be harnessed for debates about the effect of Prohibition on youth. Both Drys—Prohibition advocates—and Wets—Prohibition opponents—used arguments about young people to advance their respective causes. One of the goals of prohibitionists had been to enable generations of children to grow up without knowing the taste—or facing the dangers—of liquor. Many Drys believed that there were fewer "recruits to the army of Bacchus" as a result of the Eighteenth Amendment. But this approach brought risks as well: "[American youth] have had the temptation taken from them, but they have not been fortified against the temptation when it is offered. They have never seen a saloon, but when they [are in a setting] where the bar is a general meeting place, weak ones fall its victim as the non-immunized American people fell to the 'flu' germ a dozen years ago."[55] This comment also illustrates the complexity of American ideas about alcohol, comparing the substance to a germ—echoing the temperance paradigm—but also hinting at individual vulnerability and the importance of environmental exposure.

For their part, some Wets argued that youth's increased contact with alcohol during Prohibition was a reason for repeal. Ione Nicoll, secretary of the Women's Organization for National Prohibition Reform (WONPR), a group of upper-middle-class women who mobilized for repeal, insisted in the *North American Review* in 1930 that the speakeasy was even more dangerous than the saloon because it was not regulated, and it particularly threatened precisely those groups that had previously been protected from commercialized alcohol and vice: "If the old saloon was the poor man's club, the modern speakeasy is the club, alike, of the rich and poor, and welcomes to its bar not only men and women, but young girls and boys." Nicoll even turned temperance strategy on its head; many prohibitionists had hoped that the elimination of the saloon would eradicate prostitution as well, but Nicoll argued that new drinking establishments actually increased it.[56]

By the early 1930s, as repeal, or at least some modification, of the Volstead Act seemed likely, commentators increasingly argued that young people must learn to drink moderately. These recommendations could be especially controversial when aimed at girls as well as boys, as Eleanor Roosevelt discovered. Shortly after her husband had been elected to the presidency, Roosevelt commented that today, the average girl "faces the problem of learning, very young, how much she can drink of such things as whisky and gin, and sticking to the proper quantity." Roosevelt's remarks attracted criticism from the Woman's Christian Temperance Union as well as from others who insisted that such concerns applied only to young women in the Northeast with too much time and money. Even those who applauded Roosevelt's remarks did not advocate drinking as such. For example, Pauline Morton Sabin, the charismatic chairwoman of the WONPR, seized the opportunity to explain the true meaning of temperance, and by extension, the mission of the WONPR: To correct the excesses associated with Prohibition but not to promote alcohol consumption, especially not among children. In her response to Roosevelt's comments, Sabin suggested that they, as mothers and educators, were ideally qualified to communicate the value of temperance. This message hardly differed from that of the Woman's Christian Temperance Union, reflecting the continuing use of "Home Protection" rhetoric in which women served as moral guardians on both sides of the Prohibition debate.[57] Sabin's reliance on this language reveals the mixture of traditional and modern elements in debates surrounding drinking, and in women's roles more broadly, during the 1920s.

"Decline Relatively Greater among Women": Medicine and Alcoholism during Prohibition

Medical ideas about problem drinking and about women's health underwent similar transitions, part of wider changes in the medical profession as well as the circumstances of Prohibition itself. Although antiliquor advocates criticized the saloon as a particularly pernicious institution, their general attitude regarding alcohol should be understood as a "temperance paradigm." In this belief system, alcohol was such a powerful and dangerous substance that it threatened to ensnare anyone who drank it.[58] While some individuals might be more vulnerable than others—variations that nineteenth- and early twentieth-century Americans might ascribe to inherited flaws, weak moral fiber, or the frailty they believed to be inherent in women—the main risk came from alcohol itself. Today we do not generally conceptualize alcohol in this way, but we do tend to think of heroin, cocaine, and, more recently, cigarettes in this fashion. This comparison helps us appreciate the motivation of those who believed that eliminating alcohol from American life was the appropriate solution to alcohol-related problems, including alcoholism itself as well as poverty and domestic violence. Prominent critics at the time dismissed Prohibition as the last gasp of an embattled remnant of rural fundamentalists who were quickly losing power and influence in modern America. This critique has retained considerable staying power, shaping popular perceptions as well as some journalistic and scholarly interpretations to this day.[59] But it obscures the extent to which Prohibition, like the Pure Food and Drug Act, was intended to be a large-scale public health intervention and represented a modern, professionalizing impulse.

Many physicians during the early 1920s shared the belief that alcohol-related health problems would disappear in the new order. In this sense,

Prohibition could be seen as a "magic bullet" that would eradicate an entire class of medical problems, as the invention of the drug Salvarsan, for example, was expected to bring an end to venereal disease.[60] Reflecting this optimism, discussion of alcoholism as such almost disappeared from medical literature. One eminent psychiatrist declared in 1922, "With the advent of prohibition the alcoholic psychoses as far as this country is concerned have become a matter of little more than historical interest."[61] Such expectations, however, proved premature. Hopes that delirium tremens would become "extinct" and that charity homes for inebriates would simply close because they were no longer needed were not realized.[62] Still, important shifts were under way, including a generational transition. Many of the physicians who had been involved in the American Association for the Study and Cure of Inebriety during the late nineteenth and early twentieth centuries had retired or died, while many of the asylums they had built were closed or converted to general mental institutions during Prohibition, and the organization itself dissolved by the mid-1920s.[63] The decline of this group meant that its relatively sympathetic depiction of women's reliance on alcohol as a form of ill health consistent with femininity receded from both medical and popular awareness.

Even as rigorous medical study of alcoholism declined, the problem retained symbolic value: Doctors and scientists, as well as journalists and the lay public, posited that the incidence of alcoholism and related health problems would indicate the success or failure of Prohibition as national policy. Reports appeared in national medical and scientific journals during the 1920s and early 1930s, extrapolating from hospital admissions data at institutions in the Northeast: Boston City Hospital and the Washingtonian Hospital in Boston, and Bellevue Hospital in New York City. In his review of alcoholic admissions throughout hospitals in New York State, Horatio M. Pollock, statistician for the New York State Hospital Commission, supplied some national data for comparison.[64] In many of these reports, gender remained a fundamental organizing rubric, and commentators ascribed extra interpretive weight to rates of alcoholism among women, just as many journalists did in their descriptions of women's social drinking.

Those who sought to trace alcoholism rates during Prohibition found that methodological difficulties abounded: Hospital reports did not necessarily define "alcoholic admission," for example, leaving open the possibility that the patient could be a chronic alcoholic or simply someone arrested for drunkenness. At the same time, these tallies may well have missed other patients who were admitted under different diagnoses, especially women for whom the stigma of admitting a drinking problem could be particularly strong. The

Prohibition context also complicated such calculations, since individuals of both sexes may have avoided medical attention lest they reveal illegal activity. Prohibition also brought about new forms of collaboration between medical professionals and the legal system. For example, the admission rate at the Washingtonian Hospital in Boston fluctuated, depending on the extent to which police cracked down on speakeasies in the area.[65] Similarly, a Dr. Sears of the Boston City Hospital reported that the number of alcoholic admissions increased during the first few years of Prohibition, counter to the experience of most institutions. Sears explained that the police, fearful that anyone drunk might become violently ill (presumably because of the quality of the alcohol available), brought such individuals to the hospital for observation rather than arresting them.[66]

One consistent theme that emerges from these studies is that the Prohibition era was not monolithic; admission rates changed significantly during this relatively short period. Important variations in enforcement trends and consumption patterns characterize the later 1910s (wartime prohibition), as well as the early, middle, and late 1920s.[67] All these studies found a general decrease in alcoholic admissions from around 1910 through the early 1920s, although some identified a spike in 1916 and 1917, which most researchers attributed to wartime prosperity and unsettled social conditions related to American involvement in World War I. Despite the temporary rise in 1916–1917, then, wartime prohibition and the Eighteenth Amendment had made a difference. A physician at the Washingtonian Hospital reported in 1918 that "many hard drinkers made a serious attempt to curb their alcoholic desires, and . . . admissions were less than they had been for ten years."[68] Similarly, the New York statistician Pollock concluded that Prohibition reduced excessive drinking and thus resulted in a lower rate of patients admitted for alcoholism or for mental illness linked with intemperate use of alcohol. By the mid-1920s, however, alcoholic admission rates had begun to creep upward again, although physicians and researchers rarely speculated on the reasons for the change.[69] Weakening enforcement of the Volstead Act may have been one factor, leading to greater willingness to seek hospital care for alcohol-related health problems.

These physicians and statisticians also analyzed demographic information on alcoholic admissions, reinforcing the idea that gender mattered. Analyzing data from Bellevue Hospital, for example, Norman Jolliffe—who would become a significant figure in the post-Prohibition alcoholism movement—reported what he called "striking changes" in the admission rate of alcoholic women. During the ten-year period 1902–1911, he noted that female admissions constituted about one-quarter of all alcoholic admissions (26 percent). There was a brief upsurge during 1918 and 1919, when close to 40 percent of alcoholic admissions were women, which Jolliffe attributed to women entertaining departing soldiers, welcoming them home, or grieving their absence. By 1920, however, the proportion of female patients decreased to below one-quarter. Women represented 21.4 percent of alcoholic admissions that year and had declined to only 13.5 percent by 1933, the year of repeal. While many popular commentators believed that problem drinking among women increased during Prohibition, Jolliffe's analysis brought him to the opposite conclusion. "These figures do not support the contention that prohibition and the speakeasy increased inebriety among women," he declared.[70]

Dr. Sears of the Boston City Hospital also analyzed social factors that might affect alcoholism rates among women. He noted, "The number of women admitted for alcoholism has always been small, and it still remains so," attributing much of the difference in admission rates to women's continuing desire to hide their drinking. Prohibition may have made women even more determined to avoid the consequences of public intoxication. Sears speculated that "women who over-indulge do so chiefly at home or in the company of their friends, who take care that they escape the notice of the police." Similarly, drinking women who needed medical care preferred a private physician if possible, to avoid the hospital.[71]

While all these experts agreed that alcoholism among women decreased during Prohibition, only Pollock's studies provided detailed comparisons of demographic and sociological characteristics of male and female alcoholics. Pollock reported that the educational and class backgrounds of male and female alcoholics were similar to one another and to the general population. Immigrants were disproportionately represented among men and women, while admission rates were lowest among "native whites of native parentage" and particularly low among women of that group.[72] This ethnic- and presumably class-based variation could indicate different drinking customs and access to medical care, as well as a higher rate of hidden alcoholism among more privileged groups. Most female patients were married, which could be a sign of family support or abandonment, depending on the type of institution. Finally, the average age for women upon admission was older than that for men, although the "drinking career" leading up to the admission was shorter.[73]

Even if the number of female alcoholics remained relatively low, heavy drinking among women retained its association with other social problems, especially those related to sexuality. Physicians and others speculated whether women's sexual behavior was also changing under Prohibition. Social workers noted with alarm that younger and younger girls were forced to resort to rescue homes run by the Salvation Army and other religious organizations—"ruined" by alcohol and the dangerous sexual behavior that frequently accompanied it.[74] Dr. Sears reported that the matron of a home for girls attributed a rise in illegitimate births "to the effects of the Eighteenth Amendment." Sears acknowledged that such pregnancies could reflect a "loss of self-control on the part of the mother, which alcoholic indulgence has produced," but he reminded his readers that "the combination of an automobile, a hip-flask, and a lonely country road is not new, but what was once a sordid experience is now cloaked with an air of mystery and a spirit of adventure."[75] Here, too, actions once considered squalid or restricted to socially marginal women became normalized, even glamorized in the 1920s. Sears's language also shows that even doctors did not always define alcoholism in women as a discrete clinical entity but used the term for any drinking that might cause problems, especially when accompanied by other violations of conventional standards.

The popular press circulated scientific and statistical findings like these as part of wider debates regarding Prohibition, thereby reinforcing the idea that women's drinking had particular significance.[76] Indeed, the rhetorical power attached to assertions that alcoholism among women (and children) was on the rise proved irresistible to Prohibition opponents, especially by the late 1920s. The WONPR used such arguments frequently. The secretary of the group asserted in the *North American Review* that the Keeley Institute reported a fourfold increase in the number of patients from 1920 to 1928, requiring a new building just to treat "drink addicts among women."[77] Pauline Sabin also claimed in 1929 that the number of female alcoholics had increased during Prohibition, although she did not explain why. Lamenting the "degradation of a drunkard," whether male or female, Sabin insisted that "before prohibition there were fewer 'shes' in proportion to the number there are today."[78] These arguments implied that all women responded the same way to the stresses of modernity and war, as well as to Prohibition, blurring distinctions among women's drinking patterns that Progressive Era physicians and observers had emphasized.

The visibility of younger women who drank recreationally also changed the meaning of alcohol as a substance, recasting the medicinal use of alcohol and associated nostrums as old-fashioned and unnecessary. In 1921, a seventy-seven-year-old woman who had been arrested in New York City for possessing a flask of whiskey argued that she needed it for her health, insisting to the magistrate "I take a little drop to brace up my strength." The official did not accept this rationale as a legitimate reason for her consumption, and she was sentenced to five days in jail.[79] Recognizing that times had changed and responding to new regulatory constraints, the Pinkham company excised language about "female complaints" from the label of Lydia E. Pinkham's Vegetable Compound.[80] As women drank along with men, liquor's recreational meaning eclipsed its earlier identity as a medicine.

As the medicinal model receded, women's drinking became ever more connected with sexuality across the class spectrum. This association gained further professional endorsement when an influential article by the German psychoanalyst Karl Abraham appeared in English in 1926 (having been first published in German in 1908).[81] Abraham was a leading figure in the field who had collaborated with Sigmund Freud, and his ideas offered a professional and modern rationale for evaluating compulsive drinking within a presumption of gender difference.

Abraham asserted that people's motivation to drink was rooted in psychosexual development and sexuality. While men were apt to brag about their drinking in light of its associations with masculinity and sexual prowess, Abraham insisted that the real appeal was alcohol's disinhibiting effect, which allowed men to express emotion and affection more freely toward other men. He explained, "The same men, when sober, would call behavior of this sort 'womanish.'" Like many other professional and lay commentators, Abraham did not always differentiate between the state of intoxication and chronic alcoholism. But he maintained that "drunkards" (his term) used alcohol as a surrogate for "normal sexual activity," by which he meant heterosexual intercourse. And just as neurotics clung to their symptoms, alcoholics refused to talk about the real reasons for their drinking. As a result, Abraham called for the application of the "psycho-analytical method elaborated by Freud" to alcoholic patients.

Like many other medical and lay commentators, Abraham emphasized that men and women did not consume alcohol at equivalent rates. It is an "indisputable fact," he declared, that "men are more prone to indulgence in alcohol than women." He focused on male alcoholics for the majority of his article, noting almost in passing that alcohol's effects had the opposite meaning for women. Whereas men were rewarded for "energetic initiative" and thus had an incentive to override repressions, a woman's "sexual instinct" should be more passive. If alcohol dissolved her resistances, she would become less attractive to men. Normal women, Abraham implied, should know better and therefore avoid alcohol consumption. Furthermore, while drinking sessions among men might be "tinged" with homosexuality, the association was even stronger among women, according to Abraham, who predicted that women who "display a strong inclination towards alcohol would probably, on closer observation, always reveal a strong homosexual tendency." At this time, "homosexuality" could refer to sexual activity and to gender "inversion"—demonstrating characteristics and behaviors more commonly associated with the "opposite" sex. Here, Abraham could be referring to both object choice and comportment on the part of drinking women, suggesting that they were willing to assume a more active "sexual instinct" even at the cost of their appeal to men.

When this article appeared in English in the mid-1920s, women's drinking in the United States seemed so deeply enmeshed in heterosocial and heterosexual customs that the connection Abraham drew with lesbianism gained little attention. The clothing and manners of young, middle-class women who drank signaled an eroticized heterosexuality rather than a form of masculinity, as also happened with conventionally attractive women who participated in sports.[82] Abraham's contention that drinking had traditionally been deemed "unwomanly" and was "never a subject of boasting amongst normal women, as it is amongst men" might have seemed slightly out of date to Americans by the late 1920s but underscored the transgressive quality of women's new habits. Although the public and even the medical profession paid scant attention to alcoholism treatment during Prohibition, Abraham's claim that alcoholism, neurosis, and sexuality were closely related would influence mid-twentieth-century psychiatrists significantly. His interpretive model offered a way to explain a social phenomenon—women's new drinking patterns—in a language of individual pathology. With the authority of his professional expertise, he insisted that women's drinking violated gender differences that were fundamental to human development, mental health, and appropriate relations between men and women.

"Lit Ladies": Drinking at Home during Prohibition

While flappers, speakeasies, and ladyleggers made good newspaper copy and physicians and statisticians pondered alcoholism rates, many Americans viewed women's drinking at home to be the most threatening of all. Despite Prohibition—or, some Americans argued, because of it—liquor became a status symbol during the 1920s, converted into one more consumer good for many middle-class families. Like other matters related to food preparation and entertaining, alcohol fell under the purview of women as hostesses. By some measures, women's involvement in drinking customs even before Prohibition had domesticated alcohol, providing a genteel alternative to the saloon.[83] Women thus played a similar role in drinking culture as in sexual behavior, moderating men's baser instincts. But respectable matrons could not exercise such a stabilizing influence when they *partook* of alcohol. On the contrary, they needed their husbands to manage their consumption because they could not be trusted to know their own limits, with potentially devastating consequences for their families.

Articles in popular magazines relayed mixed messages about women's drinking. Generally asserting that it was on the rise—even though they rarely provided statistical data on consumption rates—journalists offered anecdotal evidence that could make women's consumption seem widespread and ordinary. In the past, as one journalist explained, "drinking among women was confined to those of two strata—inmates of orderly palaces and inmates of disorderly houses. There was no middle ground."[84] But Americans from different class backgrounds increasingly shared consumption habits, and now, middle-class women indulged: "The mildest little suburban wife knows enough to buy cocktail materials for her afternoon party even if it does mean that she won't be able to meet the installment on the electric washing machine that week."[85] Hostesses searched for guidelines as alcohol became more important as a sign that one was up-to-date. Even as New York–based writers might express an occasional regret at these new conventions, their detailed descriptions of how urban sophisticates entertained set standards to which their readers could aspire.

Many commentators believed that illegal drinking by men during the 1920s could not be helped; it was, they believed, a reversion to type, the expression of an essential masculine urge that had always existed. Even critics who lamented the behavior found it comprehensible and familiar. In contrast, women's drinking during these years felt new, different, and dangerous; many worried that women's willingness to violate law and custom was inspired by Prohibition itself. Women had to *learn* to drink, a behavior that presumably did not come naturally for them, and the attempts of respectable women to participate in a culture of alcohol were often dismissed as amateurish at best and a threat to social order at worst.

In fact, many women found this new landscape difficult to negotiate, as both expectations and behavior were in flux. So complete was the inversion of values during Prohibition among some social groups that women acknowledged the existence of peer pressure *to* drink. As one reporter noted, "People seem to take it as a personal insult nowadays if you don't guzzle everything they hand you."[86] Another lamented that she could not keep track of which members of her social circle drank and which did not, as many of them altered their standards with frequency.[87] While flappers came in for plenty of criticism, they projected an unapologetic, youthful exuberance. Middle-class matrons, in contrast, grappled with age-related uncertainty, even malaise, as they tried to adjust to new standards. In a 1930 article in *Harper's Weekly*, the journalist and social reformer Margaret Culkin Banning coined the term "Lit Ladies" to convey the transformative potential of alcohol for individual women and wider gender roles alike.[88] She used the term to refer to women who "get fuddled, not once or twice but, depending on their capacity for alcohol, pretty often in the year" but who are otherwise upstanding and charming. The Lit Lady was likely to be in her thirties or early forties, thus older than the stereotypical flapper. Like flappers, older women might drink due to peer pressure, to seek "new sensations," and because it seemed "almost feminist." Yet Lit Ladies also turned to alcohol for a release from "burdens" and to recapture a youthful glow: "to prolong, even through artifice, what seems to many of them their best years."[89] Perhaps because their motivations were more complicated, older women felt more conflicted. In contrast to the carefree flapper who lifted her glass without worry, Banning argued that most Lit Ladies found it agonizing. "The personal struggles which have gone on in the minds of women in regard to drinking are incalculable," she insisted.[90]

The phrase "Lit Lady" suggested that intoxication—being "lit"—did not negate a woman's identity as a lady. In some ways, the Lit Lady's consumption represented a parallel to the traditional concept of "drinking like a gentleman." But the two could not be equivalent; women were new to drinking and bound to miscalculate. Once the Lit Lady had decided to go ahead, Banning explained, she found it difficult to limit her consumption. Although the Lit Lady is not an alcoholic, she may drink more than she intends, since "the lady who decides that one cocktail will do no harm is exceedingly apt to decide the same thing about two cocktails." Banning's depiction suggested that the Lit Lady experienced a loss of control, which could spread as if contagious from one woman to the next. Acknowledging that she did not know how many Lit Ladies there were, Banning insisted that it hardly mattered: "For the lit lady is not important because of her numbers. She is important not only because of what she may be doing to herself or her family, but because her psychology, her state of mind, her relaxation of control affects even those who do not share these things. In a way, her drinking brings sober women closer to intoxication." The Lit Lady, Banning said, was here to stay, and the "twentieth century cannot be quite complete without her."[91]

The phenomenon of Lit Ladies carried important implications for American marriage and childrearing, echoing temperance discourse but with a twist: Mothers replaced fathers as the problem. For example, one journalist described afternoon cocktail parties in an unnamed small city, where wives gathered for a few drinks before their husbands came home from work. This custom demonstrates the persistence of separate spheres—these economically privileged wives did not work for wages and spent daytime hours in social and leisure activities with other women—but also a growing expectation for companionship within marriage. The reporter speculated that the husbands "encouraged" the afternoon drinks, preferring to "find their wives bright-eyed and gay, and prepared for the evening's amusement."[92]

For the most part, however, new drinking customs required husbands to exercise more authority over wives' behavior, rather than less. A husband might indulge his wife with a paternalistic attitude, counting her drinks at a party and making sure they were not too potent—especially important since Prohibition meant that alcohol could be of uncertain quality and strength. "It takes so little to make Jane's head spin," a typical husband might say. "Besides, this stuff we're getting these days is so unreliable that an inexperienced drinker doesn't know how to gauge her capacity." Far from marking equality in marriage, drinking practices could allow, even require, husbands to demonstrate their dominance. "Fortunately, a man can drink more than a woman. Under the mellowing influence of several cocktails the sense of superiority, of which modernity has almost completely divested him, returns as he hovers about his wife, seeing that her drinks are mild and that her glass is not too frequently refilled."[93]

Even if drinking increased during Prohibition, men's watchfulness over themselves and their wives reduced the number of "drunkards": "an ugly word entirely masculine in its connotation," according to one journalist. She went on to suggest that Prohibition brought a complete role reversal in which "the nagging wife of fiction has been replaced by the nagging husband who gives himself and his friends a wretched evening while he begs his wife not to forget the terrible morning that followed the last party."[94] Reducing temperance arguments to myth ("the nagging wife of fiction"), this writer insisted that men had good reason to monitor their wives closely: "women are throwing themselves into the new conviviality with utter abandon, both because they have so recently discovered the rejuvenating and care-dispelling power of the cocktail and because women, when uninhibited, know nothing about moderation."[95] In short, women's drinking hardly seemed to have ushered in a new era of companionate marriage and equality; instead, drinking practices served as convenient terrain for the ambivalence many men may have felt about women's changing roles.

Even as couples negotiated new relationships in marriage, Americans continued to believe in the importance of traditional motherhood to family stability. Temperance campaigners had grouped women with children as innocents who needed to be protected from the dangers of the saloon. But women forfeited that position when they, too, picked up a glass. Even worse, they brought liquor into the home, the safe haven in temperance rhetoric. This situation looked like prohibitionists' worst nightmare as drinking mothers became a new problem, one "strangely coincident with the Eighteenth Amendment and Volstead."[96] Although home consumption was not necessarily illegal, depending on when and how the alcohol had been acquired, most commentators agreed that it set a bad example for children and even demonstrated contempt for the U.S. Constitution. While some children had been exposed to mothers' drinking prior to Prohibition, many more faced it now. For middle-class families in particular, where mothers should embody restraint and decorum, any loss of control was especially destructive and disturbing: "Mother laughing too loudly, mother dancing grotesquely—these are distressing sights."[97] Even at home with children present, women slid inevitably to intoxication, though they should have known better. Children paid the price for their mothers' excesses, and they took the position women once had, moral critics of the drinking habits of others. As one journalist reminded readers, "There is one thing certain in all this: there is not a child who can bear the thought of his mother being even the most infinitesimal shade altered by drink, the slightest iota lit. And that is what happens to the vast majority of women if they drink at all."[98]

If drinking represented a new freedom for women, it came at a cost—the loss of a mother's unique place in her family. "Perhaps," Banning suggested, "it was only a sentimentality. Perhaps, on the other hand, it is some of the honest wages of wifehood and motherhood which she is spending for her liquor."[99] A drinking mother fundamentally compromised relationships within the family, especially with her children. Another commentator insisted, "The drinking mother knows that her children have seen her nakedness, which no garment can ever again completely recover."[100] Even in the 1920s, with substantial changes in women's behavior and with increasing numbers of Americans dismissing the temperance claim that men should abstain owing to family obligations, motherhood could not easily accommodate alcohol consumption given its promise of pleasure and release from responsibility.

Echoing Progressive Era eugenics discourse about the risks associated with women's drinking, journalists argued that, while the double standard had perhaps not been fair, women's new drinking habits represented attacks "on what were not only accepted moralities but fundamental safeguards for the race."[101] Women's drinking was not and could not be equivalent to men's: As mothers, they violated one boundary by bringing alcohol into the home, and, in not being able to drink moderately according to observers, they blurred another, that between dignified social drinking and out-of-control consumption. Clearly, these commentators did not need medical expertise or a precise diagnostic category to make the case that women's drinking was dangerous.

Toward Repeal

For alcohol scholars, Prohibition represents a black hole in some ways. Very little reliable research was conducted during the 1920s on the effects of Prohibition,[102] leaving historians to piece together fragmented, indirect, and unreliable evidence. Despite these challenges, scholars have determined that Americans' per capita alcohol consumption fell during the 1920s—contrary to many contemporary observations. Historians writing recently have concluded that women, like all groups, drank less during Prohibition simply because alcohol was less accessible.[103] But if the promise of Prohibition had been to eliminate drinking and all the problems that went along with it, then reduction was not enough. Furthermore, the Great Depression brought an economic argument for repeal: If the government could tax liquor once again, much-needed revenue would be provided without an extra burden of direct taxation. Finally, some business and civic leaders who had supported temperance became increasingly concerned about the extension of federal power that Prohibition represented. By the later 1920s, many individuals and groups began to mobilize for the unprecedented task of repealing a constitutional amendment.[104]

As in the temperance crusade, women—and ideas about women's proper roles—played important parts in assessments of Prohibition and in the campaign for repeal. Press coverage, some of which came from self-consciously sophisticated female journalists who may well have sought to normalize their own drinking habits,[105] insisted that women were drinking more than ever before and catching up with men. "Deplore it if you will," one writer declared, "the number of men who drink is scarcely in excess of the number of women."[106] Women's involvement in the repeal campaign was also shocking to many. As one journalist declared in 1931, "What an upset of preconceived notions if it turned out to be the women of America and not the men who led in repealing the Eighteenth Amendment!"[107] Revealingly, however, even as the article went on to praise Pauline Sabin and celebrated women's progress in "thinking for themselves" regarding Prohibition, no mention was made of women's drinking. Similarly, while members of the Women's Organization for National Prohibition Reform did not "demur" when others described their drinking, they did not mention it themselves, and some wets, in fact, "expressed the same shock over women's drinking as their dry opponents."[108] Thus, while female solidarity regarding the liquor question no longer seemed a given, neither were women willing to assert a right to drink as a repeal tactic. Even as reports of women's new drinking habits provided ammunition for Prohibition opponents, those who promoted repeal chose not to advertise their own consumption lest they lose respectability.

As the delicate strategy used by repeal advocates suggests, American attitudes about women's drinking remained uncertain as Prohibition ended. Had the new drinking customs been as widespread as some commentators claimed, they would have lost their power to shock. Still, the meanings assigned to women's alcohol use *had* changed. The female inebriate who turned to alcoholic nostrums out of frailty and ill health now seemed as old-fashioned as temperance campaigners who could now be dismissed as stuffy and self-righteous. Women's drinking came to look more like men's, a form of recreational consumption to be engaged in for pleasure and enjoyment. Yet as lingering concern about "lit ladies" and "drinking mothers" shows, such indulgence did not mesh easily with beliefs about women's proper roles, and Americans continued to worry that women could not be trusted to know their own limits.

Chapter 3

"More to Overcome than the Men"

Women in Alcoholics Anonymous

On a chilly April evening in 1939, Marty Mann walked into the Brooklyn home of Bill and Lois Wilson to learn about a newly formed group of alcoholics who supported one another in a search for sobriety.[1] Mann's drinking had changed profoundly since she sipped from flasks at Prohibition era dances. In the intervening years, she had married and divorced, moved to England and returned, and through it all her drinking had escalated. She found to her horror that she could not stop, not even after a devastating fall (or jump) while she was drunk led to multiple broken bones and months of painful convalescence. Unable to keep a job, increasingly alienated from family and friends, she eventually entered Bellevue Hospital in New York City as a charity patient. She spent six months on the neurology ward where she received little treatment other than occasional visits from the neurologist Foster Kennedy, M.D., but at least she did not drink. Kennedy then arranged for her to be admitted—again as a charity patient—to Blythewood, a private sanitarium in Greenwich, Connecticut, where she would be treated by Harry Tiebout, M.D., a psychiatrist.

Like Kennedy, Tiebout seemed uncertain how best to approach Mann's drinking problem. For her part, Mann feared she was afflicted with a mental disorder that was all the more destructive and terrifying for its lack of a name and treatment protocol. She remained at Blythewood for months, meeting Tiebout for an hour of talk therapy every day but still unable to control her drinking when she went on brief visits to New York. Although she insisted she never meant to drink to intoxication, she returned to Blythewood drunk multiple times. Tiebout found her case a fascinating puzzle, but he warned Mann that she could not continue this behavior and remain a patient. Around this time, the fledging organization that would become Alcoholics Anonymous (AA) circulated a manuscript in which they described their program, sending it to clergy and medical professionals for review and endorsement. Tiebout received a copy, which he urged Mann to read.

Throughout her later public career, Mann consistently identified her encounter with this text as the key moment in her recovery, an almost mystical turning point. Initially resistant to the spiritual elements of the AA philosophy, Mann nevertheless found herself transformed at a critical moment. Faced with a personal crisis, upset and desperate for a drink, she noticed a sentence in the book, which was open on her bed: "We cannot live with anger." This passage brought liberation: "The walls crumbled—and the light streamed in. I wasn't trapped. I wasn't helpless. I was *free*, and I didn't have to drink to 'show them.' This wasn't 'religion'—this was freedom! Freedom from anger and fear, freedom to know happiness and love."[2] In other accounts, she described an even more turbulent scene in which she threw the book across the room "in a fit of temper." The book fell open to the page with the sentence about anger; upon reading it, Mann fell to her knees by the side of her bed, praying and sobbing.[3] In addition to the emotional release she felt, Mann found that having a *name* for her struggle with alcohol brought tremendous relief: "I grasped the clear picture and accepted the fact that I was the victim of a progressive and often fatal disease known as alcoholism. That book made me understand that I could never again safely touch liquor if I wanted to be well."[4]

Both Mann and Tiebout welcomed the knowledge and insight they gained from the text, and he encouraged her to go to New York to meet these alcoholics. Shy and fearful, she went to the Wilsons' home but lurked upstairs until Lois Wilson brought her down to join the group in the living room. At that meeting, Mann was the only alcoholic woman—the other alcoholics were men, and the other women were nonalcoholic wives and family members. Yet in retelling this story later, Mann insisted that she felt welcome and connected as soon as she and the men started talking, for she realized that they shared an understanding of one another's behavior that she had never found before, not even with medical professionals. Returning to Blythewood, Mann's sessions with Tiebout became more effective as she continued to attend AA meetings. After six months she was discharged from the sanitarium, but she maintained her involvement with the fellowship for the rest of her life.

As Mann's experience shows, individual trajectories of drinking and recovery do not necessarily conform to a broad periodization of alcohol in American history.

She would insist later that Prohibition neither caused her drinking problem nor prevented it, and neither did Repeal. Her struggle with alcohol, like that of Bill Wilson and countless others, followed a personal, internal logic, one that was shaped but not determined by wider political events and chronology.

When Marty Mann joined Alcoholics Anonymous, the group was only a few years old. The story of the founding of Alcoholics Anonymous has taken on near-mythic status and has been discussed in detail by other scholars.[5] Bill Wilson, a stockbroker and businessman, had struggled with compulsive drinking for years when he experienced a spiritual awakening during one of his periodic hospitalizations for alcoholism. Subsequently, he and his wife Lois became involved with the Oxford Group, a movement that used small-group meetings to help members to live according to early Christian precepts. After several months of sobriety, Wilson felt that he was in danger of "slipping" into drinking again while on a business trip to Akron, Ohio. Recounting the story later, he described a powerful need to talk to another alcoholic. He called ministers at random from the phone directory, searching for one affiliated with the Oxford Group. One of them gave him the name of a woman who was involved with the group, Henrietta Sieberling. Mrs. Sieberling later described Bill's call as "manna from heaven"; she had been greatly concerned about Dr. Bob Smith, a local physician and fellow Oxford Group member who was a chronic alcoholic. Mrs. Sieberling, with the cooperation of Smith's wife Anne, arranged a meeting between the two men, who talked for hours. This conversation has been memorialized as the genesis moment of Alcoholics Anonymous, and it provided an organizational template for the group: a connection between two alcoholic men, supported and encouraged by nonalcoholic women.

Following this 1935 meeting between Bill W. and Dr. Bob, as they became known, two small groups of recovering alcoholics emerged, one in New York and the other in Akron. Today, as the Twelve Step model of addiction and recovery permeates popular culture, it is difficult to appreciate how small, fragile, and experimental the AA fellowship was at first. The early members eventually split from the Oxford Group, reshaping many of its tenets into the now-famous Twelve Step program. In 1939, the nascent fellowship published *Alcoholics Anonymous: The Story of How Many More than One Hundred Men Have Recovered from Alcoholism*. Known widely, and affectionately, as "The Big Book," the work explained the organization's philosophy and included autobiographical narratives from members. This is the text that Dr. Tiebout urged Marty Mann to read.

By defining themselves as individuals who could not control their craving for alcohol specifically, early members of AA distinguished themselves from both moderate drinkers and from drug addicts. Alcoholics Anonymous as an organization refrained from any commentary on American drinking habits and from any recommendations about alcohol regulation or policy. In this way, the fellowship contributed to the "modern alcoholism paradigm," the idea that alcohol only posed a problem for a small group of individuals. This paradigm, to which scientists, physicians, and advocates also contributed (as discussed in chapter 4), countered the logic of Prohibition that alcohol was a hazardous substance. Instead, this "modern" view held that most people should be able to drink recreationally with no ill effects, and alcohol was no longer characterized as inherently addictive or even dangerous for the majority of the population. Alcoholics Anonymous's exclusive focus on alcohol—reflected in the very name of the group—differentiated alcoholics from drug addicts. While this distinction may have reflected the habits of the founders as well as the legal status of alcohol in the post-Repeal era, it served to segregate problem drinkers from addicts who used illicit drugs (and who faced even greater social stigma than alcoholics). It also altered the pre-Prohibition "inebriety" concept that had encompassed dependence on a variety of substances.

Through the Twelve Steps, "The Big Book," and ritualized meetings, the Alcoholics Anonymous fellowship came to perform many of the functions associated with medicalization. First, although the group eschewed scientific or moral debates regarding the causes of alcoholism, AA nevertheless offered a definition of the condition, one that even sounded medical: "an obsession of the mind coupled with an allergy of the body." Second, AA principles and practices reserved to individuals the power to diagnose themselves through the Twelve Steps and made the only requirement for membership "an honest desire to stop drinking." Third, participation in the fellowship itself constituted "treatment"; after naming and accepting his or her alcoholic condition, the alcoholic practiced rigorous habits of spiritual surrender and honesty to avoid further drinking. Members also shared their experiences at meetings and reached out to alcoholics who still suffered. Central to the AA program—and exemplified by the initial conversation between Bill W. and Dr. Bob—was the belief that one alcoholic could best understand and help another, as shared experience replaced medical authority as the necessary form of expertise. All of these elements, especially the sense of identification among alcoholics, proved extremely complicated for women.

Alcoholics Anonymous offered a radical message: Alcoholics could stop drinking, and the way to do so was through mutual support. This optimistic approach, which promised that alcoholic identity and experience were more important than social status markers, has been termed "alcoholic equalitarianism."[6] But alcoholic women who approached the group in the early years faced a challenge. The structure of AA groups often replicated the heterosexual couple constellation of separate spheres, hearkening back to the temperance era: An alcoholic man was the center of attention, with his loyal wife in a critical supporting role. As suggested by the very term "fellowship," AA could also be like a fraternity. For male alcoholics, AA thus offered both a homosocial milieu and a setting in which they could be family men or, at least, husbands.[7] This situation, though, made it difficult for alcoholic women to find a place in the group. Their alcoholism branded them as fundamentally unlike the nonalcoholic wives in the group, yet the fact that they were women in a deeply gendered setting meant that they were not necessarily welcomed by the alcoholic men, either.

"They Think You're the Babe Their Husbands Went Out With": Alcoholic Women and Relations with "AA Wives"

The philosophical underpinnings of the Twelve Steps and their practical application took shape slowly, when most Americans believed that alcoholism afflicted many more men than women. As a number of scholars have shown, AA grew out of the experience of a particular group of alcoholics at a specific moment in American history—namely, white men from Christian backgrounds, many in later middle age, of middle-class status or aspiration, during the Great Depression.[8] It is not surprising that the rituals and values of the program would reflect their traditions, social customs, and drinking experiences. It is important to note, however, that AA groups differed substantially one from another. The fellowship was "structured rhizomatically, [and] growing laterally"[9] with a purposely decentralized structure.

The following account of the relations among alcoholic men, their nonalcoholic wives, and alcoholic women who approached the fellowship in the early years is based largely on documentation from Akron and a few other groups. It is not necessarily representative of all AA experiences. Despite the variation that has characterized AA, however, nearly all early groups included many more male than female members, which presented structural and philosophical challenges. In particular, members struggled with how—or whether—alcoholic men and alcoholic women should relate to and interact with each other. The relationship between alcoholic men and their nonalcoholic wives needed to be reconfigured as part of the men's recovery from problem drinking.[10] While emotionally difficult, this process made sense in social and cultural context. But since the heterosocial drinking customs of midcentury American life eroticized relations between men and women who drank, the presence of alcoholic women (often presumed to be sexually promiscuous) could threaten the capacity of the fellowship to restore alcoholic men to their marriages and even undermine their quest for sobriety.

To many participants, fundamental components of the AA program—Twelve Step practices, meeting procedures, and outreach to other alcoholics—seemed more natural and appropriate in an all-male setting where heterosexuality was presumed.[11] Alcoholics who reached the Twelfth Step spread the word about AA, visited alcoholics who were hospitalized or in jail, and simply talked with those who still struggled with their drinking. Although wives might organize Twelfth Step calls, just as Mrs. Sieberling and Anne Smith arranged the meeting between Bill W. and Dr. Bob, the essence of the encounter was understood to be the affinity between the two alcoholics, which fostered the sobriety of each. Twelfth Step calls often developed into sponsorship, an ongoing relationship in which the more senior member served as a guide to the program and a personal support system for the newcomer. These encounters and the bonds that followed could be emotionally intense, even intimate, and many early members expressed concerns about "boy-girl shenanigans" if men and women participated together.[12] In at least one case, the anxieties associated with mixed-gender sponsorship were realized. When a male AA member visited a woman alcoholic, neighbors reported it to the woman's husband who assumed that the two were having an affair. A few days later, when the AA member returned to take the woman to an AA meeting, the husband, who was hiding near the house, "blew him in half with a shotgun."[13]

Although rare, episodes like this could easily raise the question of how women should participate or even whether women belonged in the fellowship at all, for the safety of members and the well-being of the organization. This debate reflected and perpetuated derogatory beliefs about the sexual behavior of drinking women. For example, Dr. Bob felt uncertain about whether the program would even work for women, and he hesitated about interacting too closely with them himself. The wife of one early member later recalled, "The thing that bothered him was that most of the women came in with the label 'nymphomanic.' Most of the wives would back away, and the men got leery because they were afraid they would get into some situation. So, in the beginning, the woman was looked on as trouble. Nobody wanted to handle it."[14] Many early male members of AA shared this perspective; a common saying during this era warned new male members, "Under every skirt there's a slip"—a double entendre referring both to women's lingerie and to a drinking episode by one who was trying to stay sober, in this case triggered by interaction with a woman.[15] Importantly, the phrase characterizes the woman as an object—her sobriety, even if she is an alcoholic, is not a matter of concern. Furthermore, portraying alcoholic women as dangerous made it much more difficult to recognize the ways in which they might be vulnerable to unwanted advances from men, during their drinking careers and even in the fellowship.

To avoid potential sexual tensions, many men in AA, including Dr. Bob, referred alcoholic women who approached the group to the supervision of nonalcoholic wives, who assumed important roles in the fellowship during the early years. "It is no exaggeration," recalled an Akron member, "to say that there would have been no AA without those wives."[16] Wives hosted meetings in their homes, provided refreshments, and organized Twelfth Step calls. The wives of the cofounders were especially prominent. Members of the Akron group described Anne Smith as a saintly figure, a deeply spiritual and generous woman who always made new members and their wives feel welcome and who opened her home to alcoholic men. In New York, Bill Wilson and his wife Lois also hosted alcoholic men during these years. Unlike Anne, Lois occasionally expressed resentment at this "invasion" but eventually came to accept it as her part in her husband's recovery. In the early 1950s, Lois institutionalized roles for wives in the Al-Anon movement.[17]

Wives' efforts on their husbands' behalves represented an extension of the traditional role of helpmate and an application of the domestic antidote to drunkenness so prevalent in temperance rhetoric. This couple constellation resonated strongly with conventional American images of the drunkard and his family and highlighted the awkward position of alcoholic women, whose presence in the fellowship upset the equation of gender identity and alcoholic status. Wives who participated in the fellowship to support their husbands may have felt they had little in common with women who were there owing to their own drinking problems. Although some women developed rewarding relationships across this divide, mutual hostility and suspicion persisted, due in part to beliefs about the immorality about women who drank to excess and apprehension about the relative roles of the two groups of women in the fellowship.

Even as they sought to help their husbands stop drinking, wives were not immune to wider social attitudes about alcoholic women. One of the first alcoholic women to approach the Akron group was "thrown out" of AA by the wives, according to an early member: "She was so bad, they wouldn't allow her in their homes."[18] This assessment suggests a fear of contamination, especially in the intimate, home-based gatherings of early AA, as well as contempt and judgment. For their part, alcoholic women might rebuff the support and friendship wives offered. Vi S., who joined AA in Cleveland, Ohio, with her husband in 1941, recounted that every time she saw several wives together talking, she feared they were talking about her and "what a drunk" she was. "And there was no other woman I knew of in AA," she recounted. "I was scared to death of the wives. I think they really tried to help me, but I was too standoffish."[19] As one wife recalled years later, "Yes, we were mistrustful of the women who were just starting to get sober. I think we looked down on them, were not quite sure of them, because 'no lady would do a thing like that.' The women had more to overcome than the men."[20] If anything, the presence of patient, loyal, long-suffering wives could throw into sharper relief the failings of alcoholic women to live up to feminine ideals.

With their husbands newly and often precariously sober, wives might resent and fear the continuing presence of women who had shared a drinking culture with them. As one early AA woman warned another, "Be darn careful how you handle yourself around the wives. They think you're the babe their husband went out with."[21] In this situation, alcoholic women were judged, even punished, not just for having a drinking problem but for having participated in public forms of leisure and recreation with other women's husbands. This accusation shows how difficult it could be for women to interact with men as autonomous individuals in the mid-twentieth-century United States. The jealousy nonalcoholic wives felt also limited mixed-gender sponsorship, according to some accounts. In 1950, for example, panelists at an AA conference concluded that "non-alcoholic women are most intolerant of women alcoholics" and noted that many men hesitated to sponsor alcoholic women because of concern that their wives would "resent" their doing so.[22] Even as the wives retained influence, however, the growing number of alcoholic women who joined the fellowship during the 1940s and 1950s forced a recalibration, changing the meaning of woman member from sober wife to female alcoholic. Some wives may have begrudged this transformation as well, as they became less central in an organization to which their husbands devoted considerable time and energy.

For alcoholic women, as for alcoholic men, the spouse played a critical role in drinking patterns and in the quest for sobriety through Alcoholics Anonymous. While single women who approached the fellowship faced particular judgment and hostility, married women confronted challenges of their own. Some husbands prevented their wives from seeking treatment or joining AA, fearing the consequences for their own reputations. When a psychiatrist suggested that an alcoholic woman investigate AA, her husband dismissed the idea, declaring, "She's bad enough now without getting mixed up with a bunch of drunks," and for several years he did not allow her to attend meetings.[23] Even ostensibly supportive partners could complicate women's treatment immensely. One woman explained that her long-term partner "pulled me out of the gutter twice." Yet when he grew "bitter" that she "put AA first" to foster her recovery, she stopped participating.[24] Alcoholics Anonymous literature encouraged nonalcoholic wives of male members to be patient and accepting of the time and energy their newly sober husbands devoted to AA.[25] The supportive wife fostering the sobriety of her breadwinner husband did not challenge but instead reinforced traditional domestic organization. In contrast, the alcoholic woman whose recovery required that her husband play a supporting role reversed familiar patterns, upsetting both individual family dynamics and wider social standards of who should nurture whom.

Even when alcoholic couples joined the fellowship together, women still confronted the structural problem of gender-specific sponsorship, exacerbated by a double standard of judgment. In one such case in Akron, the wife found herself the only alcoholic woman present. She recalled, "They told Annabelle [one of the nonalcoholic wives] to take me under her wing, and I shall never forget how she sort of curled up her nose and said, 'They tell me you drink too.'"[26]

These examples help us appreciate how gender functions as interlocking systems of roles, attitudes, behavior, and power. Even as the AA fellowship offered a radical promise that alcoholics could stop drinking and resume productive lives, alcoholic women who approached the group in its early years found that their very presence upset an arrangement that assumed alcoholics to be men and women to be supportive wives. Many male members and their nonalcoholic wives were suspicious of the sexual habits and morality of drinking women, fearing they would jeopardize men's sobriety and thereby weaken the fellowship itself. The apparent solution of referring alcoholic women to the nonalcoholic wives served to keep female alcoholics in a kind of second-class status, not quite full members in the fellowship since they were denied the one-on-one relationship with another alcoholic that formed the centerpiece of the AA program. Adherence to conventional gender roles thus trumped AA doctrine. But even this situation did not guarantee sisterly solidarity. By serving as models of moral and loyal womanhood, these wives—by their very presence—could underscore the deviance and pathology of alcoholic women.

"She Understands Her Sister Alkies":
Sponsorship, Twelfth Step Policy, and "Our Gal Group"

At her first meeting in the Wilsons' Brooklyn home, Marty Mann remained with the men when the nonalcoholic wives moved to a different room; ultimately, Bill Wilson himself served as her sponsor. Although she was frequently the only alcoholic woman at the meetings she attended, she continually emphasized how comfortable and "at home" she felt there. As a reporter later explained, this sense of identification was crucial in her recovery: "Being able to talk plainly with no shame to others who have been through the same distress means a lot. For, she says, no one except an alcoholic can truly understand the feelings of one."[27] As a professional woman with no children, Mann perhaps found it easier to relate to the men in the group and to align her alcoholic trajectory with theirs than did women who led more conventionally domestic lives. As well, her identity as a lesbian may have deflected the concerns raised by the presence of heterosexual women, although it is not known in detail when and how she disclosed her sexual orientation in AA settings. Mann thus had her own reasons for downplaying attention to gender and sexuality, and claiming a gender-neutral category of alcoholic allowed her to access the logic of the disease model and the therapeutic support of the group.

Despite this successful experience, Marty Mann, along with other early female members, turned immediately to recruiting other alcoholic women to join the program. This pattern suggests that these women felt inherent tensions regarding their position in the fellowship. Contemporary media accounts of Alcoholics Anonymous and the recollections of women members recounted a common practice in which an early woman member might be sponsored by a man (or a nonalcoholic wife), but she would then recruit and sponsor other alcoholic women. A newspaper article on AA in Boston during the 1940s provides an example of this process, illustrating at the same time persistent assumptions regarding alcoholic women's more severe pathology. According to the article, two thousand men and women had found sobriety through AA, and many AA members attributed the program's success to the fact that they all "know what it's like" to be alcoholic. Despite this universalizing message, however, female alcoholics clearly faced a double standard, even within the fellowship: "They say there is no more disgusting sight than a drunken woman. Even male alcoholics admit that female rummies are harder to handle because they are more emotional—crack up quicker." According to the reporter, at least, the women shared these views: "The first to agree with them are the AA's reformed lady tipplers, who look upon their past indispositions with the same objectiveness that they would a case of hives. They do not mind being referred to as elbow-benders, ex-inebriates, lady-drunks." Precisely because they had been more degraded, their recovery had been all the more remarkable. The reporter noted, "Looking at these women you'd never, never suspect that very recently they were poor, sodden wrecks crying for liquor, consuming as much as a quart or two a day."[28]

The reporter devoted considerable attention to Mrs. T., the widow of a music professor, who began drinking after her husband's death and gradually lost control. For more than a decade, the reporter informed readers, "Mrs. T. reeked of whisky. Many a day she lay almost senseless on the floor of her home." Her excessive consumption threatened her social position; the "socially prominent" Mrs. T., who dressed in "chic and custom-made" clothes and sported "beautiful diamonds on her hand," was reduced to drinking with the cleaning woman, horrifying her grown daughters. Unsure what to do, her doctor hospitalized her, and she spent some time in a mental institution before her daughters contacted AA. A man ("Cooky") came to see her on a Twelfth Step call. As it happened, he and her husband had been fraternity brothers, so it was quite a shock for him to find her in such a state (presumably it could have been equally surprising for her to find out that he was in AA, but that perspective is not addressed in the story). While the social connection she shared with this man could have added to her humiliation, the familiarity it provided might also have made her feel more comfortable in the fellowship. In any event, Mrs. T. recovered and then turned her attention to other alcoholic women: "Today Mrs. T. is doing for other women alcoholics what Cooky did for her. She is taking them into her home to give them a new start. She will hold their head after a hangover and she will sit on their chests when they want to jump out the window. She understands and can sympathize with her 'sister alkies.'"[29]

Of course, woman-to-woman Twelfth Step calls did not guarantee a positive outcome, as Mann recalled in a 1948 speech: "I was the first woman [in AA] and nobody wanted anything more than I wanted another woman member, and I worked on hundreds of women the first year that I was sober, without getting any of them to stay sober. I would go anywhere, or do anything," Mann recounted. Responding to a letter a woman wrote for help with her drinking, Mann went to the address, rang the bell, and explained that she was from AA, only to be greeted with a punch in the face that sent her reeling down the stairs since the woman had changed her mind in the meantime.[30] Still, frequent pleas in the newsletter the *Grapevine* and in AA correspondence during the 1940s for more women to join the fellowship reflected women's preference for female sponsors, men's desire to avoid serving as a woman's sponsor, and the general assumption that women were best suited to helping one another.[31] Indeed, it is striking that these pioneers did not bother to explain why they wanted other women in the fellowship, suggesting that they considered society's gender divisions inviolable, even within the newly created culture of AA. This unelaborated preference shows also the strength of heteronormative attitudes and ignorance or denial of homosexuality in the belief that same-sex sponsorship, whether among men or women, would avoid any sexual tension. Same-sex sponsorship could also have been seen as especially important in promoting an image of AA as respectable, a counterpoint to promiscuous drinking customs. In practice, it may well have saved some women from being subject to sexual harassment by men in the fellowship, although that prospect is not mentioned in early AA literature—if anything, early male members and their wives characterized alcoholic women as the threat.

The publication of *Alcoholics Anonymous: How Many More than One Hundred Men Have Recovered from Alcoholism* in 1939, along with increased media coverage of the fellowship during the late 1930s and early 1940s, brought many new members and a proliferation of groups in other parts of the country. As more and more alcoholic women joined, sponsorship networks developed, especially in large cities. Internal AA evidence and news accounts of the fellowship both suggest a slow but relatively steady increase in women's involvement, at least in major cities, with a surge of attention and growth during World War II, when many Americans believed that women's drinking was increasing as a result of unsettled social conditions. Significant regional variation characterized women's participation, and many AA members believed that women found it easier to join groups in cities than in small communities. Much of this pattern, of course, simply echoed the spread of AA groups across the country during the late 1930s and early 1940s. New York City probably had the highest incidence of women members, with about forty women on its AA lists as early as 1942. Similarly, the number of women in San Francisco AA groups increased during the 1940s, according to a 1943 account. In 1947, the general secretary of AA reported that women made up 25–40 percent of the fellowship in some large cities, although in other cities, such as Dallas, the percentage of women remained lower. By the early 1950s, the gender ratio in two (unnamed) cities was reported to be equal, while Margaret G. maintained that small towns were less tolerant of female alcoholics. During the same period, however, AA members in a small town in Michigan claimed that women actually outnumbered men in their group.[32]

Growth in the number and proportion of alcoholic women in the fellowship made it more likely that prospective female members would encounter other women who had overcome drinking problems. In their AA narratives, many women emphasized the key roles other women played, inspiring the courage to acknowledge drinking problems and providing a bridge to full participation. One woman, for example, came to meetings with her alcoholic husband, which would not have been uncommon in this era for wives who were not alcoholic. Only after a young woman at the meeting asked her, "Are you one of us souses, too?" did she admit, "I'm having trouble with my drinking, too." That was the first time, this woman recalled, that she confessed her problem to another person, and she realized that night that she was "just as much a drunk as [my husband] was, if not worse."[33] Women who had once drunk together might also lead one another to AA. One woman joined, for example, after a female "drinking buddy" had achieved sobriety through the program.[34]

Women who found sobriety through the fellowship insisted that the connection it provided with other alcoholic women brought greater therapeutic power than conventional medical or psychiatric treatment. For one woman, multiple hospitalizations had made no difference; she felt that the doctors could not understand what she was going through. "But to another woman," she remarked, "the first woman I met in AA, I could talk. In all the sanitariums and psycho wards I had never met a single woman who said she was an alcoholic. They were always there because of a nervous breakdown, or for a 'rest cure'—any reason except because of drinking. (I've met some of these same women since in AA)." She explained further, "When I first came into AA, the woman who was my sponsor was the first woman I had ever met who admitted that she was an alcoholic."[35] Another woman felt a great sense of belonging when Bill Wilson asked her, "Do you think that you are one of us?" and then arranged for her to meet Marty Mann. Mann, who was "like the friends I had once had," both explained and personified the condition, bringing enormous relief: "A load weighing a thousand pounds came off my back. I wasn't insane. Nor was I the 'worst woman who had ever lived.' I was an alcoholic, with a recognizable behavior pattern."[36]

Clearly, the reception they received from other women in AA proved critical for female alcoholics. The definition of alcoholism offered by the AA program was necessary but not sufficient for many women; they needed to hear this message from, and see their own experience reflected by, other women. Many of these new members then augmented the growing female networks in the fellowship to help other alcoholic women. Mann's correspondence includes many references to such interactions; frequently, the writers asked Mann to help a friend, relative, or acquaintance who expressed interest in AA but remained tentative.[37] For example, one woman wrote to Mann's assistant in 1946, asking her to shepherd an alcoholic "prospect" to her first AA meeting in New York: "She's sold on AA and wants to attend meetings but may hesitate to go alone at first. . . . I wonder if you would be good enough to call her and give her the dope and perhaps arrange to meet her at the first meeting she attends? I'd appreciate it ever so much and so would she."[38]

These networks, which provided practical advice, logistical help, and emotional support, represented a significant success for women in the program and a critical resource for alcoholic women. Yet they also placed a burden on the pioneer women in the fellowship, especially women like Mann whose identity was well known by the mid- to late 1940s. Indeed, Mann's schedule, once she established the National Committee for Education on Alcoholism, actually precluded her continuing involvement in sponsoring women directly. Describing herself as "frantically busy" with a fundraising drive, Mann explained to a friend that she could not be consistent with visiting potential AA members and sponsorship: "I try to do some Twelfth Step work but find it is not good for the prospects since I am apt to go out of town at [a] crucial point."[39]

Mann's visibility in the popular media, however, provided a type of remote sponsorship for women who might never meet her. For example, the actress and singer Lillian Roth recalled in her memoir *I'll Cry Tomorrow* that Mann served as inspiration for her own recovery. While hospitalized for alcoholism but without specific treatment that addressed her drinking problem, Roth read an article about Mann that appeared in the *New York Times* as part of the publicity surrounding the launch of her public health campaign, crediting Alcoholics Anonymous rather than medical treatment for her sobriety. Roth became distraught: "Panic seized me. I had been tricked! If doctors hadn't helped Marty Mann, if institutions hadn't helped her, what was the good of me being locked up here?"[40] Her doctor was not willing to collaborate with AA, however, and Roth was eventually released without any support system. Humiliated by articles about her in gossip columns, isolated and unable to find work, she resolved to drink herself to death. She had climbed out onto a window ledge ready to jump, she recalled, when for the second time in Roth's story, the example of Marty Mann loomed large, this time saving Roth's life. "*Marty Mann*. The name leaped into my brain. What had the *Times* said? She lived to tell her story to Alcoholics Anonymous."[41]

Resolving to try the fellowship, Roth went to the AA clubhouse in New York. Alcoholics Anonymous members cared for her for several days and then took her to a meeting where Bill Wilson spoke. Hearing Bill, she recalled, she started to "get the message." Like many alcoholics who had experienced various treatments without success, she viewed Alcoholics Anonymous as a last resort: "If I left it, nothing waited outside but insanity or death." She became ever more committed to the fellowship: "Now I lived and breathed AA." Using the same language as Mann—indeed, the language most likely came from Mann's educational materials—Roth emphasized for her readers that there should be no stigma associated with alcoholism, a malady that, she says, is "no more disgraceful than diabetes or tuberculosis."⁴² Even without a continuing personal relationship, then, hearing the story of another alcoholic woman could have a significant impact.

Although not as well known as Mann or Roth, many other women in AA similarly aided the development of the fellowship despite their small numbers. Women played central roles in publishing the *Grapevine*, AA's newsletter, and often worked at the General Service Office in New York or in local staff positions. A woman, Bobby B., served as national secretary during the 1940s. Women helped to establish new AA groups and were also credited with playing key roles in educational and outreach efforts.⁴³ Alcoholics Anonymous members and outside observers interpreted these contributions not as individual achievement but as a form of gender-appropriate service that simultaneously marked women's recovery from alcoholism and reinforced conventional roles. Commentators as diverse as a New Jersey police chief and a Harvard psychiatrist asserted that, while alcoholic women found it more difficult than men to stop drinking, their health and femininity could be restored as they helped others.⁴⁴ Depictions like these underscored the idea that alcoholic women differed from their male counterparts in both illness and recovery. Adopting traditional female roles in supporting the fellowship, alcoholic women replicated the functions of nonalcoholic wives, demonstrating their ambiguous position as alcoholics who were also women.

In this context, some women began to form exclusively female groups, although it was not clear how, if at all, such groups would differ in format or practice. While little evidence has survived regarding early women's groups, one of the first was established in Cleveland in 1941, relatively quickly in the fellowship's development. Achieving a critical mass of women was clearly a prerequisite for an all-women's group, and some locations simply did not have enough female AA members to make this possible. In other areas, especially large cities, women's groups became increasingly feasible. During the 1940s and early 1950s, for example, women's groups developed in Minneapolis, Chicago, and Salt Lake City, among other locations.⁴⁵

Women in San Diego were especially active. There, female alcoholics formed a women's group in 1945. Initially gathering in the homes of members, the group soon rented a venue and established regular weekly meetings, as well as outreach to hospitals. Financially self-supporting, the group also held fundraisers that enabled it to contribute to other AA projects in the area. Women younger than thirty-five eventually formed their own group as well. As they explained in the *Grapevine*: "We feel that the growth of our Group is due to the rotation of responsibility, keeping business and personalities out of the meetings as far as humanly possible, and in emphasizing always that we attend our weekly meetings to help each other with a common problem and are all there for the same reason. We would be very glad to offer any help we may and when we hear that old cry 'women can't get along together' we know it isn't so."[46] In addition to demonstrating sobriety, this group felt the need to counter negative attitudes regarding women's competence and leadership skills.

In other cities, women adopted a range of strategies. In New York City, for example, women met in an all-female format every two weeks, but otherwise attended mixed-gender meetings. Similarly, Mann's correspondence included a reference to a "Women's Discussion Group of AA" that featured a "luncheon for about thirty dames and then a closed meeting."[47] In fact, some evidence indicates that women were "encouraged" to form their own groups during the early years.[48] Yet even when women-only groups alleviated some of the difficulties, especially regarding sponsorship, that women faced in mixed groups, they posed a challenge to the ostensibly universal message of AA. To the extent that the therapeutic power of AA came from embracing an identity of "alcoholic" without any modifier, a continuing focus on gender could reinforce the belief that alcoholic women were *different*, generally understood in this context to mean *worse*.

Other alcoholics who were viewed as outsiders ventured to join AA as well, with varying degrees of success. Many realms of American life were segregated along lines of race, class, religion, and gender during the middle decades of the twentieth century, so the challenges AA faced in delivering on its universal promise were hardly exceptional or unique. And as early members confronted one heavily stigmatized identity, that of being alcoholic, they sometimes sidestepped others, choosing not to acknowledge homosexual members or promote racial integration, for example. Alcoholics Anonymous's universal message about alcoholism collided with American social realities during the middle decades of the twentieth century, limiting the participation of alcoholics from a range of backgrounds.[49]

Little evidence remains regarding racial attitudes and relations in the early years of the fellowship. Even without an explicit policy of racial exclusion or segregation, however, AA groups apparently followed dominant social and legal customs, so that women (and men) of color faced even greater challenges in joining the fellowship than their white counterparts, in many regions of the country, at least. Since individual groups had significant autonomy, local conditions undoubtedly shaped the experiences of alcoholics who approached the fellowship, and African Americans often established separate groups if they were to have groups at all. In the Washington, DC, area, for example, a "colored group" met once a week in Arlington, Virginia.⁵⁰ In Cleveland, an African American woman called the local AA group during the 1940s. Members of the group (which was all white) met with her and provided encouragement and practical support, but told her that she must attend a different group. As a result, the first African American group in Cleveland formed around her. The Cleveland-area AA newsletter reminded members in 1945, "We whites, if we preach brotherly love, must practice it. And should a Negro appeal to us for help and guidance, it is our Christian duty to give the best that is in us."⁵¹ Despite these urgings, however, these white members were unwilling or unable to form integrated groups at that time. By 1950, one newspaper estimated that there were approximately "5,000 Negroes" in AA out of 100,000 members.⁵² Some of these members may have participated in racially mixed groups, while others were segregated.

Religious background and orientation could be another fault line. Numerous critics have identified AA's spiritual orientation as a liability of the program, one that excluded non-Christians or anyone unwilling to take an approach that seemed religious. In fact, the fellowship was self-consciously nondenominational, using language such as "Power greater than ourselves" or "God as we understood Him" in an attempt to make participants feel as comfortable as possible with the program.⁵³ In the early years, however, most members were probably from Protestant backgrounds, since even Catholics could not easily participate in meetings held in Protestant facilities. Some Catholic institutions, like a hospital in Akron where Dr. Bob sought to provide care for alcoholics in collaboration with a nurse, Sister Ignatia, did not want to cooperate with a religious "sect."⁵⁴

As we have seen, the very structure of AA, and particularly the practice of sponsorship, presumed heterosexuality. In fact, one psychiatrist asserted that AA wanted to keep homosexuals out of the fellowship.⁵⁵ The situation was complex, however, as lesbians and gay men, including Marty Mann herself, could participate in the program without disclosing their sexual orientation to the wider world or even within the privacy of the group. In this sense, sexual orientation differed from racial or gender identity, which was generally more visibly marked. Many early members of AA, Mann included, sought to retain the utmost respectability in every other realm of their lives, even if it required subterfuge, to protect both themselves and the fellowship. Mann's decision to keep silent about her sexual orientation even as she publicly announced her alcoholism demonstrates the continuing prejudice toward homosexuality in the middle decades of the twentieth century, as well as the complicated position of individuals who negotiated more than one stigmatized identity.

Focusing on out-of-control drinking as the primary problem alcoholics faced allowed individual members and the fellowship as a whole to evade other questions, including sexual matters, which were considered private. As we shall see, this framework contrasted with psychiatric approaches that probed "gender maladjustment" and "sexual dysfunction" as factors that then created alcoholism as a secondary condition. While critics then and now have attacked the narrow focus of AA, many alcoholics who joined the fellowship, including Marty Mann, embraced this approach with relief.

The Disease of Difference

The first step of the Alcoholics Anonymous program offered a definition of alcoholism, the equivalent of a diagnostic test, through this statement: "We admitted we were powerless over alcohol—that our lives had become unmanageable." This declaration, which an alcoholic made after "hitting bottom," could mean many things, with "powerless" and especially "unmanageable" measured in an infinite variety of ways. Yet the criteria for determining alcoholism resonated most with the image of a man who was unable to maintain employment and lost his economic position because of his drinking. When she joined AA, Mann was told that she could not really have "hit bottom" yet as such a young woman. The male members in her group defined hitting bottom as being without a clean shirt. Mann recalled, "They didn't believe that a woman in her early thirties could have hit bottom. They didn't know I had! I had been without a clean shirt often!"[56] Importantly, Mann did not offer an alternative version of what hitting bottom might have meant for a woman of her situation; instead, she accepted the standards the men had articulated and insisted that she met them in spite of her gender and age, just as she felt that she belonged in an all-male group with a male sponsor.

For many women, however, other criteria seemed more relevant or significant, especially since the question of what constituted "hitting bottom" could reflect and perpetuate a double standard of judgment. Some drunken behavior, such as sexual activity, or consequences of excessive drinking, such as a severe hangover, that might be acceptable or laughed off in a man could bring more censure or risk for a woman. One alcoholic woman, for example, explained that during the last stages of her alcoholism, she could not hold a glass in her hand because she had "the shakes" so badly; she had to sip the drink off the bar. While this situation would be embarrassing for anyone, she noted, "I was still a lady, believe it or not, and I was deeply ashamed."[57] Other encounters could be dangerous. Another woman recalled that during a wine-tasting tour of France, she passed out in a public square, then woke up to find a man leaning over her. She hit him, but he kicked her to the ground. She continued, "Bruised, and deadly ashamed, I told no one. I began, here and now, to fear the answer to the question—what is the matter with me?"[58] Alcoholic mothers described episodes related to their children to indicate their decline. One woman, for example, drank the brandy that a doctor had prescribed for her son. Another, denied access to the family car and money by her husband, robbed her son's piggy bank.[59]

However the bottom was defined, many early AA members believed that women found it more difficult to admit their dependence on alcohol. Even when they acknowledged the social disapproval alcoholic women faced, commentators blamed women for slowing the therapeutic process. In 1943, for example, the *Chicago Tribune* reported that "Miss Roe," the "charming new national secretary" of AA, had come to Chicago to discuss how women could become more involved in the fellowship. Citing women's "stronger inhibitions" and "mask of reserve," Roe explained that they are less willing to admit they need help, which is the "first step on the road to beating the liquor habit."[60] Such resistance made women harder to cure.[61] The very empowerment that came from a patient-centered movement could, ironically, work against anyone who was unwilling to admit a problem. News coverage like this perpetuated the idea of gender difference in evolving concepts of alcoholism and recovery, reinforcing a perception that alcoholic women demonstrated more severe pathology.

If alcoholic women found it more difficult to stop drinking, female success stories proved the fellowship's effectiveness. Just like late nineteenth-century inebriate specialists, AA advocates pointed to their program's promise for women as evidence of their progressive approach. The AA newsletter *Grapevine* noted in 1945, "It is encouraging to note that everywhere in the country, paralleling the steady increase in general knowledge that alcoholism is a health problem, not a moral one, women from smaller communities as well as large are beginning to come into AA a little less spasmodically and haltingly."[62] At the same time, the willingness, even eagerness, of some women to advertise their status as pioneering members of AA suggests that the persona of "recovering" alcoholic brought individual therapeutic benefit and neutralized the particularly harsh stigma that many alcoholic women faced. Both contemporary and historical accounts sought to identify the first woman in AA, as if it were a necessary counterpoint to the founding conversation between Bill W. and Dr. Bob. Given the simultaneous growth of groups in different geographic locations and a lack of membership records, we will likely never know with certainty—nor is that necessarily the best way to frame the question. We can, however, identify several early women whose varied experiences helped to structure the founding narratives of the fellowship and created templates for women's involvement: Florence, the author of the only woman's story in the first edition of "The Big Book"; Ethel M., who with her alcoholic husband joined one of the earliest AA groups in Ohio; and Marty Mann, who became a well-known public health advocate.

"A Feminine Victory"—the name itself marking the difference of its subject—was written by Florence, one of the earliest AA members, male or female. She had moved from New York to Washington, DC, to try to establish a group there, perhaps as early as 1936. Unfortunately, according to a history compiled by the Washington group, Florence became involved with a "hellion" substantially younger than she, with whom she resumed drinking. Little is known about the last years of Florence's life. Apparently she never regained consistent sobriety, although she continued to have some contact with the Washington group. In fact, when Florence died of pneumonia in 1943, two members of AA were called to identify her body. Florence's story, with its unhappy ending, was cut from subsequent printings and editions of "The Big Book."[63]

Ethel M., from Ohio, received the designation of "first woman in AA" in her obituary, which praised her "selfless help to others." Ethel joined AA with her alcoholic husband, and she was sponsored by Anne Smith, the wife of Dr. Bob, and by Sister Ignatia, a Catholic nurse who collaborated with Dr. Bob to provide hospital care for alcoholics in Akron. Although Ethel was not the first woman to join the fellowship, she reportedly had the earliest continuous sobriety of any woman. Her exemplary recovery brought her the designation of the "first woman"; claiming this status may also have allowed the midwestern groups to assert their importance relative to New York.[64]

Marty Mann became the best-known woman in early AA; a recent biography christened her the "First Lady" of Alcoholics Anonymous.[65] Although some observers argued that she forfeited first-woman status because of a brief slip in which she resumed drinking, Mann claimed that designation for herself when she launched her public health movement in 1944. Mann's references to AA as the source of her recovery and a need to clarify the relationship between AA and her fledgling public health organization helped lead to the codification of anonymity guidelines in AA's Twelve Traditions. Even after these principles had been formalized, Mann still referred in her private correspondence to her pride at being AA's first woman member.[66]

In 1957, when AA was two decades old, Bill Wilson declared that the fellowship had "come of age." Assessing the experiences of women in the program, however, he could offer only a tautology. "In the beginning," he reflected, "we could not sober up women. They were different, they said. But when they saw other women get well, they slowly followed suit."[67] Even as he emphasized the importance of identifying with other women in the fellowship, Bill left unexplained the question of how the *first* women had recovered. And even as he insisted that women, too, could recover through the AA program, the belief that women represented a distinct category of alcoholic, one particularly impervious to treatment, continued to suffuse the wider culture.

This perspective can be seen in the 1962 film *Days of Wine and Roses*, in which the fellowship figures prominently, although it was not an official production of AA. The film tells the story of a young couple, Joe and Kirsten. An advertising executive, Joe drinks heavily as part of his professional milieu and leisure time. He meets Kirsten, an attractive secretary, and on their first date he persuades her to drink a Brandy Alexander, despite her protests that she does not need alcohol to enjoy herself. Finding she likes it, Kirsten starts to drink along with him. The couple marries and has a child, and their drinking accelerates, with consequences that unfold according to a conventionally gendered script. Joe loses his job, and Kirsten neglects their daughter and her domestic responsibilities, finally setting fire to the apartment while drinking and smoking. Joe and Kirsten then retreat to Kirsten's father's home, a version of the wholesome farm cure as Joe works in the family landscaping business. Soon, however, Joe returns from an errand with liquor, and once more he prevails on Kirsten to drink despite her protests. The two become very drunk, and Kirsten tries to get into bed with her father, while Joe is humiliated trying to acquire more alcohol.

Up to this point, Kirsten's drinking and its consequences have played out at home, but Joe's public behavior lands him in an institution, where he wakes up in restraints. Fortunately for him, he is then the recipient of a Twelfth Step call and begins to attend Alcoholics Anonymous meetings with a sympathetic sponsor. These AA meetings and related scenes serve a didactic purpose for the film's audience, as various characters explain the basics of AA philosophy and practices. Despite Joe's positive experience with AA, however, Kirsten refuses to participate, and she leaves Joe and their daughter. Several subsequent scenes reinforce the stereotypical connection between women's problem drinking and heterosexual promiscuity. When Joe visits Kirsten's father to make amends, following the Twelve Steps, the father blames Joe for Kirsten's drinking and laments that now there is "always another bum" with her. Kirsten initially mistakes Joe for someone else when he finds her in a run-down motel. In the film's final sequence, Kirsten comes to the modest apartment where Joe lives with their daughter, saying that she wants to come home. Now sober, Joe wants her back but says she must not drink. She explains that she must have liquor, even at the cost of abandoning her child and her husband, in a shocking contrast to the cheerful and devoted wife and mother she had been.

The differential fates of the alcoholic protagonists plainly supply dramatic tension in the film. Although the outcome is not explained in explicitly gendered terms, audiences likely needed little help to see that alcoholism in women represented a more severe break with normalcy and health. While viewers, along with Kirsten's father, might be tempted to accuse Joe of creating Kirsten's problems, the film does not advocate this conclusion. Joe explains that he and Kirsten drink the way they do because they are alcoholics, a circular definition that does not attribute blame or even causation. Kirsten's refusal to join AA does not threaten the therapeutic promise of the fellowship; recovery is possible, but only if the alcoholic will try, as Joe does. The film thereby reinforces the idea that alcoholic women find it more difficult to admit drinking problems, and they are less likely to get well or redeem themselves as a result. Kirsten's fate represents an opposite outcome from media depictions that lauded the effectiveness of AA fellowship for women, but both characterizations underscore the idea that women constituted a distinct category of alcoholic.

The Alcoholics Anonymous fellowship—including its evolving philosophy and protocols, the official writings of the group, the genre of AA recovery narratives, and media portrayals of the program—played a fundamental role in redefining alcoholism in twentieth-century America. Although not always realized in practice, the concept of "alcoholic equalitarianism" was indeed radical, and many women—and men—found this a welcome, even life-saving, approach. Focusing on drinking as such, the program downplayed or ignored many other issues that were often associated with alcohol consumption. Alcoholics Anonymous's reliance on peers rather than experts cut against wider social trends toward professionalization, and its optimistic message that alcoholics could change their lives contradicted medical and popular wisdom about the likely fate of those who drank to excess. Yet its medical-sounding language (allergy and obsession), along with the desire of early leaders to work with the medical profession and define alcoholism as a public health problem, also helped spread an understanding of alcoholism as a disease.

Officially, AA welcomed all alcoholics and often celebrated women's recovery as proof of the program's effectiveness. While men from diverse backgrounds sometimes found it challenging to participate, women faced particular hurdles. As one early member recalled, women were "the most troublesome and, in some ways, the most unwelcome minority in AA's olden days."[68] Even naming conventions, in which AA members used their given names but not their surnames to maintain anonymity and to avoid status markers,[69] signaled gender (once again, Marty Mann is the exception that proves the rule). The role of nonalcoholic wives in the early years of the fellowship, along with pejorative beliefs about the sexual morality of alcoholic women, complicated the position of women who approached the group to confront their own drinking problems. Like the female inebriates who sought help from the Martha Washington Society or who took the Keeley Cure, women who joined AA in the early years often had to overcome a secondary social role in order to access a universalist therapeutic message.

Chapter 4

Defining a Disease

Gender, Stigma, and the Modern Alcoholism Movement

"Lady Lushes on the Loose!" screamed a 1944 headline in a New York newspaper. Accompanying the headline was an illustration of two women dressed in evening wear engaged in a fistfight; the caption read "Our women drunks are not above slugging it out."[1] Just a few years later, the *New York Herald Tribune* warned, "Women Nowadays Called 'Hard' Drinkers," while a similar article worried over "A Growing Liability: The Woman 'Bar Fly.'"[2] Even the more restrained *Life* magazine discussed the problem of "Lady Tipplers" in 1947, while *Newsweek* warned of "Mrs. Drunkard" the following year.[3] One columnist expressed alarm, even disgust, over women's drinking and the unfeminine behavior it seemed to provoke. "The lady lusher, the girlish guzzler and the woman-wowzer are among 1947's Problem People," he explained. Continuing with the alliteration theme, he decried the "Bistro Berthas, Cocktail Lounge Lorettas and Barfly Beatrices" who, he charged, "are becoming something more than sickening to people who respect womanhood." Grudgingly admitting that women's roles had changed somewhat, he still claimed that public drinking was going too far, calling for solidarity among readers who "think that women's place, while it may no longer be strictly in the home, is certainly not in the corner dive, with or without pink and white furnishings, soft music and a couple of groggy canaries."[4]

This comment perfectly illustrates the unsettled nature of American gender roles in the immediate aftermath of World War II. If women's place was no longer "strictly in the home," where was it? And who should decide? These journalists identified drinking customs as an appropriate domain for monitoring women's behavior, declaring that some spaces and privileges should remain off limits despite feminine décor. On one level, the end of Prohibition—accomplished through the unprecedented act of repealing a constitutional amendment—settled the alcohol question once and for all. But individual alcoholics and their families continued to suffer, as Bill and Lois Wilson, Dr. Bob and Anne Smith, Marty Mann, and countless others knew all too well. And although Repeal pushed prohibitionists' voices to the margins of American society, women's drinking served as a lightning rod for anxieties about social change. The belief that women's drinking meant more than men's fed into derogatory attitudes toward women who drank to excess, even within the Alcoholics Anonymous (AA) fellowship.

Marty Mann overcame this challenge to achieve sobriety. Then she ventured beyond AA as she embarked on a campaign in the mid-1940s to change American perceptions of alcoholism and of alcoholics. Articles such as those cited above—which depicted women's drinking as an annoyance, a joke, or a violation of social convention—reflected the social context she faced. The organization that Mann founded, the National Committee for Education on Alcoholism (NCEA), helped create the institutional infrastructure for the "modern alcoholism movement," as scholars have dubbed the loosely organized coalitions and research groups that investigated alcohol-related problems in the aftermath of Prohibition. With alcohol no longer generally considered a dangerous, inherently addictive substance that could ensnare anyone, experts looked to physical or psychological qualities in the person who drank to excess to understand the phenomenon of compulsive drinking. While temperance campaigners had argued that alcohol was linked to a host of social problems, many researchers in the post-Repeal era initially narrowed their focus to a concern with alcoholism, a condition that, while it could be severe, seemed to afflict only a small minority of the population.[5] Importantly, the NCEA as well as these researchers focused on alcoholism and alcoholics, not drug addiction or addicts. Alcoholism movement activists thus engaged, consciously or not, in a "politics of respectability" by creating a hierarchy among stigmatized populations.[6]

Mann sought above all to eliminate the stigma attached to alcoholism, and she believed strongly that harnessing scientific expertise was the best way to do so. Although she had stopped drinking because of Alcoholics Anonymous, she maintained that modern, scientific authority was the only antidote powerful enough to override moralistic judgments about alcoholics as weak or bad. Yet as advocates and researchers involved in the modern alcoholism movement struggled even to define the condition and to understand what it meant when women drank to excess, they discovered that the scientific authority they hoped to exercise did not exist in a vacuum but was limited by social expectations and beliefs, including their own. Similarly, clinicians found that the logic of medicalization—that the recognition of a disease should lead to treatment by medical professionals—was neither easy nor straightforward when it came to alcoholics.

As a woman who had overcome a drinking problem, Mann argued that alcoholism could afflict anyone and that the disease was the same regardless of the personal characteristics of the sufferer. These ideas had the advantage of sounding modern—making alcoholism more parallel to other diseases—and deflecting attention from areas that she and many other alcoholics preferred to keep private. But journalists, social scientists, and even modern alcoholism movement activists did not always regard women's social drinking as a benign, morally neutral counterpoint to problematic consumption. Even recreational drinking by women attracted attention as a social problem, almost as if temperance critiques now applied primarily to women's drinking. As experts sought to define alcoholism, gendered *assumptions* led to the idea that alcoholic women manifested a different, more extreme version of the condition. At the same time, the failure of social scientists and other researchers to engage in meaningful gendered *analysis* excluded women's experience as fundamental models were taking shape. As a result, the emerging disease concept of alcoholism absorbed and perpetuated postwar America's double standard regarding female behavior.

A New Era? Social Drinking and the Creation of a Public Health Movement

It is surprising that Mann is not better known today: She was named one of the ten greatest living Americans by the journalist Edward R. Murrow in 1954,[7] and her public health work has shaped what most Americans believe about alcoholism even now. Tracing the genesis and evolution of her campaign reveals that Mann negotiated a multitude of factors in her advocacy: the political context of the post-Prohibition years, especially debates about women's social drinking; strategic decisions related to organizational and fundraising imperatives; her desire to deploy scientific authority; and her own position as a female alcoholic. Mann sought above all to convey a progressive and optimistic message, which meant distancing herself from the temperance cause and invoking a disease model that could incorporate women as well as men.

By the time Mann began her formal campaign, more than a decade had passed since the repeal of Prohibition, yet political, cultural, and scientific landscapes continued to be shaped by its legacy. Despite the fears of Prohibition supporters, Repeal did not unleash a nationwide binge, nor did the saloon, with its masculine excesses, reappear in the same form. States and municipalities exercised their prerogative to regulate liquor sales and consumption, some quite stringently.[8] Moreover, drinking habits had changed, both before and during Prohibition, as Americans "domesticated" alcohol. Evidence such as cookbooks and table place settings from the late nineteenth and early twentieth centuries show convincingly that more middle-class Americans incorporated alcohol consumption into their everyday lives than temperance rhetoric acknowledged.[9] Print journalists had glamorized heterosocial drinking in new ways during Prohibition, and that trend continued in popular culture. In many films of the era, the hero and heroine were more likely to drink than the villain.[10] In the popular *Thin Man* films of the 1930s and 1940s, the charming and clever Nora Charles matches her husband Nick's witty repartee and almost matches him drink for drink. In just about every scene in the early films of the series, the couple partakes liberally of alcohol, with glamorous accoutrements for mixing and serving cocktails.[11]

Yet law, social customs, and even liquor manufacturers and advertisers—the latter groups not necessarily known for their restraint—reinforced a gendered boundary in defining acceptable consumption after Repeal. Even the sophisticated Nora Charles cannot quite keep up with Nick, suffering from a hangover when she tries. Some regulations continued to treat women (as well as youth) as a special category. For example, in 1948 in Washington State, no one was allowed to stand at the bar while drinking or to carry drinks between the bar and tables (a rule intended to avoid a return to saloon-style practices). But women were not even allowed to sit at the bar—only at tables. These regulations were not loosened until the late 1960s and early 1970s.[12] Rules like these echoed the "Ladies' Entrance" of the saloon era and continued to mark women as a separate class of patrons. Even when women's presence or behavior in drinking establishments was not limited by law, male journalists and patrons felt free to scrutinize their conduct. Echoing Prohibition themes, reporters claimed that women did not know how to drink properly and had to be coached on comportment. So deeply gendered was drinking behavior that journalists evaluated it, along with body shape, clothing, and voice, when Christine Jorgensen returned to the United States after sex reassignment surgery in Europe. Although the way she gestured with a cigarette was "gracefully feminine," according to one account, Jorgensen "tossed off a Bloody Mary like a guy."[13] But a "girly" drinking style could be wrong, too: Another journalist criticized women for ordering elaborate fruity drinks and monopolizing the bartender's time, while yet another admonished women who dared drink in a bar to sit near the door and leave after thirty minutes.[14] In short, heterosocial drinking in public settings did not represent a meeting ground of equals but a realm in which men maintained control and influence.

Although many in the liquor industry viewed women's consumption, especially within the home, as a prime area for growth, they trod carefully lest they outrun popular attitudes. Entertaining guides, women's magazines, films, and advertising (especially print campaigns for beer) helped define drinking as a regular part of middle-class life, and surveys showed that women's drinking increased, though slowly, in the decades after Repeal.[15] But survey data could easily exaggerate women's consumption rates. For example, a 1946 survey reported that three-quarters of men drank and slightly more than half of women—yet those figures referred to people who did not abstain. On further analysis, three times as many men were "regular" drinkers, while women tended to report only "occasional" drinking.[16] Similarly, many beer ads featured domestic settings, and even depicted women's hands serving the beverages, but rarely did the women take a drink.[17] The Distilled Spirits Institute, a trade group, was even more conservative; it did not feature women in advertisements until 1958—and even then women had to be dressed "tastefully." Not until the early 1960s could women be shown either holding the liquor or drinking it.[18] In this way, the alcohol beverage industry echoed the elite women who had campaigned for repeal through the Women's Organization for National Prohibition Reform. Neither constituency actively denied that women should drink, but neither directly advocated for it, either—a strategy that acknowledged the existence of ambivalent social attitudes about women's consumption. Both groups benefited from offering a flexible message that various audiences could understand as they wished.

As they had during the 1920s, Americans during the World War II era interpreted women's drinking habits as a proxy for wider social changes, and, as before, the apparently novel behavior of middle-class women drew the most attention. One group of sociologists reported that "the transformation of the traditional tea party into the cocktail party; the presence of women in public bars, cocktail lounges, taverns, and other drinking places; the phenomenon of drinking parties made up exclusively of women, all attest to a widespread change in mores." The authors found all this particularly shocking because only "in the highest and in the lowest social levels" had women's drinking been acceptable in the past.[19] Another commentator lamented the possible risk a man now faced in meeting a female family member in a drinking establishment, noting with regret that, at least before Prohibition, "a man would never meet his wife, his sweetheart, his daughter, his sister or his grandma there." Drinking, especially in public, risked collapsing class distinctions; one reporter insisted that several drunken women who got into a fight in a run-down bar were in fact identical to their "better-dressed sisters under the skin" at a swanky uptown nightclub.[20]

The lighthearted if condescending tone that had characterized at least some coverage of flappers and lit ladies was replaced during the World War II era by solemn debates over the purported links between drinking and women's urge to act like men. During the war, the beer and liquor industries promoted an image of alcohol as patriotic, and the U.S. government did not impose prohibitionary measures as it had during the First World War. Yet the war amplified the gendered meaning of alcohol use. As one newspaper reporter explained, "In this war, the fact that so many women have worked at men's jobs has played its part in stimulating drinking. Sociologists observe that when women enter a male environment, they tend to adopt the ways of men."[21] Rather than celebrating women's consumption as a form of liberation, many journalists now identified it as troubling evidence of a world turned upside down.

After the war, Americans' anxieties about reconstituting family life could be seen in concerns about excessive drinking, for men as well as women. How would men readjust to civilian life, and how would women—who may well have enjoyed certain prerogatives during the war emergency—acclimate to the domestic realm? Alcoholics Anonymous, psychiatrists and social workers (who I discuss in later chapters), and even feature films all offered a way to understand alcoholism in men as a gender crisis.[22] And while the precise line demarcating alcoholism in men was not always crystal clear, most experts and laypeople approved at least some drinking for men, including returning veterans. In fact, recreational drinking could help define and reinforce the masculinity so necessary to rebuild families in the postwar era. While nightclubs and other venues that fostered heterosocial drinking persisted, many middle-class men also created a male-dominated drinking culture after the war that was more refined than that of the saloon era but nevertheless excluded women.[23]

For all the talk of "tea parties" turned into "cocktail parties" in social science literature and the popular media, women did not create an equally robust parallel drinking world. Most women lacked the social and economic freedom to do so even if they wanted to—and if they had, critics were standing by to charge them with ignoring their duty to their families and society. One writer insisted that women's alcohol consumption—of any kind—carried unacceptably high costs: "Shattered homes, blasted lives, and an increasing drain on society are the result of the 'emancipation' that permits a women to sip a social cocktail and does not criticize her for doing so."[24] Significantly, this writer echoed temperance rhetoric that had once attacked men who imbibed, now turning it against drinking women. And while the gender crisis associated with men's drinking had to do with alcoholism, the writer here expressed outrage over a woman who might "sip" a "social cocktail."

Despite this superheated rhetoric, Americans did not universally condemn women's drinking during the 1930s and 1940s—the situation was more complicated than that. The emergence of the flapper and the involvement of women in the repeal campaign had shown that women were not a monolithic block squarely on the side of temperance—not that they ever had been. But acknowledging that abstinence was no longer an agreed-upon standard meant new lines had to be drawn, boundaries that simultaneously defined masculinity and femininity. Across the middle decades of the twentieth century, women's drinking rates trailed behind those of men, and social acceptance of their consumption lagged even further. This mattered because a new definition of alcoholism as a disease and new criteria for social drinking unfolded together as complementary processes.

In this context, Mann positioned herself deliberately, using both the cultural prestige of science and her polished and modern femininity to promote the idea that alcoholism should be regarded as a disease.[25] Although Mann later claimed that the mission for the NCEA had come to her as if in a vision, she actually harnessed existing networks and built on research and advocacy efforts that were already under way while reshaping earlier formulations so that they could more easily apply to women. During the latter 1930s and 1940s, researchers, including basic and social scientists, and a number of clinicians turned their attention to alcohol-related matters. Some were affiliated with or became attached to academic institutions, such as Yale University, while others formed think tanks such as the Research Council on Problems of Alcohol. As an early member of Alcoholics Anonymous in New York City, with social and professional connections that allowed access to these burgeoning networks, Mann, along with Bill Wilson, sought to learn more about alcoholism research and its implications. With a background in public relations, Mann became convinced that translating scientific research to the public—including the simple fact that scientists were investigating alcoholism as a legitimate problem—would help erode the stigma attached to the condition and neutralize continuing wet-dry politics. She developed an ambitious plan that would include a lecture program for professionals, such as doctors and clergy; information centers for the lay public; and improved care for alcoholics in hospitals and clinics. Organizationally savvy, she envisioned a small working committee that could then expand.[26]

To put her plan into practice, however, Mann needed a funding source. Her experience shows that this "movement" was one only in retrospect, involving as it did a range of individuals and organizations with overlapping but not identical interests and goals.[27] Mann initially approached the Research Council on Problems of Alcohol only to realize that their vision did not match her own. Turning to the Yale Center for Alcohol Studies, Mann found a welcome reception from E. M. Jellinek, a physiologist who was fast becoming a leader in alcoholism research. Mann resigned her job in New York and moved in with the Jellinek family in New Haven, where she studied the new findings on alcoholism for six months and then attended the second Yale Summer School on Alcohol in 1944. Mann and her allies considered this training essential in granting her the credibility to talk about scientific research on alcoholism. Yale University then adopted the plan that Mann had created for the NCEA, agreeing to fund the fledging organization fully for two years and then to decrease support while Mann sought other resources. Along with one secretary, Mann established an office in New York and began an ambitious program of lectures, print materials, and other publicity.

Central to Mann's campaign was a redefinition of alcoholism from a sin or weakness to a disease, a medical condition divorced from moral judgments and articulated in the language of modern medical science. The philosophy of the NCEA, as defined by Mann, contained three key elements: (1) Alcoholism is a disease and should be understood as a public health problem. (2) The alcoholic can be helped. (3) The alcoholic is worth helping.[28] To define the condition for the public, Mann relied on metaphor and analogy, often comparing alcoholism to diabetes and explaining that liquor for an alcoholic is like sugar to a diabetic—and a person should not be blamed because his or her body cannot process a benign substance in the usual way. Although she had embraced the language of "The Big Book" to name her drinking problem, she did not speak at length in public about the spiritual elements of the AA program and practices but instead framed a disease model through the lens of science. So convinced was Mann of the cultural power of scientific authority, and so important did she consider a language of disease, that she moved beyond what the scientists themselves were willing to say. She wrote to Yale researchers in 1948, "We who are meeting the public need a continuing stream of material, even if it is not conclusive or definitive material."[29]

Mann sought parallels with other health problems that had been similarly reconceptualized. Tuberculosis seemed a perfect example, one that also allowed Mann to draw on her own life story—she had experienced the illness as an adolescent—to advance her campaign and further merge her persona with her cause. Delivering the keynote address at a meeting of the National Tuberculosis Association, Mann described being sent to a "great TB specialist" in California. At that time, Mann explained, ignorance about tuberculosis was widespread, even among wealthy, sophisticated people such as her own parents. Fearing that she might reveal her condition to her friends, her parents did not tell her what was wrong, and she was not a compliant patient. When her condition worsened, the doctor violated his promise to her parents and told her she had tuberculosis. Once she knew the truth, Mann claimed, she cooperated fully with the treatment regimen and recovered. As a counterpoint to her story, Mann recounted the fate of a young neighbor named Catherine who had also been stricken with the disease but whose parents, "horrified and ashamed and disgraced," had not sought treatment for her. "They hid her," Mann recalled. "And she died. All my life I have felt that stigma killed Catherine. And it nearly killed me. So I have a strong feeling about the elimination of stigma on illness—on all kinds of illness."[30]

Invoking her life story allowed Mann to show that alcoholism, like tuberculosis, could afflict anyone regardless of background or gender. She made the case that alcoholism should follow the same trajectory as tuberculosis, that it should be viewed as a disease rather than a sin or badge of immoral behavior or "dirty" origins.[31] As a corollary, the proper response to excessive drinking should be medical care, not jail time or social sanction. Mann emphasized that alcoholism "is as prevalent a disease as either tuberculosis or cancer and one that, rightly handled is more easily treated."[32] Linking alcoholism with these other diseases carried an implicit promise that modern medicine would eradicate problem drinking, perhaps as miraculously as antibiotics conquered the tubercle bacillus. A persuasive advocate, Mann struck a balance between dire warnings regarding the incidence and severity of alcoholism and optimism about addressing it.

All alcohol researchers and advocates had to negotiate a complicated post-Repeal context, especially as they sought funding and presented their work to the public, but Mann faced particular challenges as a woman and an alcoholic. Mann's public health campaign could easily evoke prohibition efforts, and she utilized the same kinds of women's networks.[33] This strategy brought risks, however, and she sought to differentiate herself from temperance advocates. Mann likely benefited from the precedent set by the upper-class and upper-middle-class society ladies who had campaigned for the repeal of Prohibition. Press accounts during the 1920s had delighted in contrasting Pauline Sabin, the sophisticated president of the Women's Organization for National Prohibition Reform (WONPR), with the president of the Woman's Christian Temperance

Union, who was depicted as stuffy and old-fashioned.[34] Similarly, accounts of Mann's activism described her as "cultured," "well-groomed," "attractive," and "smart-looking"—in short, like a modern, sophisticated woman, not a Victorian carryover. Introducing Mann on a 1945 radio program, for example, the announcer described Mann as "a most attractive and unusual version of the lady with a cause."[35]

Mann's efforts were also contrasted with the campaign of Carry Nation, who had achieved notoriety with her "hatchetation" (as she called her campaign to close saloons).[36] One reporter wrote, for example, "No Carri [sic] Nation, Mrs. Mann, who is an ex-drinker herself, believes that a helping hand can do more to help alcoholics than all the axes in the country."[37] In a 1946 *New York Times Magazine* profile, Mann invoked Nation's reputation in order to distance herself from it: "Please don't get the idea that our committee is a crusading outfit that is going around the country with hatchets trying to smash up gin mills."[38] Even though the point was to underscore her difference from Nation, the resonance of the connection demonstrates how cultural politics related to alcohol remained deeply gendered. For purposes of comparison, media accounts did not mention Wayne B. Wheeler, the leader of the Anti-Saloon League, when describing Bill Wilson or E. M. Jellinek.

Mann's attractive and polished style simultaneously underscored her recovery from alcoholism and allowed her to sidestep lingering temperance politics. As she explained, "Those of us who are alcoholics are personal drys because we realize that we can't take liquor in moderation. But this does not mean that we believe that those who can should be deprived of it."[39] Reframing decades of prohibition debate into a matter of individual vulnerability to the substance of alcohol, Mann distanced herself from temperance leaders. Her use of the collective "we" and "us" in referring to alcoholics obscured gender identity. Nor did she qualify the category of "those who can" drink moderately. In this way, Mann asserted that the important variable in drinking practice is not gender but alcoholic status. She thus raised implicit challenges both to the continuing ambivalence with which many Americans regarded women's recreational drinking in the decades after Repeal and to the assumption that alcoholism afflicted men but not women.

Mann's careful negotiation of these complex cultural debates demonstrates how alcohol and gender remained deeply intertwined in American society well past the repeal of Prohibition. She could bring together influential women's networks with the prestige of science, all buttressed by the irrefutable proof of her own experience into a potent form of authority. Maintaining this delicate balance required that she continually demonstrate the utmost respectability in her own recovery from alcoholism—just as the nineteenth-century diagnosis of inebriety was most easily attached to women who fit the parameters of conventional femininity. Presenting herself as living proof that alcoholics can recover and deserve help in doing so meant that the stakes in her own sobriety could hardly have been higher, and the imperatives she faced as a result shaped every aspect of her public career. A brilliant strategist, Mann capitalized on the transitional quality of both gender roles and the formulation of a disease model of alcoholism in mid-twentieth-century America. At times downplaying her gender distinctiveness, Mann could also deploy it as needed to involve women's groups. Similarly, before the creation of the specialty of addiction medicine, Mann took advantage of the fluidity of the field and gained sufficient expertise through her connection with Yale that she could be a convincing spokesperson.[40]

While Mann leveraged her own story to promote her message, being a living embodiment of her cause brought challenges, particularly related to her personal and institutional position in the modern alcoholism movement. As she became better known, her prominence raised fundamental questions about anonymity. During the early years of the NCEA, Mann personified a close connection between the new organization and Alcoholics Anonymous. She relied on AA networks, including the *Grapevine* newsletter of which she had been a founder, to promote her message, and her extensive travel depended on the generosity of local AA members who hosted her and provided logistical support. In the initial years of her campaign, Mann credited AA publicly for her recovery. Then a fundraising letter from NCEA seemed to many AA members to blur the missions of the two organizations. The considerable criticism Mann faced as a result of these actions helped convince AA leaders to formulate the Twelve Traditions, principles that guide the organization (the Twelve Steps are practices for personal recovery).[41] Weathering these problems, the NCEA achieved considerable accomplishments during its first decades, including the establishment of dozens of local committees and information centers across the country, a substantial increase in the number of hospitals that accepted alcoholics, greater awareness of alcoholism as a public health problem among politicians and policy makers, and programs to help alcoholics in the workplace.[42]

Defining Alcoholism

Mann and other advocates could more easily say what alcoholism was not—not a sin, not a sign of immorality, not a lack of willpower—than they could define it clearly. Research in the post-Repeal era did not initially clarify matters, since many investigators relied on vague or circular operational definitions of alcoholism and its criteria as a diagnostic category, noting only that the subjects they studied were being treated for "alcoholism" (and were therefore "alcoholics").[43] The term itself could refer to various dimensions of alcoholism, including a compulsion to drink, drinking practices themselves, or the health effects of excessive drinking; some doctors saw only the last meaning as relevant for them to treat. For example, a major textbook in the field of internal medicine devoted only a few pages to alcoholism, in the section on "Diseases due to Intoxicants." The text focused on the effects on the body of alcohol as a poison and on the implications of chronic alcoholism for human organ systems. As to treatment, the author flatly declared, "Permanent cure of the confirmed drunkard is rare."[44]

Even when researchers hoped their work would refute pejorative attitudes about alcoholism, their agendas were inevitably shaped by social conditions and cultural beliefs. Most scientists, advocates, and physicians assumed that alcoholism occurred much less frequently among women than among men. Although a skewed sex ratio might itself be seen as a question worth exploring, relatively little investigation focused on women during the middle decades of the twentieth century. Some scholars have suggested that the physicians, scientists, and advocates involved in the modern alcoholism movement avoided the issue of women's drinking because of the particular stigma attached.[45] While some may have shied away from alcoholic women for that reason, others hoped that their efforts would especially benefit women, whose improvement would then demonstrate the applicability and value of a universalist disease model.

But popular interest in drinking women as a social problem did not automatically translate into research; scientific methodologies and conventions often excluded alcoholic women because, for example, the sample size was too small. And at the same time, the unexamined assumption that alcoholic women differed from their male counterparts prohibited their inclusion in many studies. As a result, female alcoholics could be dismissed as exceptional yet not worth analyzing in a meaningful way.

The growth of Alcoholics Anonymous and media coverage of the fellowship during the 1940s helped disseminate its definition of alcoholism to the public and shape the research agenda of scientists at the Yale Center for Alcohol Studies. As we have seen, AA offered a definition of alcoholism—a pattern of destructive drinking that continued despite the conscious desire of the person to stop—and a form of self-diagnosis, in which the person acknowledged powerlessness over alcohol and a life that had become unmanageable. The AA definition also offered a mechanism—a vaguely defined "allergy"—that could explain why some people became alcoholics while others did not. Alcoholics Anonymous narratives, both spoken at meetings and printed in the Big Book, conveyed a trajectory with recognizable turning points as a person's drinking progressed. In 1945, the *Grapevine* surveyed readers about their drinking histories. The AA fellowship then asked E. M. Jellinek of the Yale Center to analyze the findings. Jellinek acknowledged methodological flaws in the survey process, but he saw an important opportunity to use data on drinking behaviors to refine diagnostic criteria for alcoholism and to provide a corrective to what he viewed as a lack of attention to actual drinking practices by psychologists and psychiatrists, who focused instead on the personality conflicts that they believed caused the drinking behaviors in the first place.[46] While the sample size was small, Jellinek considered its source—Alcoholics Anonymous—to be a strength, because AA contained a wide variety of alcoholic "types" and because "there need be no doubt as to the truthfulness of the replies given by an A.A. to questions coming from his own group."[47] Using this data, Jellinek published his enormously influential "Phases in the Drinking History of Alcoholics" in the *Quarterly Journal of Studies on Alcohol* in 1946, where he argued that alcoholism is a progressive disease with recognizable phases, and he also called for a more refined survey instrument.[48]

While he discussed some methodological questions in the text of his article, Jellinek relegated the issue of sex differences to a footnote, explaining that he excluded the fifteen questionnaires returned by women "because on the one hand the number was too small to be analyzed separately, and on the other hand the data differed so greatly for the two sexes that merging the data was inadvisable."[49] Since 158 surveys were returned (out of 1,600 copies of the *Grapevine*), women represented almost one in ten of the responses.[50] Although precise figures for AA membership during this period are not available, as we have already seen, women were estimated to be anywhere from one-quarter to 40 percent of members, at least in larger cities. Meanwhile, the general sex ratio as calculated by various researchers varied widely but tended to cluster around 6:1 (that is, six male alcoholics for every alcoholic woman).[51] Offering a "tentative revised questionnaire form" at the end of his article, Jellinek recommended separate forms for men and women "in order to avoid awkwardness in the formulation of questions." It is unclear whether he meant grammatical clumsiness or something more substantive, since, significantly, "Only the form proposed for men is shown here."[52] Jellinek thus dodged the question of gender difference even as he acknowledged it, failing to capitalize on alcoholic women's participation to inform fundamental research in the field.

Investigators who focused on alcoholic women also grappled with methodological challenges. For example, a few years after Jellinek's "Phases" article appeared, a graduate student in sociology at Texas Christian University named Twila Florence Fort developed a different survey instrument to study alcoholism in women. Only limited research had been conducted on alcoholic women, Fort explained, which "may seem surprising" given the "great interest that attaches to the problem of the alcoholic woman." She noted that the shame that prevented alcoholic women from seeking care voluntarily also had implications for knowledge, since the limited data that were available came from female patients with alcoholic psychoses, contributing to the belief that alcoholic women were more pathological than their male counterparts. As more women joined the Alcoholics Anonymous program and sought out other treatment, Fort hoped that they would become more accessible to researchers as well. Her thesis, encouraged by Jellinek himself, was meant to help define a research agenda that would support future work by the Yale Institute for Alcohol Studies in the Southwest.[53]

Like Jellinek before her, Fort collected information on drinking histories. Her study included fifty alcoholic women from AA groups in three Texas cities, who completed a new questionnaire that Jellinek had developed with AA members as well as Fort's survey instrument. Fort also interviewed thirty-four of the women. Despite Jellinek's earlier recommendation that separate questionnaires be produced for men and women, his revised version could be used by either, with a space for the subject to designate whether male or female and items about the "wife or husband's attitude toward drinking." Some questions seemed intended for men (item 111 about "diminishing sex potency," for example) while others were explicitly designated for men ("Only men answer: Ever supported by wife or wife's family? Ever have to turn over finances to wife or wife's family?"). This survey did not include questions about neglecting children specifically, only about whether the subject had ever been "reproached" by spouse for being a "bad example."

In contrast, Fort's survey included items that aligned more with women's conventional roles. For example, item 18 asked, "Did your alcoholism have any effect on your children (child)?" and parsed the question into such realms as "your neglecting them"; "their fear or dislike of intoxication"; effects on their schooling or social life; and "change in their affections." For each part of the question, the woman could answer on a spectrum from "Worried me" to "They never knew of it." Fort also asked questions about the woman's family of origin, schooling, hobbies and social activities, and employment (questions in this area included the wording "If employed . . ." and "If you had vocational ambition . . . ," indicating a presumption that women would not necessarily work outside the home).[54]

Fort's study seemed designed to provide insights into sex differences in drinking and into how alcoholism affected women's lives specifically, and she highlighted such variations in her discussion of findings. For example, job loss, brawls, or jail time could indicate loss of control over drinking for men, whereas women were more likely to experience social ostracism (which could extend to their children); they also faced other risks, including "sexual humiliation." The location of the woman's drinking—whether at home, in "semiprivate" locations such as others' homes, or in public—and whether she was accompanied by her husband could determine the consequences she faced, even more so than the duration of her alcoholism, which Fort and others had presumed to be a critical variable. Fort concluded, "The severity of these social repercussions in women cannot be measured by the same standards as in men."[55]

Fort also found that women moved through the stages of alcoholism more quickly than men, so fast that "some of the phases were to all appearances practically simultaneous."[56] This finding also appeared in other research and clinical reports during the post-Repeal period. As such, it rearticulated an older idea, going back to the nineteenth century at least, that drinking women were more troubled and debased than their male counterparts because the condition itself represented an aberration for them. The new definition of alcoholism as a progressive disease with distinct stages meant that this belief could be reinscribed with a precise quantitative vocabulary that sounded objective and modern.

Rather than simply accepting the assumptions that shaped other assessments of alcoholic women's trajectories, though, Fort offered a more complicated analysis, emphasizing differences within her sample of women: Some had "pre-alcoholic maladjustments" such as a "neurotic character" that contributed to their drinking, while others started drinking in response to a stressful life event. She concluded that fewer women than men were "pampered drinkers," those who "develop their alcoholism in the absence of neurotic tendencies or strong emotional stresses."[57] Even as she identified these differences, however, Fort pulled back from a full-fledged comparison, which she deemed "not feasible at this time,"[58] and she did not propose that the Jellinek model be reconceptualized for women. Just as Jellinek excluded the surveys returned by women due to methodological concerns, so, too, the conventions of social science research led Fort to gesture toward gender difference, even presume its importance, but not explore it in detail. As a result, research like hers reinforced the idea that women deviated from standard alcoholic patterns just as important models for understanding the condition were taking shape.

The research findings of Jellinek and Fort appeared in scholarly journals and professional publications. As part of her campaign to popularize scientific findings, Mann wrote a trade book called *Primer on Alcoholism: How People Drink, How to Recognize Alcoholics, and What to Do about Them*, which was included in Book-of-the-Month-Club materials upon its publication in 1950.[59] In this text, Mann like Fort acknowledged that women might manifest alcoholism in particular ways, but Mann departed from scholarly conclusions when she insisted, "I personally do not believe . . . that this is due to some peculiar difference in the kind of alcoholism women are subject to, or that it is actually any different from the alcoholism of men." Instead, Mann blamed a double standard. "It is still not *as* acceptable for women to drink (at least more than one cocktail, or one highball, or preferably sherry or other wine) as it is for men. And it is nowhere acceptable for women to drink to drunkenness."[60] Mann here pointed to the complicated position of female alcoholics in the modern alcoholism paradigm; even as men's alcoholism was defined in opposition to normal drinking, ambivalent social attitudes about women's drinking made it harder to draw the line for them. It was thus more challenging to argue that alcoholism among women was a disease entity for which sufferers should not be blamed. The stereotypes and judgmental beliefs about women who drank to excess carried over into the diagnosis itself, influencing the experiences of alcoholic women as well as the ways their condition was evaluated by professionals and the general public. Mann worked to counter this situation through her rhetoric as well as advocacy, using "alcoholic" as a noun rather than as the modifier of "man" in the central statements of the NCEA. This wording made the diagnosis the key, now not just an adjective but the identity itself.

Mann also followed Jellinek in emphasizing the progressive quality of alcoholism. Unlike Fort who pointed out gender differences in how the phases unfolded in women as opposed to men, Mann likened the disease to a gravitational force that is ruthless and oblivious to the characteristics of the afflicted person. As she explained in her *Primer on Alcoholism*,

> It is this inevitable progression, along with the striking similarity of the signs and symptoms marking the progression—both of which appear in identical forms in all kinds of highly differentiated individuals—which mark alcoholism for the disease it is. Background, environment, race, sex, social status—these make no appreciable difference when once

the disease takes hold of the individual. For all intents and purposes he might just as well then be labeled with a number: he has become just another victim of the disease of alcoholism.[61]

According to Mann, the fact that alcoholism can afflict anyone, and afflicts diverse people in the same way, shows that it is a disease. And not only does the disease of alcoholism not respect individual characteristics or status markers, it has the power to erase them.[62] Mann was not the only person to make this claim, nor did it arise only from the study of female alcoholics. Still, Mann herself embodied the message in a way that the white, male leaders of the modern alcoholism movement never could. Her charismatic manner meant that she crafted and disseminated a persuasive fusion of the "alcoholic equalitarianism"[63] of AA with a modern understanding of disease that emphasized the uniformity of the condition rather than the characteristics of the sufferer. Understanding alcoholism in this way, Mann believed, was consonant with the most progressive medical thinking and brought the greatest potential to reduce stigma for all. To that end, she articulated this view forcefully, whether it could be supported by scientific research or not.

An Alcoholic Housewife on the Silver Screen: *The Smash-Up* (1947)

Mann energetically promoted her public health message through personal appearances, print, and radio. When possible, she also sought to influence depictions of alcoholism in film and, later, television. During the middle decades of the twentieth century, a number of movies featured alcoholic characters; some were serious "social problem" films of the era, while others were more sensationalistic.[64] *The Lost Weekend* (1945), one of the most well known of these films, contributed to a familiar narrative in which a devoted female partner remained loyal to a male alcoholic protagonist whose return to a productive career marked a successful recovery. *The Smash-Up: The Story of a Woman* was released two years later, serving in a sense as a female counterpoint to *The Lost Weekend*. *The Smash-Up* was co-written by Dorothy Parker, a well-known writer who was herself an alcoholic and a board member of the NCEA; Mann served as a consultant on the film.[65] It is difficult to know the extent of Mann's involvement from available evidence, although dialogue regarding the disease model of alcoholism certainly suggests her strong influence. Given the participation of two prominent alcoholic women, neither of whom was a conventional wife and mother, the film's ambivalent portrayal of domesticity provides important insights into the evolution of the disease model of alcoholism in the context of mid-twentieth-century gender-role expectations.

The film tells the story of Angie, a professional singer who leaves a thriving career when she marries and has a child, only to become an alcoholic. The audience learns that Angie had begun drinking in order to cope with stage fright and shyness. As her husband Ken grows more successful in his own singing career, Angie increasingly relies on alcohol as she is marginalized socially, professionally, and even within her marriage as Ken's manipulative secretary Martha takes on responsibilities that would more appropriately belong to Angie. Like the mothers in the short stories and the Washingtonian narrative discussed in chapter 1, Angie abstains from alcohol when caring for her sick child, but her husband's absences and the pressures of entertaining drive her to drink. Brought up short by her own behavior when drunk at a party, Angie asks Ken why she seems different from other people who are able to drink without problems, thus clearly articulating the modern alcoholism paradigm. Hardly the counterpoint to the supportive girlfriend in *The Lost Weekend*, Ken says that Angie's drinking will ruin their marriage and that he has had enough. The argument escalates and he packs a suitcase and leaves Angie, who drinks to the point of passing out.

The plot then turns on Angie's capacity to mother, reflecting long-standing concerns on this issue as well as particular challenges in conceptualizing how any woman could have both a career and children in this historical moment. Angie wants to care for their daughter, but she is also determined to sing again to achieve financial self-sufficiency and a sense of worth. Ironically, the only way she can reclaim her child is to earn enough money to hire domestic help just as Ken does, illustrating the difficulty she faced in combining the roles of professional and mother. Ken disapproves of her plans, insisting he will support her even if they are separated. When Angie resumes her career, now performing under her maiden name, Ken changes the locks and forbids her from seeing the child. A devastated Angie starts drinking again and falls asleep on a stoop. She awakens in bed in a lower-class apartment where she has been cared for by a kindhearted couple but has risked her class status and respectability, as well as her physical safety.

Desperate for her daughter and seeing no other recourse, Angie takes the child from the park while the nanny's back is turned. The fears expressed by other characters that her drinking compromises her ability to mother are realized when Angie absently drops a cigarette after singing her daughter to sleep. The film cuts between the smoldering cigarette as it catches fire and Angie drinking and arguing with Ken in her imagination. Finally the child's frantic cries rouse Angie, who rescues her daughter but is badly burned herself.

In the aftermath, Ken and Angie turn to Dr. Lorenz, who embodies wide-ranging medical expertise and wisdom. Although his vaguely European accent hints that he could be a psychiatrist, he also served as a family physician by caring for the sick daughter. Dr. Lorenz's explanation of Angie's drinking combines several elements, including the disease model—complete with a diabetes analogy—psychological motivations, and the Alcoholics Anonymous concept of "hitting bottom." Ken, with the best of intentions, gave Angie everything she wanted but took away her sense of responsibility. The doctor does not explain whether he means her maternal and domestic obligations, given the household staff the couple employed; her role relative to Ken, which was usurped in many ways by Martha; or her financial contribution to the family, which vanished when she stopped singing. For her part, Angie uses the "made-up belief" that she had lost Ken to Martha to justify her drinking. Angie then says to Ken, "I needed to hit rock bottom before I could change. Now I'm never going to be afraid again." Angie does not refer to drinking or abstinence; there has been no treatment, and the cure, such as it is, is not psychiatric, not even medical—even though Dr. Lorenz serves as the authoritative voice. Moreover, the cure does not involve a feminist analysis of Angie's life circumstances. Instead, a language of courage, love, and honesty, presumably inspired by the trauma of "hitting bottom" through the fire, evokes AA narratives, including Mann's own, even though AA as such is not named in the film.

Like Mann's self-presentation, the film both highlights and minimizes the gender of the alcoholic protagonist, reflecting the complex intersections of gender roles and disease model advocacy at this time. For much of the film, Angie's identity as a woman seems almost beside the point. Her drinking is not interpreted as resistance to her marginalized position but as a coping mechanism that she proves unable to control because she is an alcoholic. Yet the film's subtitle, *The Story of a Woman*, marks its inversion of the typical pattern of alcoholic man and supportive female partner. Further, the narrative arc, in which Angie's self-esteem plummets and her drinking escalates when she leaves behind a successful career for family life, could provide an interpretive opening into the potentially destructive effects of domestic constraints, although the film does not pursue this theme.

Juxtaposing the character of Angie with Mann's life and advocacy shows important tensions. Angie's commitment to live with courage rather than fear at the end of the film has an inspirational quality, but the lack of details about any regimen that could be used to accomplish this goal suggests how difficult it was to convert disease model rhetoric into effective treatment models (though at least moviegoers were spared horrific hospital scenes like those in *The Lost Weekend*). Angie's struggle to find fulfillment in her family life, the dilemma of whether she should sing again, and the greater power her husband assumed in their marriage as his career success surpassed hers—all replicated the issues faced by many women, if in a more glamorous setting. Yet Mann's own standing as a career woman and her public health strategies did not highlight these matters, complicating how other women might or might not fit into diagnostic categories and benefit from treatment opportunities.

Although she continued to use the title "Mrs." throughout her life and presented herself as the epitome of feminine propriety, Marty Mann hardly represented conventional womanhood. In fact, her public narrative echoed a typically male story in key ways. Mann had no children, and although this circumstance could have marked her as a failed woman in a postwar setting characterized by the Baby Boom, at least she could not be accused of neglecting children because of her drinking. Her ability to hold a job—indeed, to craft a successful career that brought prestige and fame—signified her recovery, just as it would have for a man. Lest her determination appear unfeminine, however, she built on a female reform tradition, offering herself as an exemplar of selfless advocacy who only came forward to help others. Mann transformed her professional ambition into a form of social motherhood, a status that could be understood as compensation for her biological childlessness.[66]

Occupational stability had long been viewed as a sign of a disciplined, sober life, and Mann's frequent assertion that most alcoholics were not skid row bums but people from all walks of life who could contribute significantly to society if only their alcoholism could be arrested built on temperance arguments about the social dividends that would come from abstinence. The personal, familial, and economic implications of job loss could be easily understood by the general public and quantified by social scientists. Items about the effects of excessive drinking on occupational status appeared frequently in diagnostic questionnaires, making it more difficult for those with the occupation "housewife" to fit into alcoholic categories. Under Mann's leadership, the NCEA developed strategies to assist alcoholics in the workplace, forerunners of what came to be known as employee assistance programs. In this way, Mann helped institutionalize the equation between occupational productivity and successful recovery from alcoholism. This approach undoubtedly resonated with her own experience—after all, she had worked professionally almost her entire adult life—and also buttressed her central message that alcoholism should be considered a public health problem, one in which all Americans had a stake whether they or their family members were alcoholic or not.

As she did in the AA fellowship, Mann again served as the exception that proved the rule—her career success and recovery mapped onto this model of occupational adjustment as barometer of health, but the experiences of many other women did not. Although Mann's insistence that the disease could strike anyone, regardless of personal characteristics, was itself a potentially radical statement that gender (as well as other markers of identity) did not matter, she did not pursue this aspect of her argument overtly. Nor did she address directly the implications of this approach for women; after all, her goal was not to remake gender roles but to alleviate the stigma associated with alcoholism. Even as her public demonstration of recovery implicitly promised that other women could follow in her footsteps, her trajectory did not provide a road map for women who may have struggled to articulate a link between the challenges of domestic life and their drinking problems or who had to cope with children or other family obligations as barriers to seeking treatment.

In the decades following the repeal of Prohibition, social scientists, physicians, advocates, and alcoholics all sought to define and explain the condition, to facilitate treatment, and to reduce stigma. In all these domains, alcoholic women seemed to be a self-evidently separate category. Despite claims in the popular media and in some scholarly research that drinking and alcoholism among women were on the rise, methodological conventions in the social and natural sciences excluded the experiences of alcoholic women from newly articulated definitions of the condition. Alcoholic women served a rhetorical purpose but did not garner systematic attention. E. M. Jellinek's rationale in discounting a small number of surveys returned by women perfectly captured the dilemma many female alcoholics faced in the middle decades of the twentieth century: They were too small a minority to merit equivalent attention, yet they were presumed to be different enough to forestall inclusion with men. As a result, alcoholic women were omitted just as important new models were taking shape.

American ambivalence about women's social drinking undercut the purportedly clear divisions fundamental to the modern alcoholism paradigm. And yet beliefs about alcohol and about gender roles had changed so much that the nineteenth-century definition of the female inebriate as a frail creature deserving of sympathy could not be resurrected. This apparently paradoxical consequence of a move toward medicalization was especially unfortunate as biases about alcoholic women became embedded into the diagnosis, with the growing prestige of scientific medicine making them that much harder to dislodge.

Chapter 5

"A Special Masculine Neurosis"

Psychiatrists Look at Alcoholism

In 1949, readers of the professional journal *Psychiatry* encountered the case of a thirty-two-year-old woman who sought help after several years of heavy drinking.[1] This anonymous patient was a "career woman" holding an "important executive post," but her intimate relationships had been marked by failures. Her mother disapproved of her ambition, and although her father had helped advance her career, she feared that he now resented the fact that her salary topped his own. The patient admitted to several previous episodes of "emotional illnesses," all precipitated by romantic disappointments, family turmoil, or both. As a six-foot-tall woman, moreover, the patient felt that she had never fit in with existing standards of femininity.

Following a complicated entanglement with a married co-worker, she had sought psychiatric treatment. The affair and her drinking were closely linked as they had begun almost simultaneously. Only after drinking could she have sexual intercourse, and even then she suffered "extreme guilt and depression." Seeking to terminate the relationship, she moved in with her brother and her drinking decreased. But when her brother moved, she reconnected with her lover; her drinking resumed and ultimately led to her being fired. Although she hoped her lover would leave his wife for her—she even loaned him money to help with divorce costs—he abandoned her after she became pregnant and had an abortion.

In contrast to Alcoholics Anonymous (AA) and medical regimes that focused directly on drinking behavior, Dr. Noble, the psychiatrist in this case, "did not advise . . . against drinking at any time," though he noted with apparent relief that "on her own initiative she reduced her drinking considerably soon after treatment began." In Dr. Noble's view, the therapist's function was to help his patient address the psychic conflicts and ambivalence she felt toward her parents. Just as nineteenth-century inebriate specialists had blamed women's drinking on "female complaints," Dr. Noble now saw her drinking as merely a symptom of deeper emotional problems. Rather than describing his patient's drinking behavior, he chronicled her upbringing, love affairs, work history, dreams, and emotional state, looking for triggers for her drinking episodes. Citing comments from the patient's mother such as "I would rather see you dead than alcoholic," Dr. Noble asserted that the patient drank to excess in order to exact revenge upon her parents.

As this patient's life trajectory clearly illustrates, not all American women in the post–World War II era conformed to conventional domesticity.[2] Although Dr. Noble did not criticize her directly for having a career, he did not acknowledge how social norms complicated her situation within her family and at work. As this woman had made important life choices, she had received conflicting messages from the women closest to her. Her mother indicated that a desire for financial security had motivated her own marriage, which was strained by frequent quarrels and infidelity. Yet she disapproved of women who sought careers, a criticism which even extended to her own daughter. As an alternative, the patient had looked to a female employer as a possible role model. But this supervisor had also been disappointed in love and "had given up hopes of happiness in life," advising the patient "to seek satisfaction in working 20 hours a day." While the patient's father had encouraged her in masculine pursuits ever since she was a child, her mother had repeatedly cautioned her about the limitations and vulnerability of her body, warning her about sexual problems as well as "the agonies of menstruation and the horrors of childbirth." As a result, the patient had developed considerable anxiety about sexual intercourse and pregnancy, and these fears had been reinforced when she resorted to an abortion. After her abortion, she began drinking more heavily than ever. Facing such contradictory pressures about how to manage her life as a modern woman, she turned to a psychiatrist.

The author of this article, Dr. Douglas Noble, had worked at the Johns Hopkins University Hospital and other facilities on the East Coast while also maintaining a private practice. He offered this case review, he explained, in light of the absence of medical literature on female alcoholics. The patient had been hospitalized for brief stretches as well as spending longer periods in outpatient therapy. By the 1940s, the field of psychiatry had evolved; psychiatrists had rejected the nineteenth-century title "alienists" and moved away from the institutions where they had cared for disturbed patients in custodial asylums. Both psychiatrists—medical doctors with specialized training beyond the M.D.—and psychologists—those who held a Ph.D. degree and conducted clinical psychotherapy as well as lab-based research—played important roles in the mobilization of the American military during World War II, resulting in significant cultural authority in the postwar era.[3]

Alcoholism, a more common and "everyday" malady than a disorder like schizophrenia, provided an ideal opportunity for psychiatrists to intervene in a vexing behavioral problem while clearly demonstrating their expertise to the lay public. Articles in prestigious medical journals such as the *Journal of the American Medical Association* and in specialized publications like the *Quarterly Journal of Studies on Alcohol*, along with popular magazines and books, now focused significantly on the problem of alcoholism. Since many of these professionals were affiliated with major institutions for alcoholism treatment, their views shaped the care that many patients received. In accordance with established professional hierarchies, social workers and psychologists, as well as the popular press, now adopted the language of psychiatric expertise.

As they sought to explain women's drinking, professional and lay commentators shared a powerful engagement with issues of gender and sexuality, matters particularly resonant with the general public as Americans faced widespread social, economic, and political changes during World War II and after. As we have seen, writers in the popular media criticized women's liquor consumption and fueled a fear that rates of alcoholism among women were increasing, all of which contributed to a sense that traditional standards of behavior and family organization were eroding. Even as psychiatric models reinforced the focus on individual vulnerability that lay at the center of the modern alcoholism paradigm, psychiatrists' willingness to engage directly with wider cultural meanings attached to alcohol consumption—an issue that AA and modern alcoholism movement advocates often chose to avoid—meant that psychiatrists also emerged as expert commentators on the matter of problem drinking as a *social* problem. As a result, psychiatric authority mediated the border between normal drinking and alcoholism, reconstituted in the wake of Repeal.

Psychiatric Authority and the Process of Medicalization

Tracing psychiatrists' role in medicalization shows how complex the process could be. Like the Alcoholics Anonymous fellowship and disease model advocates, psychiatrists sought to clearly and qualitatively differentiate between alcoholism and social drinking. Yet as Dr. Noble's assessment of the career woman at the beginning of this chapter shows, psychiatrists did not necessarily focus on excessive drinking as the primary problem. Instead, they generally identified underlying emotional conflicts or weaknesses to which excessive drinking was a maladaptive response or symptom. Alcoholism was not the only disorder that they characterized in this fashion; influenced by the ideas of Sigmund Freud, psychiatrists in the middle decades of the twentieth century understood many behaviors and psychological states as reactions to, or symptoms of, underlying drives and conflicts that were not easily understood by the affected person. But this approach meant that psychiatrists differed from AA and other constituencies in the modern alcoholism movement who considered excessive drinking the most important variable in identifying the condition and those who suffered from it.

Psychiatrists admitted, at least among themselves, that alcoholism was a perplexing disorder, one complicated by assumptions and stereotypes. Doctors at the private McLean Hospital in Massachusetts emphasized their modern, rational, scientific approach in the pages of the *New England Journal of Medicine* in 1937, even as they acknowledged the lack of consensus in the profession:

> Perhaps in no other division of psychiatry are the prevailing ideas as to etiologic factors and therapeutic methods and results so obscured by controversy, prejudice, ignorance and commercialized charlatanry as in the general field of alcoholism and drug addiction. . . . Is one dealing with sin or economic maladjustment or latent homosexuality or oral eroticism gone rampant and must the clinical picture be formulated in etiologic concepts of this or that particular bias, or is it possible for the time being to approach the problem profitably from an empirical and purely objective point of view?[4]

These remarks show the wide range of explanatory models in circulation, including the continuation of long-standing ideas that associated alcoholism with sin as well as more recent, specialized concepts that had originated from the field of psychiatry itself.

As part of a broader effort to standardize their vocabulary and nomenclature, the American Psychiatric Association produced a handbook in 1952 called the *Diagnostic and Statistical Manual: Mental Disorders* (*DSM-I*). This publication built on earlier work by military psychiatrists during World War II while also incorporating and adapting material from the World Health Organization. The *DSM*, like the internal medicine textbooks discussed in the previous chapter, sought to enumerate health conditions caused by alcohol intoxication and alcohol poisoning such as hallucinations or delirium tremens or other brain impairments. The authors of the *DSM* grouped alcohol along with other toxins, such as lead and mercury, that could lead to brain damage. Neither this kind of poisoning nor "alcoholic intoxication (simple drunkenness)" constituted the condition of alcoholism, however, which the *DSM* categorized under "personality disorder."[5] Even here, the authors differentiated between alcohol and other substances: "alcoholism" and "drug addiction" each received a separate diagnostic code. This division, which reflected political and cultural circumstances as much or more than pharmacology, contrasted with the ideas of many nineteenth-century inebriate specialists who had emphasized continuity across alcohol and other drugs. It also reinforced the tendency of AA and modern alcoholism movement advocates to avoid association with other drugs.

For alcoholics, psychiatrists' focus on problem drinking brought advantages but also risks. On the one hand, attention from a segment of the medical profession whose prestige was increasing could legitimate alcoholism as a medical issue. On the other hand, psychiatry as a field could bring another layer of stigma—one linked with mental illness. For their part, some psychiatrists, like physicians in other specialties, preferred to avoid alcoholic patients. As both doctors and family members reported, alcoholics could be obstinate and noncompliant. Denial, evasion, and lying proved particularly formidable obstacles in the "talking cure," and physicians and family members, especially those who paid for care, often lost patience with alcoholics who would not cooperate. As one family member complained after her nephew had spent hundreds of dollars on treatment for his alcoholic wife: "How can psychiatrists help her when she spins yarns about herself!"[6]

The diversity of treatment approaches during the mid-twentieth century indicates a lack of agreement on the causes of alcoholism; experts struggled to explain why some people became alcoholics and others did not. As the *DSM* indicated, psychiatrists and other mental health experts insisted that alcoholics suffered from specific constellations of underlying psychological problems—personality disorders—that were related to psychosexual development and gender-role identity. In contrast to Marty Mann's insistence that personal characteristics of the sufferer were irrelevant, psychiatrists underscored differences between alcoholic women and alcoholic men.

During the middle decades of the twentieth century, psychological development meant learning the appropriate gender role in childhood and then fulfilling it as an adult; many mental health professionals considered the ability to follow gendered rules an important marker of health and normalcy. While most nineteenth-century Americans had believed that social roles followed automatically from biological sex differences, that straightforward equation no longer held true. Now, psychiatrists spoke of an "adjustment" to conventional standards of behavior, a process mediated by a person's attitude and psychological state. Unlike biology, which had seemed "natural" and inevitable, the concept of "adjustment" allowed for some degree of will and agency—and alcoholism signaled that that adjustment had gone awry. Dr. Noble did not count the number of drinks consumed by the career woman described at the beginning of this chapter; instead, he offered a way to understand her behavior in the context of her search for meaningful work and for successful relationships. This type of approach aligned neatly with the desire of many Americans to reconstitute family life in the wake of the Great Depression and the upheavals of World War II.

"Mom in a Bottle": Alcoholism and the "Crisis of Masculinity"

Psychiatrists maintained that their proficiency in assessing healthy masculinity allowed them to distinguish the normal male drinker from the alcoholic.[7] In this way, they helped to renormalize men's recreational drinking in the wake of Repeal: A man had a beer with his buddies in the "manly" atmosphere of the bar or saloon. Learning to "hold one's liquor like a man" was an important coming-of-age ritual, and a man's drinking capacity was often linked to his sexual prowess.[8] As one physician explained, "One of the most powerful attractions in drinking is the *demonstration of masculinity*. To drink someone under the table, to carry one's liquor well, has always been held in high estimation."[9] Yet men who relied on alcohol in the hope that its masculine connotations would compensate for feelings of confusion and inferiority risked becoming alcoholics.

Psychoanalytic theory led psychiatrists to interpret alcoholism in men as resulting from a failure to achieve psychological and sexual maturity. One doctor maintained that alcoholism was a "special masculine neurosis" because the "excessive use of alcohol makes it possible to realize, in a fantastic subjective way, the primitive solution of the oedipus complex."[10] Drawing on similar themes, most psychiatrists located the origins of alcoholism in early family relationships. The typical male alcoholic, according to psychiatrists, had an overprotective, indulgent mother and a remote father. Such men were dependent on their mothers, passive, and unable to form a masculine self-image. Instead, they identified with their mothers and developed feminine constitutions.[11] Adolescence represented a danger zone, during which these young men would feel caught between "passive, childish, feminine wishes" and the "masculine strivings inculcated by the father and by the cultural ideology absorbed from schooling and from conflicts with other boys," according to Robert Knight, M.D., a psychoanalyst at the well-known Menninger Clinic in Kansas. Drinking appeared to resolve this conflict, offering "implicit gratification of passive oral wishes" even as it promised "the illusion of being masculine."[12] Excessive drinking as a strategy to feel more masculine ultimately and inevitably failed; psychiatrists explained that alcoholic men were unable to realize that the masculinity they sought in this way was "superficial," "spurious," and "distorted" and could not resolve their conflicts, only leaving them, in the words of one psychiatrist, "as frustrated as ever."[13]

In this interpretive framework, homosexuality was closely linked to alcoholism; both were considered to be symptomatic of psychosexual immaturity that was itself caused by an exaggerated dependency on one's mother. While the medical literature on alcoholism contained relatively few examples of homosexual behavior—one study of alcoholics treated at a state-operated outpatient clinic, for instance, reported only two active homosexuals out of sixty-three patients[14]—psychiatrists nevertheless discussed the issue extensively, citing frequent examples of latent homosexuality, sexual maladjustment, and marital failure among male alcoholics.[15] Doctors reported that many alcoholic men had difficulty sustaining relationships with women and seemed to prefer the company of other men. Echoing Karl Abraham, whose influential article had been translated into English during Prohibition,[16] psychiatrists in the post-Repeal era continued to emphasize how the male-dominated setting of bars, in which alcohol lowered inhibitions, provided the ideal environment for alcoholic men to express their unconscious desires in a socially acceptable manner. Knight described one patient: "He showed the typical behavior of alcoholics toward men friends in drinking and getting tenderly affectionate with them, swearing eternal friendship, becoming lovingly demonstrative toward them, thus acting out strong and thinly disguised homosexual attraction. When he was sober, on the other hand, he feared he would be regarded as a 'sissy' or a 'fairy.'"[17] Another doctor, while acknowledging that the "stage of direct genital homosexual acts is omitted, due to the remaining resistance," nevertheless insisted that bar fights and even "paying another man's debts in the bar" represented a "direct manifestation" of homosexual drives.[18]

This psychoanalytic language may seem odd today, but it reflected underlying ideas circulating in mainstream American society. Analysis of the potentially negative consequences of the mother-son relationship resonated strongly during and after World War II, when prominent psychiatrists and others warned that the mothers of America were ruining the next generation by emotionally smothering their children.[19] This phenomenon, termed "Momism," was discussed in great detail by Edward A. Strecker, a well-known psychiatrist who also treated alcoholics, in his book *Their Mothers' Sons: The*

Psychiatrist Examines an American Problem, first published in 1946. Drawing on his experiences as a consultant to the military during World War II, Strecker argued that mothers should be blamed for the high incidence of "the so-called psychoneuroses" displayed by soldiers. Strecker went on to argue that, even in peacetime, "moms" posed a threat, since their sons frequently developed significant emotional problems and did not become productive citizens who could handle the responsibilities of living in a democracy. In a chapter entitled "Mom in a Bottle," Strecker proclaimed, "Alcohol is a mom that can be poured into a glass." He insisted that immaturity represented an alcoholic's fundamental weakness and reported that in "about eighty percent" of the alcoholic cases he had studied, "momism in childhood was the basic, underlying cause."[20]

In treating alcoholics, then, psychiatrists addressed the neurosis or underlying emotional problems that in their view caused excessive drinking. Some psychiatrists treated patients in outpatient therapy sessions, while others cared for alcoholics in institutions. At private hospitals like McLean in Boston, Bloomingdale in New York, and Rocky Meadows Farm in Rhode Island, initial treatment included general medical care to ease patients' symptoms during withdrawal from alcohol and to address any other medical problems.[21] During the second phase of treatment, which might last six months to a year, psychiatrists sought to "reeducate" patients, helping them gain insight into personality characteristics and situations that triggered drinking episodes.[22] The therapeutic mission of Rocky Meadows Farm, for example, included not only abstinence from alcohol but also a new approach to life, encouraging growth "in maturity and self-wisdom," according to its director, Charles H. Durfee.[23] In mid-twentieth-century psychiatry, "maturity" often served as a code word for appropriate gender roles, and psychiatrists emphasized a range of activities that provided structure and therapeutic benefits for patients. Doctors hoped that encouraging appropriate masculine expression would circumvent patients' misguided attempts to seek it through alcohol. Exercise offered opportunities to practice managing aggression, while organized sports provided a way for male alcoholic patients to express latent homosexual drives in a more positive way.[24] Dances encouraged heterosexual interest, and male patients participated in carpentry and metal work as occupational therapy.[25]

Psychiatrists also used the psychotherapeutic encounter to encourage their patients to restructure their behavior and relationships, especially within the family, to conform to more traditional gender role patterns. Claiming that male alcoholics often duplicated with their wives the dependency relationship they had had with their mothers, therapists attempted to change the interactions between spouses. One psychiatrist described the wife of a forty-year-old alcoholic: "She was a remarkable individual, vigorous in all her movements and masculine looking. She breathed domination, although it was somewhat tempered by a fine intelligence." Attempting to break the "vicious cycle" of the husband's dependency in this relationship, the therapist instructed that the "wife was no longer to pay the bills or perform any of the household duties of the man."[26] Echoing Strecker's concern about the threat posed by "Momism," this psychiatrist suggested that any woman, if she were too dominant or powerful, might destroy a man's masculinity and thereby drive him to drink.[27]

Alcoholism among Women as a Failure of Femininity

Like other medical professionals, psychiatrists devoted much less attention to female alcoholics, sharing the consensus view that the condition afflicted fewer women than men. When they did turn to women, they used the same general framework of an underlying personality disorder that led to excessive drinking. But because psychiatrists recognized the social meaning of drinking as a masculine act, this diagnosis could not parallel that of men. Even though more women engaged in social drinking by the middle decades of the twentieth century, the practice did not reinforce femininity (as recreational drinking signaled healthy masculinity for men) but remained in tension with it. As a result, drinking as a symptom retained a very different meaning for women compared to men. This was not a new idea, of course, but it took on new significance in the post-Repeal era. In the late nineteenth century, Dr. Agnes Sparks had insisted that women's unique motivation for consuming alcohol (to cope with "female complaints") should lead to an especially sympathetic view of inebriate women. In contrast, now that Americans understood alcohol in primarily recreational terms, alcoholic women's drive to drink indicated particularly severe pathology.

Dr. Benjamin Karpman published one of the most detailed studies to appear during this period, a 1948 book called *The Alcoholic Woman*. In the preface, Karpman recalled being asked to give a paper on alcoholism in 1934—only a year after the repeal of Prohibition—and his interest in the topic had grown after that. Trained as a psychoanalyst as well as a physician, Karpman practiced at St. Elizabeth's Hospital in Washington, D.C., and published prolifically. When he died in 1962, he was hailed in the *American Journal of Psychiatry* as "among the most articulate and dedicated champions of the psychiatrically 'dispossessed.'"[28] Like Dr. Noble, Karpman viewed alcoholic women as an important and understudied phenomenon, modestly offering *The Alcoholic Woman* as "a minor contribution to a major social problem."[29] Publication of the book was sponsored by the Washington Institute of Medicine Research Foundation, which sought to provide "actual case studies in the psychodynamics of alcoholism" to professionals working in such fields as medicine, law, psychology, social work, education, and pastoral care.

Karpman agreed with other professionals that alcoholism appeared less frequently among women than among men, putting the ratio at 1:5. Yet, in a memorable turn of phrase, he insisted that "what alcoholic women seem to lack in quantity, they certainly do make up in quality." Clinical observation proved that alcoholic women "are much more abnormal than alcoholic men"; as he helpfully explained, "when an alcoholic woman goes on a tear, 'it is terrific.'" Karpman's explication of why this was so illustrates how psychiatric models could lead to a questioning of conventional gender roles. According to Karpman, even in modern America, in this "sophisticated age," as he put it, women still faced more "repressions" than did men and a narrower range of acceptable outlets for managing those conflicts. Because excessive drinking violated conventional standards for women even more so than for men, he insisted, women who engaged in this behavior must be especially disturbed. Rather than challenging the double standard that limited women's development and behavior, Karpman embedded it into the diagnosis itself. He even warned his colleagues of the therapeutic consequences, concluding that, "as alcoholic women are more abnormal than alcoholic men, they are, by the same token, more difficult to treat."[30]

In the text, Karpman offers three case studies—Elizabeth, Vera, and Frances. All three of the women were white, and their ages and marital status varied. Karpman treated the women at St. Elizabeth's Hospital, although each had had numerous encounters with the medical establishment and the judicial system as a result of her drinking. Elizabeth had voluntarily committed herself to a state hospital following a rape; Vera had been arrested for "delinquency" and had been institutionalized several times; and Frances had experienced multiple hospitalizations in both public and private facilities and had been jailed for drunkenness. While he acknowledged that there were other types of alcoholic women, including some who remained faithful to their husbands, Karpman nevertheless implied through his selection of these three that they exemplified women who drank to excess.

In stark contrast to what these women might have encountered in Alcoholics Anonymous, Karpman's account did not focus on their drinking habits; instead, it revealed a litany of promiscuity, rape (for which he blamed the victim), abortion, and even a rare example of lesbianism. Indeed, in his 234-page text, he provided scores of pages on the "Sex Life" and "Dream Life" of his patients but only five pages total on alcoholism per se, an approach consistent with the idea that alcoholism was the result of neurosis. Interestingly, he offered virtually nothing on treatment besides dream analysis, and even there he downplayed the importance of drinking. When Frances, for example, reported a dream about whiskey, Karpman insisted that the real subject of the dream was her "father hatred."[31]

Karpman, like other mental health professionals, interpreted female alcoholism as the result of a lifelong failure to adjust to the feminine role. Women who became alcoholics had not been adequately prepared for their adult roles as wives and mothers, whether because of the death of a parent, a divorce, "ungiving" or "ignorant" parents, or even frequent instability that could result from precarious class status.[32] Karpman blamed one patient's parents for not telling her about sex, calling her the "victim of stupid parental mis-education"; similarly, the five alcoholic women cited in another study had been ignorant of reproductive matters in their youth.[33]

Although psychiatrists' call for improved sex education appeared to be progressive, their goal was to ensure that women were better prepared for their roles as wives and mothers.[34] They emphasized that a lack of parental guidance had disastrous consequences, as many alcoholic women formed an early pattern of masculinity, displaying tomboy-like behaviors including tantrums when they were young. For example, "G," a thirty-year-old alcoholic woman who "walks with a somewhat masculine stride" according to her therapist, had been a "tomboy" as a child, doing "all the stunts that the boys did, and a few more to prove she could outstrip them even though she was a girl."[35] In this case as well as others, experts did not bother to explain a connection between playing boys' games and growing up to be an alcoholic, suggesting that they considered the gravity of such gender nonconformity to be self-evident.[36]

While childhood patterns laid the psychological groundwork for alcoholism, most experts maintained that stressful experiences or emotional difficulties later in life, almost always related to sexual and reproductive matters, precipitated the development of alcoholism in women.[37] Dr. Noble identified this pattern with the career woman described at the beginning of this chapter. Yet psychiatrists did not view this dynamic as a straightforward cause-and-effect relationship. Instead, underlying psychosexual adjustment problems led both to alcoholic women's drinking and to their failure to fulfill conventional responsibilities of motherhood and domesticity in a contented manner.

As part of this focus on adjustment, mental health experts reassessed women's reliance on alcohol to treat female complaints—the pain and discomfort that could accompany menstruation, pregnancy and post-partum recovery, and menopause. This drinking pattern had once helped define the female inebriate, and it continued into the twentieth century. As late as 1949, for example, one author found it necessary to warn against the many "popular remedies used by women to relieve painful menstruation" because they "usually contain a high concentration of alcohol." Women should avoid these, not least because any "apparent relief" was in fact the result of the "dulling of the brain and the production of a mild intoxication."[38] By the late 1940s, this "dosing" seemed old-fashioned; the women who relied on Lydia E. Pinkham's Vegetable Compound into the post–World War II era tended to be older, of minority races, and working class.[39]

Psychiatric parlance shows as well that the meaning attached to this sort of dosing and drinking had changed profoundly by the middle decades of the twentieth century. Nineteenth-century doctors had viewed women's drinking for this purpose as a direct, if misguided, response to pain that was an expected part of the female experience. Now, psychiatrists and other researchers dismissed alcoholic women's complaints of physical discomfort, maintaining instead that women's *emotional* conflicts regarding these processes led to alcoholic drinking.[40] In one oft-cited 1937 study of alcoholic women, for example, forty out of fifty patients suffered from dysmenorrhea, reporting pelvic discomfort and "premenstrual depression of spirits" and expressing annoyance with this "periodic physiological dysfunction." But the psychiatrist was unwilling to accept these women's complaints, and he arranged for them to be examined by a gynecologist, who found "no pelvic pathology to which the pain could be attributed." The psychiatrist explained, "Careful psychological investigation revealed deeper motives behind the symptoms and emotional attitudes toward menstruation."[41] A female psychologist echoed this theme more than two decades later, suggesting that, while menstrual pain and premenstrual tension, post-partum depression, and menopause might be linked to alcoholism in women, the primary cause was probably "the woman's emotional adjustment to and acceptance of these feminine physiological functions."[42]

Experts also reshaped ideas about motherhood and drinking to align with the post-Prohibition view of alcohol. In a striking reversal of many of the ideas of the Progressive Era, scientists and physicians denied many previous conclusions about the reproductive consequences of alcohol use and the role of heredity in alcoholism.[43] Environment was the more important factor, reported the author of a study of children of alcoholics who had been raised in foster homes.[44] The question-and-answer column of *Hygeia*, a magazine published by the American Medical Association and aimed at a popular audience, dismissed the idea that alcohol damaged the sperm, egg, or embryo, despite previous claims, which had been "greatly exaggerated."[45] The *Journal of the American*

Medical Association denied that drinking during pregnancy posed any danger, reassuring a physician who inquired about a woman who had drunk a significant amount of beer before she knew she was pregnant, "The patient need have no worries about the effect of her beer debauch on her unborn baby."[46] The tone and placement of this coverage suggests that experts saw a need to correct persistent lay beliefs about alcohol's reproductive harm.

Alcohol might be considered a benign substance in the post-Repeal era, but psychiatrists and other experts did not stop scrutinizing drinking women's maternal behavior. Just as these doctors regarded gynecological problems as emotional rather than physical matters, so, too, did they emphasize the psychological and environmental—rather than the biological and genetic—aspects of motherhood. No longer as biologically reductionist as their predecessors, these experts expanded the realms in which women's behavior could be judged. Through the middle decades of the twentieth century—even as increasing numbers of women, including mothers with young children, worked outside the home—most Americans assumed that becoming a mother marked a woman's emotional and even sexual maturity. The belief that all women should want to be mothers took on the quality of a medical truism: "Women totally lacking the desire for children are so rare that they may be considered as deviants from the normal," proclaimed the *Journal of the American Medical Association* in 1951, the height of the Baby Boom.[47]

If alcohol was no longer a race poison, motherhood at midcentury was not a simple matter of biological reproduction. Instead, it required careful management of maternal emotions. A mother must love her child, of course, but not too much lest she reduce him or even her to dependence and neurosis, as Dr. Strecker warned with his accusations of "Momism." A mother must cultivate an ideal balance of love, obligation, and autonomy in order to produce well-adjusted children. Mothering in this context could not be reduced to biology or even behavior. Rather, it required an ongoing psychological vigilance; a mother needed to be constantly available to her children without expecting the emotional rewards and gratitude mothers once received as a matter of course. Such expressiveness now seemed sentimental at best and psychologically harmful at worst.[48] While many American women failed to measure up to this standard, alcoholic women's behavior could be particularly egregious in this context. Their maternal shortcomings provided a way to measure their drinking problems and to underscore their deviance as women.[49]

Psychiatrists noted with concern that a substantial number of alcoholic women did not seem to want children. One psychiatrist reported the case of a thirty-eight-year-old married woman who began drinking after her marriage:

"[She] had an abortion as she 'did not want to be bothered with children.' ... She was a poor manager and housekeeper and engaged in none of the domestic arts. ... Sexually she was frigid."[50] The career woman mentioned at the start of this chapter had had an abortion, although the doctor did not overtly criticize her for doing so presumably because the circumstances surrounding her pregnancy were hardly ideal. Karpman noted that one of his patients "had upon her conscience the fact of a most distressing abortion" and that she was otherwise "an incompetent and unsatisfactory mother."[51]

Alcoholic women shared some of these beliefs about the importance of motherhood and its implications for their drinking. One alcoholic woman explained that her three miscarriages "made her feel rather inferior and an incomplete woman,"[52] implying that she might not have started drinking otherwise. In another example, a suburban housewife who was newly married and hoping to become pregnant began drinking during the day while she devoted herself to cooking and other domestic tasks, then greeted her husband each night with a martini. Gradually, her drinking intensified, and she drank secretly at night from a bottle she hid in the dresser. When she consulted a psychiatrist, he told her that her problem was not alcoholism but childlessness: "If I had a baby," she recalled him saying, "my drinking would stop." Although she shared his view at the time, she found that having two children did not lead to abstinence—hospitalization and Alcoholics Anonymous were necessary several years later.[53] The notion that having children would effect a recovery from excessive drinking was a notable reversal from the views of nineteenth-century inebriate experts who had advocated sterilization.

Psychiatrists' discussions of alcoholic women's domestic frustrations implicitly acknowledged the limitations of women's conventional roles. One doctor described an alcoholic woman who began drinking heavily after her first child was born: "She showed little interest in the child, and was bored and irritated by the other young mothers who were naturally her companions. ... Drinking commenced."[54] But psychiatrists, consistent with their professional training and orientation, blamed women's dissatisfactions not on social conditions but on their lack of preparation for, and their failure to embrace, traditional domestic responsibilities. In *The Alcoholic Woman*, for example, Karpman simply urged his patients to conform to social expectations and resolve their feelings through psychotherapy.[55] Similarly, in his study of alcoholic women, James H. Wall attributed one patient's drinking at least partly to her previous frustrations with housework, yet he noted with approval her participation in cooking classes while in treatment. Her restoration to femininity and domesticity became central to the therapeutic process, as important as her abstinence from alcohol.[56] Just as Marty Mann constantly demonstrated her sobriety through her attractive feminine style and comportment, alcoholic women could only gain access to the promises of medicalization, such as they were, by conforming to a traditionally narrow view of female behavior.

Motherhood had long been an important theme in how Americans thought about alcohol, with the purity of the domestic realm serving as counterpoint to male excess elsewhere. Women who drank upset this equation, threatening the family in fundamental ways. By the middle decades of the twentieth century, the danger no longer seemed to come from alcohol itself, as it had during the Progressive Era. And although drinking mothers set bad examples and could endanger their children through neglect, as in previous decades, they posed a new risk by midcentury: their own neuroses, which compromised their ability to meet modern standards of motherhood. Because of the kind of mothers they had and the kind of mothers they were, alcoholic women interrupted the transmission of femininity and family stability across the generations. Their maternal missteps served simultaneously as a medical diagnosis and a social indictment.

"A Futile and Mad Career of Promiscuity and Drunkenness": Sexuality, Marriage, and the Woman Alcoholic

As demonstrated in the case of the career woman cited at the beginning of this chapter, psychiatrists also addressed the sexual behavior of alcoholic women. Sex, like maternity, represented a perpetual theme in discussion of female alcoholics, but the links between sexuality and drinking took new forms in the mid-twentieth century. Just as social drinking became more acceptable for women over time, so, too, had sexual exploration become more common, even for young middle-class women. While the ideal of the nuclear family remained largely unchanged, Americans increasingly believed that marriage should bring sexual fulfillment to both partners. These new attitudes, which historians have named "sexual liberalism," brought more freedom for some kinds of sexual expression but at the cost of greater scrutiny, now often phrased in psychiatric language, of the sexual behavior of all women.[57] Commentators recognized that alcohol and sexual activity could be a volatile mix, but they were less likely than their predecessors to acknowledge that women lacked economic, social, and sexual power relative to men. Tracing these shifts demonstrates that new midcentury standards and expectations did not create sexual equality between women and men. Even when women's behavior, whether erotic activity or alcohol consumption, started to resemble men's, it carried different implications and elicited an unequal standard of judgment.

As during Prohibition, women reported that they were initiated by men into both drinking and sexual behavior, sometimes with destructive consequences. One woman in Karpman's study recalled, for example, that she began drinking so that she might understand the appeal it held for her older, married lover, who was an alcoholic. Karpman speculated that another patient was drawn to the man who became her husband because he could obtain liquor for her. Some men also used liquor to make women more sexually available or vulnerable. Frances, another of Karpman's patients, began drinking at the insistence of her male companion. She recalled, "I started drinking home brew and brandy and rum. I acquired a taste for alcohol. He thought that alcohol would break down my resistance to his demanding lust." Drunk for the first time, she felt "too happy and affectionate," and eventually she had sexual intercourse with him, just as he had hoped.[58] Frances, at least in retrospect, identified the man's intention and understood how the mind-altering effects of alcohol increased her vulnerability. The man who plied her with liquor recognized the implications of her intoxication all too well. Yet Karpman was unwilling to address the ways in which social or pharmacological forces shaped his patients' experiences, instead focusing relentlessly on what he considered underlying neuroses.

For women, public intoxication brought vulnerability, as other studies reported. "Cecily," for example, experienced a "[humiliating] sex advance" when a strange man followed her from a phone booth to her car. Although the man had apparently threatened her, *she* was jailed and fined for drunken and disorderly conduct before her husband arrived to take her home.[59] In another case, Karpman blamed his patient who had been raped, claiming that a "normal woman" would have resisted more and suggesting that she may have received some gratification from the experience since she was "most unattractive physically." He maintained that the same psychological and sexual problems that produced her alcoholism also made her want to be raped.[60] In a clear contrast with nineteenth- and early twentieth-century discourse, he did not use terms like "seduction" but instead used medical language to insist that she had, at some psychological level, "desired" sexual activity. His assessment reflects the uneven and transitional quality of attitudes about gender and sexuality during the mid-twentieth century, here refracted through the explanatory categories of dynamic psychiatry. No longer able to view her as an innocent victim, he lacked a vocabulary to articulate the constraints and dangers she faced and so deployed his professional expertise to assert that the outcome was somehow her fault.

As social expectations for emotional and sexual compatibility shifted during the mid-twentieth century, psychiatric models connected alcohol use with the most intimate realms of family life. The erosion of the temperance mandate eliminated a class-based presumption that wives should inspire their husbands to abstain through example. But if women no longer exerted moral influence from a pedestal, some men felt *they* had lost power under new marital standards and might even drink more as a result. As one sociologist explained bitterly, "So-called egalitarian marriage, which tends to subordinate the husband to the ambitions of the wife, may result in an attempt on the part of the husband to re-establish himself in his traditional role of master in his own house through the status-giving effects of alcohol."[61]

Not all married couples would have agreed with this assessment, but many accounts indicate that men now shaped their wives' drinking habits in an inversion of the temperance model. Some women reported that they had begun drinking at their husband's urging. One alcoholic woman, for example, recalled that her husband "taught her to drink and then shamed her as a prude until she drank with him."[62] Even in these relationships, however, the husbands had strict standards that they expected their wives to uphold, criticizing them if they became intoxicated at a party or if they drank at home alone. For some husbands, a wife's alcohol consumption became a variable to manage not just in the context of their relationship but also as part of the entertaining and socializing that might be essential to his career advancement.

These husbands were less patient than those of the Lit Ladies during Prohibition, perhaps reflecting a sense that women's grace period for learning to drink was over. In a typical example of this, a wife began drinking with her husband, and they "frequently got drunk together." But when he found out that she "continued drinking when he was not at home," he "resented" it. Another husband liked his wife to drink socially but was "shocked" and "upset" to learn that she was drinking privately (as he discovered when the nursemaid found her unconscious).[63] These examples suggest that many husbands retained the authority to monitor and regulate their wives' drinking, as they might have done in other realms of married life such as family finances, work outside the home, or social participation. Although Americans increasingly viewed alcohol as a consumer good, it was not under women's purview as securely as other foodstuffs.

Alcoholics' narratives showed that marital problems could be both a cause and effect of excessive drinking. Some alcoholic women reported that they had begun drinking as a result of a husband's infidelity or a divorce, while in other cases couples separated or divorced because of one partner's drinking. For example, "Laura," a thirty-six-year-old alcoholic, had taken her first drink after she saw her husband check into a hotel with another woman, confirming her suspicions that he was having an affair. To cope with the resulting turmoil, she drank heavily and took sedatives prescribed by a doctor, explaining that she "tried to keep herself unconscious with liquor and sedation." After three more years of "sexual and emotional incapability," the couple divorced.[64] In general, alcoholics had high rates of marital disruption, and separation and divorce were especially common among women alcoholics. Of course, some men devoted themselves to helping their wives address drinking problems,[65] but husbands were more likely to leave their alcoholic spouses than the reverse.[66] The loyal wife who covered up for and stood by her alcoholic husband had no obvious counterpart for men in terms of social role or cultural representation, and a woman who committed infidelity would face even more social stigma than an unfaithful husband.

Just as mainstream Americans no longer needed to abstain from alcohol but should not drink to excess, so a "good" marriage included enough sexual activity to satisfy both partners. But here, too, alcoholic women could not seem to get it right; psychiatrists criticized them for having (or at least wanting) sex too little or too much. While frigidity might seem more respectable than promiscuity—after all, a housewife who drank all day at home and then failed to respond to her husband's advances certainly presented a different image than a working-class woman who frequented bars with multiple sexual partners—psychiatrists simply saw frigidity and promiscuity as different manifestations of sexual dysfunction.[67] This framing also reinforced the idea that alcohol activated or disrupted women's sexual behavior. In fact, promiscuity was often interpreted by psychiatrists as an attempt to flee from a homosexual identity (as in the case of Karpman's patient Frances) or, more commonly, as an effort to compensate for frigidity. With the addition of alcohol, one woman, even an apparently "respectable" one, might demonstrate both frigidity and promiscuity. One physician relayed the case of a "young woman, of good family background and fair educational training, married to a bank official, and the mother of three children, who indulged, while under the influence of liquor, in indiscriminate sexualities with strange men; under the same conditions she was rejecting and frigid in her relations with her husband."[68]

Lillian Roth admitted in her memoir that her periods of particularly heavy drinking sometimes included "one-night romances," and she also recounted a string of failed marriages, with graphic descriptions of violence. But this checkered sexual history was balanced in her sobriety by her devoted marriage to Burt, a man she met in Alcoholics Anonymous who supported her desire to stop drinking and facilitated her career comeback. Roth demonstrated recovery from both alcoholism and heterosexual promiscuity, but her example reinforced the linkage of the two.[69]

As we have seen, during Prohibition and World War II, journalists and social commentators, as well as physicians and psychiatrists, interpreted women's drinking as a manifestation of the desire to act like men. This association could have led to the assumption that alcoholic women were lesbians, the mirror image of the effeminate male alcoholic in psychiatric literature who was described as a latent homosexual—and certainly Karl Abraham had drawn this connection earlier. However, American psychiatrists reported few, if any, lesbians among the alcoholic women they studied in the decades after Repeal.[70] This finding is surprising in some ways, especially since historians have documented the existence of a vibrant lesbian bar culture during this period.[71] The relative lack of attention to lesbians in the literature on alcoholism stemmed from the ways in which homosexuality came to be defined, as well as the intensely heterosocial and heterosexual context surrounding women's drinking in the United States.

During the late nineteenth and early twentieth centuries, experts debated various definitions of homosexuality, which might include gender inversion—the expression of traits and behaviors generally associated with the "opposite" gender—as well as sexual object choice. Definitions were very much in flux, and individuals might engage in erotic acts with a person of the same gender without assuming an identity as a homosexual. Male homosexuals, who generally had more autonomy and geographical mobility than women, gradually attracted more attention as they created a lively urban culture and the concept of homosexuality as an identity (rather than discrete acts) consolidated.[72] The separate spheres doctrine of the nineteenth century and associated social practices that divided women and men meant that even the saloons and other drinking establishments frequented by heterosexual men had a homosocial atmosphere, a situation that contributed to claims by psychiatrists that men's drinking patterns provided camouflage for latent homosexuality.

But this spatial organization of saloons and bars meant that most women encountered alcohol (at least for recreational drinking) in settings where men were present. Compared to homosexual men, lesbians remained less visible overall, and their bar culture was even more hidden. As we have seen, journalists commented on women-only drinking practices such as afternoon tea parties that included cocktails, but even they were understood as a prelude to husbands' return. Liquor consumption was deeply embedded in heterosexual courtship practices and marriage, as seen in customs ranging from Progressive

Era treating, to sipping a flask during Prohibition, to cocktail hour in postwar middle-class homes. As a result, men usually controlled access to alcohol or at least monitored women's consumption. Researchers debated whether female alcoholics preferred the company of other women or of men while drinking,[73] but they did not translate a preference for women-only drinking settings into "latent lesbianism," nor did they necessarily recognize the risks that women faced in mixed-gender settings.

One notable exception to the general lack of attention to lesbians was the case study of Frances, from Karpman's *Alcoholic Woman*. Frances attributed her alcoholism to fear, explaining that the "greatest fear of all was that of my homosexuality being found out." Karpman described her situation this way: "Realizing her homosexual tendencies and fearing them, she embarked on a futile and mad career of promiscuity and drunkenness. When she wasn't seeking an escape from homosexuality in the embraces of some man, she was seeking it in alcohol and often she sought it simultaneously in both." Interestingly, and perhaps naïvely, he believed that she greatly exaggerated the social consequences she would have faced if her homosexuality had been known.[74] He observed, "In trying to avoid the accusation of lesbianism, she became lower and more despicable than almost any homosexual."[75] He refused to allow that her alcohol consumption might have been an understandable response to social discrimination, insisting instead that psychological flaws formed the common denominator behind her drinking and her sexual promiscuity. In Karpman's telling, the behavior of all three of his subjects illustrated the close connections between alcoholic and sexual excess.

In her public health career, Marty Mann worked hard to avoid these associations. She acknowledged that she had been divorced, assimilating that event, which had occurred almost twenty years before, into a narrative of recovery and forgiveness. Mann spoke fondly of her ex-husband, who served on a U.S. Navy ship in the Pacific during World War II after he, too, stopped drinking. Her husband's return to full emotional health was also demonstrated by his remarriage. Lacking the stamp of propriety that a heterosexual marriage would have added to her persona as a recovered alcoholic, Mann had to prove her respectability in other ways. Intriguingly, Mann continued to use the title "Mrs." for the rest of her life. In a letter, an old friend (who apparently had been long out of touch) expressed surprise over this version of her name and asked if Mann found it better in her work to go by "Mrs.," but unfortunately Mann's answer is not available.[76] That she used "Mrs." along with her maiden name and her androgynous nickname underscores the extent of her self-creation.

In fact, Mann lived in a decades-long relationship with another woman, Priscilla Peck.[77] Although her intimates knew of this relationship, neither it nor Mann's sexual orientation was revealed publicly during her career as a health advocate, in contrast to her almost belligerent outspokenness about her alcoholism. Mann undoubtedly believed she had good reasons for keeping silent. Beyond the general social disapproval of homosexuals during this era in American history, the belief that alcoholism was linked to psychosexual adjustment problems complicated the position of gay and lesbian alcoholics. Mann's writings suggest that the focus of Alcoholics Anonymous on drinking as such, without reference to sexual orientation or emotional issues, proved crucial to her personal recovery.[78] Similarly, the disease model she advocated allowed her to sidestep any question of sexual behavior or orientation. Revealing this second stigmatized identity, one she was not willing to relinquish in the way she abstained from alcohol, threatened to undo the carefully calibrated life story that supported her public message of the worthiness of all alcoholics.

The more common view that drinking women were heterosexually promiscuous probably made it easier for Mann to deflect attention from her sexual orientation. Even the hallucinations alcoholics experienced reflected this connection: While alcoholic men frequently heard voices accusing them of being homosexual, alcoholic women were much more likely to be called "prostitute" in their hallucinations.[79] This belief had important implications for treatment and research, shaping the reception alcoholic women found in early Alcoholics Anonymous. It could also amplify other pejorative attitudes. Although African American women received very little attention in the alcoholism literature generally, the way they were portrayed perpetuated negative beliefs about their sexual behavior. In one study of fifty alcoholic women, only eight were "colored," but they were disproportionately represented in the group that had "conscious knowledge of sexual relations before puberty." Another study that reinforced and reflected both racial and gender stereotypes reported that more alcoholic women than alcoholic men were infected with syphilis, but of the women, more black than white women were infected.[80] Accusations of promiscuity thus underscored the deviance of alcoholic women relative to other women as well as to alcoholic men, making recovery a multifaceted challenge.

Many psychiatrists considered themselves self-consciously modern, viewing sexuality and gender identity as fundamental elements of human development for both men and women. The psychiatric framework for understanding alcoholism resonated with wider concerns in mid-twentieth-century American society about an apparent breakdown in conventional behavior and family stability. Chronic, compulsive drinking violated Americans' belief that familial and social stability depended on unselfish, pure, and nurturing women, but even casual consumption, which entailed pleasure and a possible loss of control, could undermine women's obligations, making it harder to characterize alcoholism as a specific clinical diagnosis as opposed to a troubling social phenomenon. Although they did not advocate temperance or abstinence as social policy, psychiatrists insisted that only severe pathology would prompt women to drink excessively in violation of social taboos. This view reinforced popular judgments of alcoholic women as especially disturbed while simultaneously incorporating different degrees of judgment into the diagnosis of alcoholism. Psychiatric explanations for alcoholism demonstrated the malleability of American concerns about women's behavior as persistent anxieties previously framed in biological or moral terms reemerged in an ostensibly modern and objective psychological language. Although psychiatric expertise contributed to medicalization, this approach complicated the efforts by other disease model advocates to extract the diagnosis from fraught associations with sexual comportment, psychological development and vulnerabilities, and judgments of mental health.

Chapter 6

"The Doctor Didn't Want to Take an Alcoholic"

The Challenge of Medicalization at Midcentury

In 1939, Wilma Wilson, a young waitress, dancer, and actress from Los Angeles, was committed to Camarillo State Hospital as an alcoholic. After Wilson had engaged in a severe drinking binge that lasted a week and culminated in her taking a large dose of sleeping pills, Wilson's mother initiated the necessary legal steps to have her committed. Wilson recounted her hospital stay in *They Call Them Camisoles*, a rare first-person account from this era.[1] The title refers to the restraints some patients had to wear, and while Wilson describes some of her encounters with psychiatrists humorously, her commitment was no laughing matter. Her account of the powerful regulatory structure that put her in the hospital and the circumstances she found there is chilling even decades later.

Unlike many narratives by alcoholics, Wilson's book does not describe her drinking in detail, nor did she write from a secure position of abstinence. Rather, she described some of her drinking episodes as if they were merely hijinks before explaining that she developed into a "spree," or periodic, drinker. The bulk of the book centers on her time in the hospital, ending as she is about to be released. The reader does not know what will happen to her upon discharge. Although she did not deny her drinking problem, her lucid and sophisticated authorial voice hints that she did not belong in the hospital.

Like other alcoholic memoirs, *They Call Them Camisoles* was intended to educate the reader as well as recount a life story, and much of the narrative details Wilson's observations of the patients around her. Being confined with mentally ill patients made her and other alcoholics doubt their own sanity. Yet alcoholism could bring even more stigma than mental illness, and as an alcoholic woman, Wilson had few legal rights. When Wilson petitioned for a jury trial to contest her commitment, she was told that only insane patients were entitled to that procedural step. A staff physician "recoiled in horror" when told that the patient he wanted to hire to care for his young daughter had been admitted for alcoholism, not mental illness, as he had presumed. Upon release, Wilson was effectively on parole, forbidden to work anywhere where liquor was served (though she had earned her living as a waitress) or even to enter any home that contained alcohol. In addition, her fiancé informed her that he would leave her if she drank again.[2]

Wilson emphasized the lack of specialized or effective treatment provided to alcoholics inside the hospital, in contrast to the expectations of alcoholics and family members. "Well," she explained sarcastically, "an alcoholic is given a dose of salts and a Wasserman [test for syphilis]. And then the alcoholic is given a mop or a polishing block used for waxing floors. If these cure drinking, then commitments are not in vain." She also described a double standard in practices and attitudes. Male patients received more privileges in the hospital; they were, for example, allowed to smoke in more settings than women and granted more access to outdoor spaces. The male hospital attendants admired the alcoholic men "for having the physical stamina, money and perseverance to drink to the point of needing hospitalization." The contrast was stark for the "female of the species," according to Wilson, since "women attendants apparently thought girls who drank were too depraved to be worthy of courtesies." Harsher judgments and stigma followed alcoholic women even into such institutions.[3]

Wilson gained more notoriety upon her death than she experienced while alive. In 1943, only a few years after the book was published, Wilson was found dead in her apartment, apparently murdered by a soldier. Newspaper accounts from the murder trial indicate she was drinking again. In fact, one neighbor reported that Wilson had stood outside asking for help the night of the murder, but no one responded because she seemed to be drunk. Wilson went back into her home, where she was later discovered with a fractured skull. The soldier was found guilty in a military trial, but the precise circumstances that led to her death remain a mystery.[4]

Wilma Wilson's experiences illustrate important elements in how alcoholic women were treated in the years following the repeal of Prohibition; like her, many female alcoholics faced greater discrimination and had less autonomy than their male counterparts. During these years, doctors, hospital and clinic administrators, legal experts, social workers, and alcoholics and their advocates developed treatment protocols and policies. The logic of medicalization held that alcoholics, as victims of a disease, should be treated by sympathetic and knowledgeable health care professionals, but realizing that vision was not easy. Simply articulating a lexicon of sickness did not lead automatically to a standard treatment regimen or even an agreed-upon diagnosis or definition of cure. The medicalization process could not erase biased ideas about women who drank to excess, nor could it fully accommodate differences in their drinking experiences, family roles, and social position. As a result, medicalization had a different effect on women than on men, amplifying rather than reducing the significance of gender in the emerging disease model.

Although popular media sources suggested an "epidemic" of drinking women during the World War II era as well as a growing population of women who drank at home—"housewives with the secret sickness"—in the postwar years, a deeply skewed sex ratio among alcoholics shaped treatment opportunities just as it influenced sponsorship patterns in Alcoholics Anonymous. This lopsided ratio, whether genuine or an artifact of the additional stigma that alcoholic women faced, raised questions of quantity *and* quality, to paraphrase Dr. Benjamin Karpman.

This chapter assesses a sampling of treatment protocols during the post-Repeal years in order to explore the implications for alcoholic women of a medical model. Women's experiences differed from men's in diagnosis, access to care, and hospital commitment. Doctors brought unexamined beliefs about drinking women into the most cutting-edge and ostensibly objective forms of medical care. They consistently reported that women did not respond well to treatment. Although this finding could draw the entire disease model into question, it instead reinforced the idea that women were a particularly intractable subset of alcoholics. In contrast to medical regimens overseen by physicians, programs in jails and hospitals that focused on women, often run by social workers, provided a wider range of support services tailored to women's particular needs even as they drew on the prestige of medicine to do so.

The complicated landscape that alcoholics encountered shows that medicalization involves fundamental questions of power, as Wilma Wilson learned all too well. Various types of health professionals jockeyed for authority relative to one another and with the criminal justice system, with a diagnosis like alcoholism or insanity shaping legal rights as well as medical care. Medical care could be seen as an adjunct to—or in competition with—Alcoholics Anonymous or reliance on clergy. While many alcoholics benefited from these alliances, such a mix complicated the process of medicalization. Alcoholism illuminated how physicians and policy makers could expand their jurisdiction over patients and over ideas about health and illness, but experts also retained the power to say no, to deny not just treatment but the cultural sanction of a medically defined diagnosis—as some potential patients found when they sought help for this perplexing condition. While some, like Wilson, were subjected to institutional discipline against their will, others searched in vain for any care or attention at all.

An alcoholic's behavior profoundly affected family members and friends, a truism that many Americans realized through direct experience and a message that was reinforced through temperance rhetoric, Alcoholics Anonymous (AA) and Al-Anon literature, psychiatric case studies that were published, and even Hollywood films. Medicalization, including such specific elements as the alcohol information centers established by the National Committee for Education on Alcoholism, offered the allure of a cure to families who hoped to gain assistance for a loved one. Yet the structure of the twentieth-century family meant that access to treatment differed for women and men. An alcoholic husband and father could devastate a family financially and emotionally, but social conventions and cultural scripts, not to mention economic dependence, encouraged a wife to stay with her drinking husband even in difficult circumstances and to facilitate his rehabilitation. An alcoholic wife and mother inverted this scenario, leaving even supportive husbands in a confusing familial and social situation. And just as men often mediated women's access to alcohol, so, too, did husbands exercise considerable control over alcoholic women's access to medical care. An alcoholic woman's path to treatment unfolded in a dense web of caretaking obligations and financial dependence that replicated the life circumstances of most women, whether alcoholic or not. Although they may have preferred to focus on a narrowly defined disease, those who diagnosed, treated, and advocated for female alcoholics found that they inevitably confronted the question of what it meant to be a woman in mid-twentieth-century America.

"They Didn't Have to Tell Me That Alcoholism Was a Sickness": Disease, Shame, and Stigma

Alcoholism advocates believed that doctors' acceptance of alcoholics as patients would reduce the stigma attached to problem drinking and encourage alcoholics to seek help. But to achieve this outcome, both doctors and alcoholics had to adopt new attitudes. Even when they suffered from acute physical symptoms, many alcoholics still hesitated to ask for relief. One woman recalled such an episode: "I lay across the bed on my stomach with nothing but pain and sickness." Although medical attention would seem warranted, she was reluctant to pursue it. "I was scared to death to call a doctor," she explained. "I thought when people did what we did that they just locked them up. I didn't know that anything was ever done for them in a medical way."[5] When they consulted doctors, alcoholics often encountered an unhelpful or even hostile reception. Those who had achieved sobriety through AA after unsuccessful attempts at medical and psychiatric treatment could be especially critical of physicians and frequently incorporated this litany of failure into their recovery narratives. For example, when one alcoholic woman decided she should see a psychiatrist, her husband found one, but, she explained, "the doctor didn't want to take an alcoholic. He called me that because I was drinking too much. So I got drunker and drunker, and then, suddenly, I woke up in the booby-hatch."[6] Her experience shows how the lack of medical help along the way could lead to institutionalization as the only alternative. In another case, an American doctor in Paris told a wealthy expatriate woman that she had an enlarged liver. She recalled that "he also said, 'You are an alcoholic and there is nothing I can do for you.'"[7]

While the Paris doctor turned this woman away because he did not think he could help, other physicians freely expressed their frustration with patients who drank to excess. One doctor commented on the difficulties involved in caring for alcoholics in the *Pennsylvania Medical Journal* in 1946, characterizing them as "the most uncooperative, nasty, mean, dirty, vulgar patients that the physician is asked to treat. That is the reason," he insisted, that "many conscientious and hard-working doctors decline to handle such patients." The alcoholic patient "wastes the time of a busy doctor" and "seldom, if ever, follows advice." This profile conflicted with expectations that women especially would be meek and obedient patients. The family posed another problem, according to this doctor: "Shamed by the presence of such a disease in their household, fearful lest the neighbors know, frequently terrified by the patient's accusations, worried over the mounting costs of treatment, the family usually detains the busy doctor to pour in his ear all the latest misdeeds of the suffering miscreant."[8] The phrase "suffering miscreant" captures the challenges of converting problem drinking into a medical condition, as does the doctor's observation that family members are "shamed" by the "disease." Advertisements for specialty hospitals that treated alcoholics were interspersed with the text of this article. Presumably directors at these institutions hoped to capitalize on physicians' unwillingness to treat alcoholics in private practice.

Even as advocates argued for a disease model and desperate families turned to medical experts for help, alcoholism as a health condition did not conform to a standard medicalization script. Doctors did not always play the role of benevolent and all-knowing professionals, nor were patients necessarily compliant and grateful. Even defining the condition and identifying those who suffered from it proved challenging. The AA fellowship, alcoholism researchers, and psychiatrists all tried to differentiate alcoholics from "normal" drinkers, but none produced a standardized and definitive diagnostic test, and certainly not the sort of lab-based evaluation that was increasingly becoming orthodox practice in identifying diseases. This lack of clarity complicated efforts to provide treatment or even to determine whether intervention was necessary or appropriate. Diverse sources including medical literature, published AA narratives, and letters Marty Mann received from alcoholics and their families show ambiguity; language could be clumsy and unable to align excessive drinking and its consequences within the narrow constraints of a disease model. For example, one woman recalled her situation before contacting AA: "I had been drunk for nine days, sick and alone and desperate. They didn't have to tell me that alcoholism was a sickness."[9] Yet the husband of another woman admitted confusion in interpreting his wife's drinking. "Whether or not my wife is alcoholic or not I don't know," he wrote to Marty Mann. Significantly, he did not attempt to quantify her consumption or describe any health problems she had; instead, he pointed to the behavioral consequences of her drinking, especially on her family. "But I do know," he declared, "that when she drinks she gets into trouble, neglecting the children, etc."[10] How—and even why—should doctors address a complex situation like that?

Hospital Care, Commitment, and Power

One place to begin was with the health consequences of excessive and chronic drinking. Mann and other advocates pushed for hospital access for alcoholic patients as a top priority since it would demonstrate that alcoholics deserved medical care. Relieving pain and addressing physical complaints seemed squarely in doctors' domain; as we have seen, medical textbook authors considered alcohol poisoning and the effects of chronic drinking on human organ systems to be within doctors' jurisdiction even when they did not believe they could arrest compulsive drinking itself. Furthermore, the act of going to the hospital could be easily understood by the general public and reinforced the idea that alcoholism was a health problem like any other.[11]

Yet doctors and administrators debated whether general hospitals should even accept alcoholics, with some arguing that they drained resources that could better serve other, worthier patients. In 1939, physicians at the Haymarket Square Relief Station, a branch of the Boston City Hospital, insisted in the prestigious *New England Journal of Medicine* that alcoholism must be recognized as a public health problem, comparing it to tuberculosis and syphilis, even as they acknowledged that the cost of admitting alcoholic patients was "disproportionately high."[12] Similarly, the Council on Medical Education and Hospitals, responding to a resolution released jointly by the New York Academy of Medicine and the Research Council on Problems of Alcohol, published a statement in 1947 recognizing the "importance of improving the standards and facilities for the hospitalization and care of alcoholic patients."[13]

These declarations were important, but admission policies still varied greatly. As a result, the experience of an individual alcoholic could be shaped by something as simple and serendipitous as which doctor she encountered when she went to a hospital, as well as by variables such as gender, class status, race, and region. Fewer than one-third of six thousand hospitals cited in a 1947 survey reported that they accepted alcoholic patients for treatment, although the fact that this survey was discussed in the *Journal of the American Medical Association* indicates increased attention by mainstream physicians toward alcoholism. Calculating accurate numbers was very difficult: While restrictions and stigma prevented some alcoholics from being admitted, patients who received care for other health problems or accidents while intoxicated might not be diagnosed as alcoholic even if they were. And in spite of warnings about an epidemic of drinking women in the popular media, this report did not break down statistics on available beds or admission rates by gender, making it difficult to assess women's treatment opportunities.[14]

We will never know how many patients admitted for other reasons were also alcoholics. For example, AA co-founder Dr. Bob Smith cooperated with Sister Ignatia, a nurse administrator at a Catholic hospital in Akron, Ohio, who used creative diagnoses to admit male alcoholic patients during the 1940s. Sister Ignatia later recalled her maneuvers in a letter to Bill Wilson: "I, personally, put them in under varied diagnoses, such as medical observation, nervous breakdown, or if they had a black eye, I would use 'possible head injury.'"[15] In this way, advocates could provide care for at least some alcoholics when hospital policies did not allow or encourage their admission. Yet even this limited access depended on medical professionals' ingenuity and commitment to treat alcoholics.

Doctors who advocated for medical treatment for alcoholics often depicted their involvement as a necessary addition, even corrective, to the spiritual approach of AA and the interference of temperance advocates. Typically, one physician applauded the efforts of the AA fellowship but then urged his colleagues that "it is the responsibility of individual doctors and of the medical profession as a whole to contribute the scientific approach to the problem [of alcoholism]."[16] Although they had no "magic bullet" or treatment protocol that unequivocally brought relief and long-term abstinence to alcoholic patients, doctors emphasized their expertise and progressive approach, especially with each new technology. One female physician, reporting the successful application of the psychotropic drug Thorazine in the treatment of alcoholics, concluded in 1955 that "modern treatment methods . . . make it possible to handle alcoholics in a general hospital."[17] Mann encouraged this shift in attitude, noting in 1950 that unfortunately "many hospitals still feel that alcoholics are not their responsibility, that their facilities are 'for sick people, not for drunks.'" She declared that her organization and its local branches were helping to change this "antiquated and inhumane treatment."[18] By midcentury, more and more doctors and medical organizations demonstrated their willingness to care for alcoholics. The American Hospital Association issued a series of resolutions asserting that community general hospitals should provide alcoholism treatment. Similarly, the American Medical Association declared that alcoholic patients should not be denied hospital admittance and that the alcoholic should be regarded as a sick person.[19]

These successes in reconfiguring alcoholism as a public health matter both echoed and extended the work of the inebriate specialists of the late nineteenth century. Like their predecessors, mid-twentieth-century advocates insisted that compulsive drinking could be treated in a medical setting. This optimistic and progressive attitude aligned neatly with a general confidence in science and technology in the post–World War II era—but this context also brought new standards and expectations regarding the power of medicine compared to what inebriate specialists had faced. Twentieth-century medical and public health triumphs such as control over infectious diseases through immunizations and antibiotics, the steep decline in infant mortality, and the standardization—even bureaucratization—of many aspects of medical care underscored the lack of consensus regarding the causes of alcoholism and the best means for treating it. Short-term hospital stays to manage acute physical symptoms were one thing; the prospect of longer-term treatment highlighted the intractability of alcoholism and the difficult behavior of many alcoholics, adding to the frustration and discouragement many doctors felt.

Mid-twentieth-century plans for specialized inpatient care also built on a complicated legacy of asylums and raised important issues of patient autonomy. Longer-term treatment might be simply custodial or a form of punishment; it also could involve questions of power and family relations, as in the case of Wilma Wilson. Mann and other advocates presented modern hospital care as an unalloyed good, for men and women alike. But other forms of evidence, including hospital data and letters Mann received after her *Reader's Digest* profile,[20] show that the reality was much more complicated, illuminating the challenges involved in defining alcoholism and providing treatment for women in light of family obligations and economic dependence.

Like the man who wondered whether his wife was an alcoholic, those who wrote to Mann frequently described the effects of women's drinking on their families and expressed uncertainty over what to do. One mother wrote, for example, "I have just read your story in the readers digest [sic] and it is the life of my daughter. She is now a hopeless alcoholic—we have all tried to help her. I have comdemmed [sic] her for neglecting her husband and children." Despite her anger, this mother would not abandon her daughter: "She was such a good person before this got ahold of her, where are the hospitals located . . . where she can get help, and what would it cost."[21] Even as they worried, mothers and sisters often yielded to the husband of the woman in question; the husband's attitude frequently made the difference in whether an alcoholic woman received care. Some husbands supported their wives' attempts at treatment, even accompanying them to AA meetings or "going on the wagon" (avoiding alcohol) themselves. One husband mortgaged the family car so that his wife could have the "wonder cure"—a version of aversion therapy—at an institution in the Cleveland area, without success. The woman explained her return to drink: "After they made me puke for three days and three nights, I just had to have some whiskey to settle my stomach."[22]

In cases like these, it can be difficult to know where support ended and coercion began. The husband of one alcoholic woman treated at the Washingtonian Hospital in Boston, for example, threatened to institutionalize her if she began drinking again, while another man contacted the police while his wife was on a five-day drinking binge.[23] At the Haymarket Square Relief Station, physicians who analyzed the patient population concluded that the majority of male patients were unmarried, while the majority of female patients were married.[24] Since the facility represented a last resort, the admission of married women could mean that their husbands were no longer willing or able to care for them at home, as wives might have done for alcoholic men in similar situations. Mann explained in her *Primer* that husbands were more likely to abandon alcoholic women than nonalcoholic wives were to leave their drinking husbands.[25]

Even as husbands walked away and health care professionals rejected patients who drank excessively, female alcoholics like Wilma Wilson and many others received treatment under pressure from family members or state imperative, and these instances require careful interpretation. Institutional records suggest that alcoholic women were generally more likely than men to be committed for treatment, sometimes against their will. At a state mental hospital in Kansas, for example, fewer than one-quarter of the female alcoholic patients had been admitted voluntarily, as opposed to almost half of the male patients. In one study of fifty alcoholic women treated at a New York hospital, only fifteen patients had sought admission voluntarily, while the rest were committed. Yet those patients were not completely powerless: Most of these women petitioned for their own commitment after the hospital staff discussed it extensively with them and their families. And even then, the average length of stay for committed patients was not that much longer than that of voluntary patients.[26] The greater proportion of commitments among women is therefore difficult to evaluate: The definition of commitment was not standardized, many doctors believed that commitment was more likely to bring improvement, and the alternative could be no care at all.

Hospital data show that fewer women than men received treatment under any circumstances. For instance, Bellevue Hospital in New York City, the McLean Hospital in Massachusetts, and the Haymarket Relief Station in Boston all reported many fewer female alcoholic patients than male.[27] At the Haymarket Square Relief Station, women constituted fewer than six hundred out of approximately ten thousand patients treated for alcoholism from the late 1920s through the late 1930s. In addition to alcoholism per se, alcohol-related problems were a factor in the admission of a smaller number of female than male patients. The sex ratio among alcoholic patients at the Haymarket Relief Station was thus calculated as 18:1, much more skewed than the sex ratio among all patients there and also much higher that the general estimate of the sex ratio among alcoholics, generally considered to be around 6:1 during this period. The number of alcoholic women admitted to Haymarket had, however, increased following the repeal of Prohibition, supporting the common belief that alcoholism among women was on the rise.[28]

The ability to pay for one's care made a difference as well, and "housewife"—the most common occupational designation for women hospitalized for alcoholism reported in these studies—obscured class backgrounds. The structural layout of some treatment facilities, with few beds or rooms for women, made monetary issues all the more important. For example, Knickerbocker Hospital in New York City started an innovative regimen for alcoholics in cooperation with AA during the mid-1940s. While the program accepted women, only a few double rooms were reserved for them, and the ward was exclusively for men. Such an arrangement presumably meant that alcoholic women who could pay for semiprivate facilities had a better chance of receiving treatment, while women who could only afford the ward had no options.[29]

Unraveling the interactions among alcoholic women, family members, and professionals is difficult. Reflecting their relative lack of power in the family and in society, female alcoholics may well have been more likely than men to be committed for treatment rather than admitted to a hospital voluntarily. Many medical professionals and the general public, however, tended to assume that alcoholism was not a women's problem, and treatment often required a sacrifice that not all families were willing to make, especially when women's drinking could be hidden or understood as willful misbehavior rather than as a medical disorder amenable to cure.

"Applies Also to the Women": Medical Treatment and the Problem of Difference

By the middle decades of the twentieth century, calling something a disease promised medical treatment and the possibility of cure. Unlike infectious diseases, however, no "magic bullet" emerged to eradicate addiction. Lacking this standardization, doctors and other professionals who cared for alcoholics offered a bewildering array of modalities. Medical treatment regimes, like drinking practices, became a domain where beliefs about gender difference could be enacted and debated. During the late nineteenth century, the notion that female inebriates represented a distinct class meshed seamlessly with widespread sex segregation in American life, and treatment facilities were structured accordingly, as the Keeley Institute showed. But in the post-Repeal era, women and men mixed in many more settings, including drinking culture. Moreover, the logic of medicalization now pushed toward uniformity, as Mann insisted in her *Primer*. We have seen that gendered social practices coexisted uneasily with alcoholic identity in Alcoholics Anonymous. As they developed medical treatments, even those doctors who insisted that female alcoholics differed from their male counterparts seemed unsure whether treatment should differ as well.

Lillian Roth's memoir, *I'll Cry Tomorrow*, demonstrates the wide range of treatments that many alcoholics tried; in her case, these included hospitalization, dietary changes, a primitive form of aversion therapy, and psychoanalysis. Family members and Roth's marital status also shaped her treatment over time. When Roth's drinking first accelerated, her mother wanted her to enter a sanitarium. Roth refused but agreed instead to hire a nurse who would administer a "salt water cure" in an isolated country cottage. Roth soon rejected that regimen and returned to New York City, where she tried other forms of medical treatment, including "vitamin injections, fruit juices, bromides, sleeping pills." Perhaps not surprisingly given this haphazard approach, she continued to drink heavily. Married to a soldier during World War II, Roth saw army doctors who diagnosed her health problems as "colitis and a liver ailment—a polite way of saying that I suffered from acute alcoholism."[30] Roth's condition deteriorated, and she consulted with the prominent psychoanalyst Dr. A. A. Brill, who recommended that she be hospitalized immediately. Roth entered Bloomingdale Hospital in Westchester, New York, where she went through detoxification. Once she had completed that acute phase, she experienced a routine that seems largely unchanged from that provided by institutions in the late nineteenth century: light household chores, exercise, wholesome meals, "community therapeutic shower," and crafts, along with psychiatric counseling, the one element that looked new and modern.[31]

Even as she abstained from alcohol, Roth could use other drugs to manage her emotional and physical state. When he discharged her from the hospital, Roth's doctor gave her a bottle of sleeping pills, warning her not to "make a habit" of them.[32] Alleviating withdrawal symptoms and managing alcoholic patients' emotions remained important tasks for which twentieth-century physicians increasingly turned to pharmaceutical tools. Such practices reveal important shifts from the late nineteenth century, when many inebriate specialists had regarded alcohol as a drug on a spectrum with other substances such as opium and caffeine. In contrast, by the mid-twentieth century, physicians as well as other Americans were more likely to regard liquor as a benign recreational beverage, divorced from both pharmaceutical medicines and from street drugs. In fact, by the 1950s, sedatives, tranquilizers, and other psychotropic drugs became a modern replacement for the medicinal use of alcohol,[33] with some physicians concluding that tranquilizers were more effective in alleviating symptoms of alcohol withdrawal in female patients.[34] For their part, some women requested sedatives,[35] even as some alcoholics and clinicians viewed these drugs as dangerous substitutes for liquor.[36]

The understanding that some classes of tranquilizers could lead to dependence and addiction emerged slowly, in part because of a profound division between "medicine" and "dope" by this period.[37] But pharmaceuticals offered another lesson in how alcoholism might be understood and treated. The efficacy of tranquilizers in alleviating anxious mood helped create the diagnosis of anxiety; if a pill could cure it, the condition looked biological.[38] In aversion therapy for alcoholics, doctors similarly hoped that combining a drug with behavioral therapy could remove an alcoholic's craving to drink.[39]

Designed to make liquor itself repugnant to the alcoholic, aversion regimens were known by various names, including the "conditioned reflex" and Antabuse, a trade name for the substance administered to the patient. Physicians at the Shadel Sanitarium, an institution near Seattle devoted exclusively to the treatment of alcoholics, developed a form of conditioned reflex treatment that Mann lauded as "modern and scientific."[40] Staking their claim to expertise, Shadel doctors explained that alcoholism was more than "a weakness of willpower," as many laypeople assumed. Yet treating alcoholism as a neurosis, which many psychiatrists did, was not successful. Following the modern alcoholism paradigm, Shadel physicians distinguished between alcoholics, who reacted abnormally to alcohol, and everyone else. Treatment should produce "a reflex aversion to the sight, smell, taste and thought of alcoholic beverages." Patients following the protocol drank an alcoholic beverage, preferably one of their favorites, and then the doctor injected the patient with a drug that made him or her violently nauseated. Patients underwent a series of treatments during the first week, along with counseling, then returned for "refresher" courses at intervals of several months. In 1942, Shadel doctors reported that "[patients] under 30 years of age, professional men (including doctors) and women were especially difficult to treat, as drinking in these patients represents a more severe break with normalcy than in the average patient."[41]

Like an antibiotic to eliminate infection, a regimen like the conditioned reflex gained credibility if it worked on anyone diagnosed with alcoholism. The Shadel results showed the weakness of a one-size-fits-all approach, demonstrating instead distinctions among alcoholics and highlighting those who contradicted the stereotype of an older man on skid row. Even as they considered subtypes among male alcoholics, however, Shadel doctors considered women to be a category of their own.

Dr. C. C. Turner, a physician who used the Shadel method in his private practice, also asserted that female alcoholics were less likely to recover than their male counterparts, offering detailed case reports in the *Memphis Medical Journal* in 1942. Mr. H. was thirty-three years old and reported that he had been drinking heavily for the past five years. A spree drinker, he was a "dependable, conscientious, thoroughly reliable man—a good husband and father" between drinking bouts. When the doctor described the regimen to him, Mr. H. "showed good insight into his condition" and "seemed earnestly and conscientiously desirous of obtaining a cure if such was possible." After five treatments, he was tempted with whiskey but became nauseated immediately.

In contrast, Turner's discussion of a female patient focused on her relationship with her husband, a businessman twenty years her senior. Although Mrs. W. indicated that she "adored" her husband, the marriage was difficult. The couple drank together, and the doctor reported that "during the sprees physical violence is evidenced by both parties." Turner described Mrs. W. as a "fine, modest, and excellent young woman" when sober, but she had attempted treatment frequently without success before she agreed to the conditioned reflex. He did not provide details regarding the mechanics of her treatment, only describing the outcome: She went home in a "state of exhilaration," proclaiming her happiness that she had finally "conquered demon liquor." After two days, however, she called the sanatorium, obviously intoxicated according to the doctor, who did not explain why her treatment failed, noting only that fewer women than men achieved abstinence.[42]

Like Turner, other physicians pointed to gender differences without exploring their implications, if any, for treatment. For example, psychiatrist James H. Wall published two separate articles on alcoholism in medical journals, one focusing on men and the other on women, using data from the Bloomingdale Hospital. Dividing his reports this way suggests that he considered gender a fundamental factor, but when it came to treatment he simply stated, "What has been said concerning the treatment of alcoholism in men applies also to the women."[43] Yet he also emphasized that proportionately more of the female alcoholics developed psychoses and that "deterioration was more frequent" in women. Wall thus highlighted a greater degree of pathology among female alcoholics yet did not propose any particular strategy for addressing it. This mismatch reinforced the idea that women were the wrong kind of alcoholics, just as they were deviant women.

The responses of Turner, Wall, and other doctors to their female alcoholic patients echoed the rhetorical and methodological choices made by E. M. Jellinek and other researchers who identified or assumed differences between male and female alcoholics but failed to analyze them in a nuanced, meaningful way. These conceptual gaps paralleled a myriad of practical constraints that limited care for alcoholic women, including institutional barriers and economic and logistical factors in women's lives. The additional stigma alcoholic women faced could also cause them to delay treatment even more than men, with the result that their drinking and its negative effects had become more pronounced by the time they saw a doctor—a phenomenon that contributed to doctors' conclusion that alcoholic women deteriorated faster than their male counterparts. Beyond these variables, the disconnect between the claim that women did not respond as well as men to treatment and a failure to envision alternative protocols for women shows the universalizing pressure of the medical model as well as inconsistency regarding the meaning of gender difference in the middle decades of the twentieth century.

The "Greatest Humiliation": Jail and State Hospitals

Although middle-class status did not guarantee access to compassionate and effective medical treatment, it generally protected alcoholics of both sexes from some of the consequences of excessive drinking, including arrest. Conversely, poor and marginalized women as well as men found themselves caught in a web of interlocking institutions where medical and legal jurisdictions overlapped. As in the case of Wilma Wilson, coercion could play out quite differently in this context. Since individuals could be arrested for a single episode of drunkenness, it is impossible to know how many women who found themselves in state facilities for drinking-related crimes were truly alcoholic. Institutionalization thus differed sharply from modes of authority such as the *Diagnostic and Statistical Manual* that aimed to delineate alcoholism as a chronic condition distinct from intoxication or alcohol poisoning. As during the Progressive Era, prison authorities and other experts judged the overall comportment and habits of women who were arrested, in contrast to medicalization proponents who tried to extract drinking problems from other traits and behaviors and to distinguish precisely between those individuals who manifested a specific condition and those who did not. Incarceration and other forms of institutionalization often represented a last resort for alcoholic women with few resources, and the experience could mark them as especially deviant. But in some circumstances at least, these facilities provided a multifaceted response that was more attuned than most forms of medical treatment to the complex circumstances of women's lives.

Alcohol-related crimes included drunk driving, public intoxication, prostitution, public lewdness, and disorderly conduct. A significant number of incarcerated women were jailed for these offenses. At the Reformatory for Women in Framingham, Massachusetts, for example, more than 40 percent of the inmates during the mid-1930s were considered to be alcoholic, and the number of alcoholics committed increased during the 1940s. According to one prison report, alcoholic inmates often had long drinking histories, up to forty years in some cases, with frequent arrests. Parole was only granted to first or second offenders, since the board of parole believed that those with long-standing drinking problems had little chance of improvement.[44]

One woman described her arrest for driving while intoxicated as "the greatest humiliation, to think that I'd finally landed in jail."[45] After having a car accident while under the influence of beer, another woman was committed to a state hospital, even though her family could afford to send her to a psychiatrist and her husband was willing to attend AA with her.[46] Another desperate woman wrote to Mann from jail where she was awaiting trial for attempted burglary. She explained her dilemma this way, "At the time of this so-called crime, I was drunk, I don't remember a thing of what happened, I had a blackout. And the reports of the Doctors are in my favor. This has happened to me before, and that is what frightens me. I know I need help very badly, and the only one that can help me is someone who really understands and knows the problem." Her plea suggests the power of Mann's alcoholic identity to surmount class lines. Although Mann did not come to the prison as the woman had hoped, the National Council on Alcoholism (NCA) office arranged for an AA member to visit her there.[47]

Working-class women were more likely than their middle-class counterparts to be arrested for "morals" offenses, which often meant public or sexual transgressions. Once women were imprisoned, psychiatrists, social workers, and other experts scrutinized their behavior closely. "Dora," for example, was arrested in New England numerous times for drunkenness, for being "idle and disorderly," for "lewd and lascivious cohabitation," and finally for "common night walking" after being found "in the company of two strange men from whom she had got some 'moonshine.'" Those who evaluated her case emphasized how her drinking influenced her sexual behavior. Dora was only "occasionally immoral," they explained. "She had no particularly strong sex urge, but when very drunk would yield to her friends."[48]

With their lives devastated by alcoholism, some women found themselves in jail or state hospitals simply because there was no alternative. "Laura," for example, served several sentences in the Framingham Reformatory during the 1940s. One report summarized her life this way: "Failure of marriage, onset of alcoholism, arrest, divorce, suicidal attempt, mental hospital observation, Reformatory commitment, and loss of child by the order of the court all occurred in quick succession."[49] In 1963, one woman wrote to Mann to describe the situation of her neighbor, Mrs. K, who was divorced and lived alone. Mrs. K. had one son who "will have nothing to do with her when she is drinking." Local women intervened when Mrs. K. disappeared for several days and did not answer her phone; entering the house, they were unable to rouse Mrs. K. and found the temperature to be thirty degrees. Given Mrs. K.'s propensity to call them without reason, the police were reluctant to become involved, but at the insistence of the neighbor women, they took action. Mrs. K.'s doctor would not admit her to the state mental hospital, and an AA member found her unreceptive to the fellowship. After that, Mrs. K. was taken to the county jail.[50] Her story illustrates how family and community resources could eventually wear thin, leaving alcoholics with no option but incarceration.

While her neighbor hoped that Mrs. K. could be transferred to the state hospital, those who spent time in such facilities found them not much better than jail; often they provided nothing but custodial care. One woman wrote to Mann, "To sum it up—my mother has a life sentence to a state institution for nothing except alcoholism." While the writer lived on the West Coast, her mother had spent the previous decade in a state hospital the Northeast. The daughter explained, "Even the hospital authorities do not consider her as mentally ill; they simply have no other place for her to live. She has a long history of arrests and hospitalization due to acute alcoholism, has neither family nor friends [there]." According to her daughter, the mother could be "most obnoxious" when drinking, whereupon "the landlady or the neighbors call the police, and Mother is back in custody." While sympathetic, Mann's assistant urged caution regarding the daughter's plan to move her mother across the country and urged her to consult her mother's physician: "You have not seen your mother in many years, and the tragic progression of the disease after such a prolonged period of time may have left her greatly changed." Deferring to medical authority, the NCA also provided the address of a family service agency near the daughter.[51]

By the late 1940s, a growing network of referral services, including the National Council on Alcoholism, community clinics, and Alcoholics Anonymous, had made a significant difference for women in jails and state hospitals, those who often had the worst stigma with the fewest resources. For example, one woman found arrest to be the "wake-up call" that she needed after she had been drunk for "sixty days around the clock." Family members asked a doctor what to do, and he suggested AA; she was sent to a sanitarium to be "defogged" and decided to go to AA upon her release.[52] Some judges took such initiative into account when allocating punishment; one woman, for example, received probation as long as she attended AA meetings.[53] An alcoholic woman who had been sentenced a reformatory for being "idle and disorderly" later became secretary of the local AA group and even went to the Yale Clinic for training to assist other alcoholics.[54]

Many of these facilities accepted women only or were organized as single-sex wards with female staff. This arrangement did not guarantee a positive outcome, but it brought more attention to women's particular needs, compared to hospitals or other treatment settings in which the vast majority of alcoholics were men. One advantage was that female social workers, prison matrons, and reformers showed much more awareness of the sexual danger that alcoholic women faced than did male psychiatrists, who often implicitly or even explicitly blamed alcoholic women for any sexual activity, including rape. In 1947, for example, the League of Women Voters in Massachusetts criticized the treatment of women who were imprisoned for moral crimes, arguing that some female "criminals" were actually alcoholics who "became victims of unscrupulous men" during drinking episodes.[55] While many psychiatrists in private practice paid little attention to lesbianism among alcoholic women, mental health workers who treated alcoholic women in prison devoted considerable attention to the subject, reflecting the political pressure they faced to prevent sexual "irregularity" among inmates. At one Massachusetts institution, case reports included one woman whose alcoholism was "complicated by a homosexual involvement" and a recommendation that another alcoholic be watched so that any "evidences of abnormal sexual tendencies with other inmates" could be recorded promptly.[56]

During the late 1940s, the Reformatory for Women in Framingham, Massachusetts, implemented a pilot program for alcoholic inmates, including physical care as necessary, psychological counseling, academic and vocational classes, organized recreation, and work placement when the alcoholic was released.[57] This endeavor reflected the goals of alcoholism advocates like Mann: a nonjudgmental definition of alcoholism as a disease, efforts to alleviate the stigma associated with alcoholism, and practical aid to help alcoholics achieve and maintain sobriety. The social workers involved in this multifaceted project adopted the psychiatric terminology associated with the Yale Clinic, but they also devoted significant attention to the environment alcoholic women faced both before and after their incarceration. Ironically, even as imprisonment could be the "greatest humiliation" that an alcoholic woman might face, programs like this may have come closest to realizing the goals of the modern alcoholism movement.

Shifting Roles as Strategy: Social Workers and Alcoholism Treatment

To diagnose alcoholism without a clear-cut laboratory test, professionals, family members, and even individuals concerned about their own consumption evaluated whether the person in question could carry out his or her sanctioned role. For men, employment served as a key indicator; for women, domestic responsibilities represented an important benchmark.

Marty Mann noted in her *Primer* that, "if the alcoholic is the wife, it means that dinner is not ready, with feeble excuses as to why it isn't."[58] As we have seen, the strong belief that drinking is antithetical to the maternal role has proven remarkably persistent and flexible in American society, articulated in terms of biological damage to offspring, physical danger of children due to neglect, and psychological risks. In AA narratives and sociological questionnaires, alcoholic women, too, invoked this language to show the depths of their illness and also the scope of their recovery.

But only rarely did alcoholic women at midcentury identify housework and the limitations of the domestic role, including the intense responsibility of caring for children, as a cause of their drinking. One alcoholic woman explained her drinking this way, recalling that the "kids' washing and ironing got me down." When a doctor told her that she needed rest, she entered a state psychiatric hospital, hoping to recover her strength and "break myself of depending so on liquor." Yet she did not find the respite for which she had hoped: She was assigned to manual labor in the laundry facility of the hospital.[59] Some alcoholism researchers, treatment professionals, and advocates feared that the life of a housewife, which they perceived as lacking structure and perhaps even purpose, could facilitate a slide into alcoholism.[60] Even though few alcoholic women articulated their situation in these terms, debates about women's drinking resonated with a growing unease in the United States that domesticity could breed discontent.[61]

In this context, the Washingtonian Hospital in Boston, a facility that specialized in the treatment of alcoholics and drug addicts of both sexes, developed a novel program that addressed directly whether strains associated with being a housewife and mother might contribute to alcoholism and what to do about it. Founded in the mid-nineteenth century to treat male inebriates, the Washingtonian Hospital grew out of the Washingtonian mutual-help movement. By the mid-1950s, the facility reflected the professionalization of the field, offering a wide range of treatment modalities for both inpatients and outpatients: conditioned reflex, injections of adrenal cortex extract, psychotherapy, assistance from social workers, and a plan that allowed patients to live in the hospital while they worked at outside jobs. In 1954, Dorothy Jean Deex completed a master's thesis at the Boston University School of Social Work in which she examined seventy-five women who were alcoholic inpatients at the hospital from April 1951 to June 1953. Criticizing the lack of systematic, scholarly research on alcoholic women, she explained the rationale for her work this way: "There seems to be a popular notion that women who drink must do so because they have ample free time; hence the housewife can more readily become addicted to alcohol. Implied also in this notion is the further idea that housework is drudgery and therefore women who become bored with the daily routine of the housewife might more readily drink excessively."[62]

Deex's study reveals challenges in defining alcoholism, as well as dynamics inherent in the hierarchically organized helping professions. Although she used a definition from the World Health Organization—demonstrating attempts to standardize the diagnosis by mid-century—she admitted that it was impossible to determine retrospectively whether all the women in the study actually met the criteria for alcoholism. She further explained that the goal of treatment was generally understood to be abstinence from alcohol, although that measure meant "the condition is arrested and not cured."[63] Moving beyond abstinence as the only criterion for assessing outcomes, Deex defined "improvement" as "complete or nearly complete abstinence (i.e., less frequent relapses)." She also incorporated other measures such as productive work, more social engagement, and reduced tension.[64] Some of these indicators would be difficult to quantify, and the variety indicates an understanding of alcoholism as a multifaceted condition, demonstrating yet again why it could be difficult to fit problem drinking into a particularistic disease framework. In her analysis, Deex focused on casework, or intervention and support from social workers, whose role she contrasted with that of psychiatrists. Only the doctor "recommends" medical and psychological treatment, while the social worker "offers the patient reassurance and clarification concerning her attitudes toward treatment." As well, the social worker "assists the patient to adjust the social factors necessary to enable her to continue treatment."[65]

Deex divided her patient sample into two groups: "housewives," which included all women who performed housework even if they worked outside the home, and "all others," who were not housewives. Almost two-thirds of the subjects fit into the first group; as Deex emphasized, "for the largest number of patients the role of housewife is a day to day reality." She was especially interested in the types of treatment that the two groups of women accepted and the question of whether housewives pointed to either domestic responsibilities or their housewife status as primary factors contributing to their drinking. In fact, only about one-third expressed "negative concern" about being housewives, about the same proportion as those in the other group who identified their occupational status as a problem. Housewives also listed other factors that precipitated their drinking, such as conflict within their marriages, excessive drinking by the husband, a death in the family, and "individual insecurity in social relations." And while housewife status could interfere with treatment by making it harder for women to be hospitalized for long periods, it also facilitated care because of a greater investment by relatives. Deex even suggested that housewives might have a better prognosis overall.[66]

Although the majority of these women did not blame their drinking on domestic responsibilities, those who participated in a role-shift protocol—an intervention that encouraged female patients to engage more fully with the outside world through paid work, hobbies, and structured social activities—found that their condition improved, according to Deex.[67] For them, moving away from traditional roles facilitated recovery from alcoholism.

Some patients who participated in the role shift had expectations for domestic life that did not match the reality they found. Mrs. D., for example, reported that she had "wanted to stay home and make a home for herself and her husband" and so quit her job just two months after their marriage. But she found herself bored and isolated, which she believed contributed to her drinking problems, although economic uncertainty and her husband's heavy drinking were also factors.[68] Mrs. F., in contrast, initially found the housewife role "satisfactory" but became overwhelmed with responsibilities when her husband deserted her shortly before their second child was born. Interestingly, Deex characterized Mrs. F. as now facing a "dual role"—that of housewife and mother—which "became increasingly difficult to perform the longer she had to perform it by herself." Mrs. F's case report included contradictory details about her children: Although Mrs. F. provided "good supervision, attention, and physical care," they were later placed in foster care. And while she said she wanted to be reunited with them, social workers concluded that "she actually preferred to be relieved of the responsibilities of their care." Her treatment therefore included "environmental manipulation," helping her to find a job as a waitress. These new circumstances—work she found satisfying and relief from maternal obligations—facilitated her rehabilitation and abstinence.[69]

Mrs. L. also experienced a positive outcome from a role shift. Mrs. L. was forty-one years old, married with two young children, and had struggled with "excessive periodic drinking" for seven years when she was admitted to the Washingtonian Hospital. While her husband participated in hobbies and social outings with friends, Mrs. L. remained at home, spending much of her time on housework, caring for extended family members, and even taking in boarders. The strains associated with these efforts, especially a "compulsion to perform perfectly within the housewife role" contributed to Mrs. L.'s alcoholism, Deex reported. While Mrs. L. tried many treatment approaches, including Antabuse, injections of adrenal cortex extract, and group therapy, as well as Alcoholics Anonymous meetings, the role shift brought the greatest improvement. As Deex explained, "Following therapeutic suggestions Mrs. L. herself manipulated her environment to secure outside interests and a job."[70] Deex's analysis equates finding a job and developing hobbies with medical interventions as therapeutic agents. While Antabuse and injections could be seen as gender-neutral, scientific tools aimed at a disease, the "environmental manipulation" approach raised questions about the circumstances of women's lives.

Although Deex used "housewife" as the defining occupational category in her study, she concluded that the responsibilities of motherhood specifically proved too much for these alcoholic women to handle, defaulting to psychiatric language that defined them as "immature" and "dependent." She explained, "It would seem that these women could hold jobs adequately but they could not be adequate parents."[71] It is difficult to tell from the study whether coercion was involved when children were removed as part of the role shift. For example, Mrs. A.'s children were placed in foster homes after she had a significant relapse, a situation that Mrs. A. was eventually "able to accept." What is clear is that the social workers believed themselves to be supportive of women who could not cope with the pressures of motherhood and sought other arrangements, even when such preferences violated a renewed cult of motherhood. In the case of Mrs. H., for example, "treatment discussions reassured her by supporting her desires to be relieved of the care of her children."[72]

Assessing the overall role-shift protocol, Deex concluded that these alcoholic women "needed considerable support in seeking outside interests and in manipulating their environment instead of participating in alcoholic bouts."[73] While Deex may have meant to convey that the women required assistance owing to psychological vulnerabilities, it may well have been that the invitation to manage their lives differently was equally important—if not more so. As this program shows, social workers generally looked beyond intrapsychic factors to address social context, and Deex emphasized that American women faced an uncertain transitional period in cultural expectations. As she explained, "If some women take the work drive seriously, an almost completely new and different way of life, for which they have no pattern and few precedents to follow, has to be developed. Under these circumstances dissatisfactions could not be unusual or unexpected."[74]

Just as the diagnosis of alcoholism provided an increasingly authoritative way to name a drinking pattern that had gotten out of control, the role-shift protocol—originating as it did in a hospital—offered a medically sanctioned means of acknowledging domestic discontent. The experimental quality of this program and its small size are not surprising. Its gender-specific focus harkened back to older models even as it presented an alternative to mid-twentieth-century domestic expectations. It also contradicted other approaches in the alcoholism field—even that of other social workers who urged the wives of alcoholic men to fulfill a feminine, supportive role as part of their husbands' struggle for sobriety.[75] For their part, psychiatrists urged their patients to align their interior psychological state with social expectations rather than inviting them to change their external circumstances, as the Washingtonian social workers did. Likewise, nothing inherent in the approach of modern alcoholism movement advocates would lead to questioning traditional standards for how men and women should behave. Alcoholics Anonymous as an organization and individual alcoholics such as Marty Mann had every reason to emphasize that alcoholics could be typical in all realms except their drinking and therefore capable of restoration to full respectability when they achieved sobriety. These social workers, in contrast, offered a different perspective on the causes of alcoholism and simultaneously helped their patients imagine an alternative way to live as women.

As the experiences of many alcoholic women demonstrate, the modern alcoholism movement failed to deliver on an important promise of medicalization, that all who suffered from the condition would be treated equally and offered access to care without judgment. All alcoholics confronted considerable hurdles, but beliefs about gender roles exacerbated the challenges that alcoholic women faced. If, as Mann argued, the disease was the same regardless of the characteristics of the sufferer, then treatment should be the same as well and lead to similar results. For Mann, individual variation among alcoholics meant that a range of modalities should be available; women, like men, might respond differently to any one treatment, in her view. But many professionals continued to harbor the belief that female alcoholics as a group represented an aberration; they were innately more clinically ill and morally questionable than their male counterparts. This pejorative attitude not only prevented some women from even seeking treatment, it also compromised the care that women received.

Ironically, it was not the modern and ostensibly objective treatment methods following from a narrowly defined disease model that helped women the most. Rather, the efforts of social workers to address women's domestic situations, and outreach programs in jails and state hospitals, seemed most responsive to alcoholic women's needs—perhaps because these programs were more attuned to women's life circumstances, not attempting to fit them into a gender-neutral category that contradicted the social reality experienced by both doctor and patient.

Epilogue

"How Could a Mother Drive Drunk?" asked a headline in the *New York Times* on August 5, 2009,[1] referring to the tragic car crash in which thirty-six-year-old Diane Schuler drove the wrong way on the Taconic Parkway for almost two miles before colliding with another vehicle. The crash killed Schuler, four of the five children in her minivan, and the three passengers in the car she hit. This horrific event initially seemed a mystery: How could an attractive, white suburban mother behave so erratically with a van full of children? Although some observers may have wondered about alcohol or drugs, the police did not initially suspect intoxication, and the media coverage focused simply on the funerals that occurred amid an outpouring of grief and compassion for the families involved.[2] But when Schuler's toxicology results became public a few days later, coverage of the event shifted sharply. Schuler, who had had a blood-alcohol level of 0.19 percent, "and even more still in her stomach, so fresh that it had yet to be metabolized," was now vilified. Her blood was also reported as having "high" levels of the psychoactive ingredient in marijuana. Equally damning, the press focused on a vodka bottle found in the van (the *Times* even noted the size and brand: 1.75 liter, Absolut). The director of the toxicology lab described Schuler's blood-alcohol level as "the equivalent of 10 shots of 80-proof liquor." Reporters concluded that the mystery had been solved: "The real reason" for the crash "was stark in its tragedy and simplicity: She was drunk."[3]

But these toxicology findings, so definitive on the surface, only raised further questions and debate. According to family members and friends, and even the owner of the campground where the family frequently stayed and who saw the van depart that day, such intoxication was completely out of character.

Investigators sought to retrace Schuler's journey using cell phone and toll booth records, but they were unable to determine when and how, let alone why, she consumed so much alcohol and marijuana. Her husband denied that she would have used these substances, insisting instead that she must have had a stroke or similar episode that made her lose control. For their part, the family whose relatives had been in the vehicle that Schuler hit said the news made them "victims all over again."[4] Despite multiple lawsuits among the families, an HBO documentary, and even a book by Shuler's sister-in-law, whose three daughters were killed in the crash, Schuler's actions remain as incomprehensible as ever.

Observers and reporters have repeatedly focused on the fact that Schuler was a mother. The woman who lost her father and brother in the second vehicle denounced Schuler for making "that choice," yet simultaneously depicted her as a chronic alcoholic. "How do you put five children in a car when you're a mother who's a drunk?" she asked. "We're mothers. I would never do something like that. It's crazy."[5] For *New York Times* columnist Lisa Belkin, the toxicology findings likewise transformed Schuler from an object of sympathy, even identification, into an alien being whose intoxication overrode maternal feeling that should have been primal. "Like so many of you," Belkin wrote, "I had been haunted by the story from the start, horrified by the thought of a poor woman, the victim of a stroke, or diabetic shock, or something debilitating and out of her control, speeding frantically toward death. Now I am even more horrified that the cause was her own doing, driving a weapon down the highway, slaying innocent people." Belkin reminded her readers that the three men in the second car were also innocent victims, but noted that the deaths of children are especially poignant: "There is an extra jolt of pain in the fact that a biologically based hard-wired warning failed to flash through the alcoholic haze in this mother's head as she took the wheel with five children buckled in the back of her minivan."[6]

This episode would have been searingly tragic, no matter who had been driving and under what circumstances. But the public reaction demonstrates that American ambivalence, even censure, toward women who drink remains close to the surface. We still lack a precise vocabulary that can accommodate blame, volition, victimization, and the mind-altering effects of alcohol—perhaps especially for mothers.

Publicity and Shame in the 1970s and 1980s:
From the Women's Alcoholism Movement to Betty Ford

Diane Schuler had not yet been born when Marty Mann appeared in *Reader's Digest* in 1963,[7] and considerable attention had been directed at women's drinking and alcoholism during the intervening decades. Beginning in the early 1970s, physicians, therapists, and scholars increasingly turned their attention to alcoholism among women, calling for more research and treatment opportunities. Literature reviews demonstrated the dearth of studies on alcoholic women to that point.[8] Once they began to look, some researchers declared they had found an "epidemic" of alcoholism among women. Indeed, this flurry of attention is sometimes called the "women's alcoholism movement,"[9] as if it constituted the counterpoint to the efforts of Alcoholics Anonymous, research scientists, public health advocates, and physicians of the 1930s and 1940s to redefine alcohol-related problems in the aftermath of Prohibition. During the 1970s, Mann's organization, the National Council on Alcoholism, for the first time created an Office on Women; a female alcoholic created Women for Sobriety as an alternative to Alcoholics Anonymous (AA); and a staff aide, Nancy Olson, helped organize special congressional hearings on "The Female Alcoholic's Special Problems and Unmet Needs."[10] Many of the women involved in these efforts knew each other through personal or professional networks, and their interconnections sparked much of this activity.

In an important continuity, these advocates and treatment professionals focused on alcohol, not other drugs. This specialization reflected an institutional reality since the federal government created the National Institute on Alcohol Abuse and Alcoholism (NIAAA) in 1970, a division distinct from the existing National Institute on Drug Abuse.[11] But it also reinforced divisions among women by substance, which increasingly paralleled categories of class, race, and age. In this way, addiction treatment and advocacy created a hierarchy of stigma, with alcoholics—who were more likely to be older white women—continuing to differentiate themselves from addicts who used illicit drugs and who were more likely to be women of color. These developments also recapitulated and exacerbated divisions in second-wave feminism.[12]

Advocates in the "women's alcoholism movement" defined women as a "special population" of alcoholics. This categorization reflected institutional and strategic imperatives, since federal grants used this nomenclature for funding formulae. But it contradicted the universal disease model advocated by Marty Mann and the "alcoholic equalitarianism" that had once characterized the Alcoholics Anonymous fellowship. By this time, women-only groups had become much more common in AA. Even so, some alcoholic women rejected AA completely, claiming that its philosophy of "surrender" harmed alcoholic women who already suffered from low self-esteem. As an alternative, Jean Kirkpatrick founded Women for Sobriety, an entire organization devoted to alcoholic women.[13]

These efforts hearkened all the way back to the nineteenth-century emphasis on fundamental sex differences and rejected—whether explicitly or implicitly—the ostensibly gender-neutral disease model of the mid-twentieth-century alcoholism movement. The very public addiction and recovery story of First Lady Betty Ford—probably the most famous alcoholic woman in the twentieth century—illuminated this continuing tension.

Often described as a breath of fresh air, Betty Ford brought a welcome informality and directness to the White House when her husband assumed the presidency upon the resignation of Richard Nixon in 1974. She spoke frankly about political issues, including the Equal Rights Amendment, as well as the challenges of parenting during the turbulent 1960s and 1970s. When Ford was diagnosed with breast cancer, her disclosure of her illness and the details of her treatment won admiration and affection. Her political outspokenness complicated some aspects of her husband's unsuccessful campaign in 1976, alienating some voters as it endeared her to others.[14] Ford thus already had a well-established reputation for candor when she found herself in the news again when she sought treatment for addiction to painkillers and alcohol in 1978.

Ford's drug use and her mental state had attracted attention as part of the intensified press coverage that accompanied her husband's ascendance to the presidency. The *Washington Post* explained that a pinched nerve had led her to take "tranquilizers to relieve the pain which was aggravated by stress," and Ford "sometimes drank to relax." Seeking professional help, Ford "finally went to a psychiatrist to help her over the bad times."[15] The implication in 1974 was that she had resolved any psychological problems and overuse of medication, and this storyline was soon overshadowed by her breast cancer. After the 1976 election, the Fords moved to California. The former president continued to travel extensively for political fundraisers and speeches, and Betty Ford went with him to the Soviet Union in 1977, where she—a former dancer—narrated a performance of "The Nutcracker Suite" ballet for NBC television. Her presentation, particularly her slow and slurred speech, attracted criticism.[16] By the spring of 1978, her family concluded that she had worsened considerably and staged an intervention, in which they urged her to enter treatment for substance abuse.

Today, it can be hard to appreciate the magnitude of Ford's health-related disclosures. With pink ribbons a common accessory, we risk overlooking how courageous she was in revealing her breast cancer. Similarly, now that "intervention" is both a reality television show[17] and an overused joke in popular culture, it can be difficult to appreciate the significance of the family of a former president of the United States publicly divulging that they had staged an intervention—and not for a youthful user but for a wife and mother, a former first lady. In April 1978, with the support of her family, Ford checked herself into the alcohol and drug rehabilitation center of the U.S. Naval Hospital in Long Beach, California, where she remained for several weeks. Again, the media praised her courage and honesty and expressed the hope that her frankness would inspire others to seek help.[18] Like Mann and other women who came before her, Ford and her family imbued her disclosure with a wider social meaning.[19]

Significantly, however, Ford and her family did not reveal her addiction to pills and alcohol simultaneously. Rather, the initial announcement stated that she was seeking treatment for dependence on prescription medications. "Former First Lady Betty Ford has shown commendable courage in facing up to a problem of drug dependency, seeking medical help to overcome it—and acknowledging the difficulty publicly," announced the *Chicago Tribune* in April 1978.[20] Her announcement was used to educate readers about a perceived "epidemic" of prescription drug use by women. Meanwhile, in the hospital, Ford also confronted her drinking problem. The treatment protocol she experienced in 1978 included both medical care and mutual-help meetings with other addicts, although Ford did not name the particular fellowship program. Both her doctors and other female alcoholics who worked with her came to believe that Ford needed to admit a dependence on alcohol as well, and they staged a second intervention. At the time, Ford resisted: "I wouldn't say I was a drunk. . . . I could *not* say I was alcoholic,"[21] but she then issued another statement: "Through the excellent treatment I have had here at the Long Beach Naval Hospital, I have found I am not only addicted to the medication I have been taking for my arthritis but also to alcohol, so I am grateful for this program of recovery."[22] Even then, for some time she and her family tended to refer to her drinking as though it was only a problem because of interaction with her pills.[23]

Ford did achieve sobriety, and then she, like Mann, turned her attention outward. As a former first lady, Ford had a built-in audience for whatever message about alcoholism and addiction she might put forward, but this brought risks as well. While she collaborated enthusiastically in creating a new treatment center in Southern California, she feared the responsibility of having it bear her name.[24] One result of her identification with the treatment center was that her advocacy stayed closely tied to the medical model.[25] Ford, like Mann, relied on the cultural prestige of biomedicine to alleviate the shame associated with addiction. Yet if a medical definition neutralized derogatory stereotypes that had deemed alcoholic women in particular to be unworthy, it also disallowed any analysis of social or political reasons for women's drinking. The diagnosis itself served as a closed, circular explanatory framework: Identifying oneself as "alcoholic" could be sufficient to explain why one drank to excess. By the late 1980s, Ford found that this definition existed in tension with a gendered, even feminist, analysis of women's drug and alcohol use.[26]

The combination of substances Ford had used and the different interpretive possibilities inherent in her use of them meant that she combined the earlier inebriate model with post–World War II anxieties that domestic pressures could breed discontent. Ford's social position as the wife of a high-ranking politician and the relative respectability of a reliance on prescription medications may well have allowed her rhetorical freedom to point to possible connections between domestic constraints and women's addictions. In 1973, for example, she explained that she had visited a psychiatrist, who acknowledged the strain she was under due to her husband's demanding career and frequent travel. As she explained, the psychiatrist encouraged her to move beyond a strictly domestic role: "The idea was to make me realize I must think of myself and not be so concerned with my family."[27] This recommendation echoes the "role shift" at the Washingtonian Hospital described in the previous chapter.

Ford criticized doctors for relying too frequently on medications for women instead of taking the time to listen to their concerns.[28] In this way, she exemplified the "Valium Panic," a campaign against the overprescription of tranquilizers and sedatives to middle-class women without acknowledging the dangers of dependence and withdrawal. Women like Ford represented descendants of female inebriates like Mrs. C., the Iowa farm wife described in chapter 1. Instead of physical "female complaints," however, late twentieth-century housewives suffered from psychological and social malaise. Like other debates connecting women's substance use with their domestic lives, concern about Valium could lead to a harsh judgment of women or to a social critique. Was the problem maladjusted housewives, or domestic life itself? Despite the feminist ferment and other social movements of the 1970s, Valium critics did not link their analysis to debates about other drugs and social inequalities—both reflecting and reinforcing a stark social, cultural, and medical divide between pharmaceuticals and illicit drugs.[29]

The Valium Panic also shows how alcohol as a substance and alcoholism as an addiction occupied categories of their own during the later twentieth century. Had Betty Ford developed a dependence on heroin or cocaine, she would have lost considerable public sympathy. Although alcohol was less threatening than illicit street drugs, it could not be as easily assimilated to the Valium narrative as it had been aligned with patent medicines or even opiates in the nineteenth century. In her ground-breaking book *The Invisible Alcoholics*, journalist Marian Sandmaier asserted in 1980 that the problems faced by alcoholic women were the same challenges that all women faced.[30] Yet this assertion of sisterly solidarity did not gain the same cultural currency as the Valium story, perhaps because no clear outside villain—like overzealous physicians—could be identified. After all, no doctor had forced Ford to drink, and neither scientists nor the general public considered alcohol inherently addictive, as Valium came to be seen at this time. It was hard to escape the view that women who became alcoholic had only themselves to blame.

Motherhood and Alcohol in the 1980s and 1990s: Fetal Alcohol Syndrome and Mothers Against Drunk Drivers

Two other major developments in this era showed that neither Ford's celebrity nor her advocacy was enough to transform medical and social attitudes toward drinking women. The nearly simultaneous appearance of Fetal Alcohol Syndrome (FAS), first named in 1973, and Mothers Against Drunk Drivers, founded in 1980, shows that the veneer of a disease model could easily erode when the fate of children was the counterweight. Through the middle decades of the twentieth century, scientific experts insisted that alcohol was a relatively benign substance and did not cause reproductive harm. Yet doctors, social scientists, and the lay public consistently feared the transmission of alcohol-related problems through the generations, recognizing that alcoholic families suffered emotional and psychological consequences even if not biological damage.[31] In this context, new findings in the early 1970s about alcohol-related birth defects helped tip the balance back toward the idea that alcohol could be a toxin.[32] Not surprisingly, this conclusion greatly intensified social disapproval of women's drinking.

Over the next few years, evidence mounted that chronic, severe binge drinking caused Fetal Alcohol Syndrome. Yet public health messages and advice to women insisted that no level of alcohol consumption could be shown to be safe to the developing fetus, so women should abstain completely. In fact, experts warned that women should avoid alcohol if they were even considering pregnancy. During this same era, experts also sounded the alarm over so-called "crack babies" and newborns who underwent withdrawal from heroin presumably owing to their mother's use of the drug. Women of color who were drug addicts suffered particularly harsh penalties, often losing custody of their children and facing incarceration themselves.[33] In all of these "moral panics," both scientists and pundits accused women of violating their maternal role for their own selfish pleasure. Like their predecessors, twentieth-century experts asserted that maternal love and duty should be enough for even addicted women to overcome their dependence.

It is worth remembering that by the late twentieth century, alcohol, unlike cocaine or heroin, was legal and had been normalized as a consumer good, and the modern alcoholism paradigm was forty years old. Yet the FAS phenomenon undercut any division between recreational and problem drinking, as illustrated in a Minneapolis newspaper article of 1999: "Here in the land of 10,000 Treatment Centers, it's almost as easy to find an AA meeting as a bar. Yet too many pregnant women, it turns out, are skipping the meeting and opting for the bar. Some drink a lot, some only a little. Some drink because of addiction, others out of ignorance. Very few have stopped to think that a night on the town might mean permanent brain damage to a child. If they could be made to think, they might be coaxed not to drink."[34] Such admonitions evoked nineteenth- and early twentieth-century fears that alcohol threatened the health of the (white, native-born) American "race." The failure to differentiate among women's reasons for drinking—lumping together addiction, ignorance, and a "night on the town"—implied that women's lack of knowledge must be alleviated and, if necessary, their behavior controlled by physicians, public health experts, the media, or even the general public who, one reporter suggested, could simply "use the time-tested technique of looking askance whenever we pass a pregnant woman sipping Chardonnay."[35] Even as clinicians and feminist activists insisted that pregnant women who were alcoholic needed treatment, not punishment, the popular media continued to exclude women from the disease model: "Mothers' Vices during Pregnancy: Drinking on Rise despite Risks to Fetus" declared a headline in one Cleveland newspaper in 1998.[36] In short, female alcoholics were not at the vanguard of converting excessive drinking into a disease, as inebriate specialists had hoped a century before. Instead, debates about women's drinking contributed to *de*-medicalization, providing an entry point for disbelief and resistance as Americans questioned whether alcoholism was a disease at all.[37]

Mothers Against Drunk Drivers (today renamed Mothers Against Drunk Driving), or MADD, was organized in 1980, just as Americans were becoming familiar with the recently named Fetal Alcohol Syndrome. Founded by Candy Lightner, a woman whose daughter had been killed by an intoxicated driver, MADD evolved from a "handful of grieving mothers" to more than two million members and supporters.[38] The organization lobbied successfully for changes in the legal drinking age and in legal standards for blood alcohol content. Today, the organization provides a range of victim services, youth programs, and public awareness programs. The MADD campaign echoed nineteenth-century temperance rhetoric that granted women moral authority because they, along with their children, were innocent victims of men's drinking. That this argument remained so effective and familiar for more than a century helps us understand why many Americans could condemn "FAS mothers" so easily. The centrality of maternity to the feminine gender role also allows continued scrutiny of the drinking habits of all women of child-bearing age, whether pregnant or not and whether alcoholic or not. The activism of MADD and FAS warning labels mutually reinforce the imperative that good mothers do not drink—rather, they fight against drinking.

Alcohol and Vulnerability: Binge Drinking, Date Rape, and "Closing the Gap" Today

While maternity defined FAS and MADD, Americans also continued to link sexual behavior with women's drinking patterns, especially those of young women. During the 1990s and 2000s, social scientists, activists, journalists, and college administrators devoted considerable attention to "binge" drinking among young adults, especially college students, and to the apparent connection between heavy drinking by women and "acquaintance rape." The typical account, in which a young woman is intoxicated and then is manipulated or coerced into sexual intercourse by her male companion, evoked late nineteenth-century fears about the vulnerability of naïve young women alone in the city. These accounts were often characterized by the same mixture of pity and blame found in nineteenth- and early twentieth-century accounts of drinking women.

In one case, for instance, a sorority woman accused three members of a University of California, Los Angeles, fraternity of sexual assault after a party in Palm Springs in 1996. Prosecutors declined to press charges, partly because the young woman refused to testify. Yet the *Los Angeles Times* explained that the "case was further complicated by the woman's use of alcohol and marijuana, and her participation in a sexually explicit party game before the alleged incident."[39] Such attitudes can be widespread: One poll of five hundred Americans during the 1990s found that more than one-third of respondents (and more than one half of those over the age of fifty) believed that a woman who was raped was "partly to blame" if she had been under the influence of alcohol or drugs.[40] A constellation of cases at the University of Montana—and the reactions of university administrators, area law enforcement, and the wider community in the 2010s—sounded remarkably similar.[41] With the female victim stripped of her innocence, the male "seducer" comes to be relieved of responsibility. Further, just as a pregnant woman today may be criticized for ordering wine in a restaurant, so one episode of intoxication can be enough to prove the unworthiness of sexual victims; whether or not they are alcoholics is beside the point. Having claimed male prerogatives, these young women have only themselves to blame if things go wrong.

Both maternal and sexual issues seem more urgent because of a recurrent fear that both drinking and alcoholism among women are increasing, "closing the gap" with men's rates of consumption and addiction. A presumption that gender makes a difference, even if we are not sure how or why, underlies this discussion. For example, national media coverage of a 1996 study by the Center on Addiction and Substance Abuse at Columbia University reported with alarm that consumption rates among women were converging with those of men. Largely ignoring the magnitude of male substance abuse, these commentators reserved their consternation for the fact that women seemed to be "catching up." As the *New York Times* proclaimed, "Gender Gap in Drug Abuse Said to Close."[42] As in previous decades, journalists insisted that women's use should be viewed as a harbinger of widespread social crisis. Sounding remarkably like their early twentieth-century predecessors, reporters in the *Wall Street Journal* insisted that the "surge" in women's substance abuse had affected "a whole host of other social problems such as illegitimacy, welfare dependency, health care, and crime."[43]

Recent research even seems to validate fears that women are more susceptible than men to the psychoactive qualities of alcohol and that women deteriorate faster through the disease trajectory, offering new evidence for these long-standing beliefs about women drinkers. During the early 1990s, scientists asserted that the relatively lower amount of a particular stomach enzyme in women explained sex differences in how the human body metabolizes alcohol. First reported in the *New England Journal of Medicine* in 1990, this finding was discussed widely in the popular media, from the *New York Times* to *Glamour* magazine. As the *Times* explained, "Women become drunk more quickly than men because their stomachs are less able to neutralize alcohol, scientists have found." In alcoholic men, the enzyme becomes less efficient, but in alcoholic women, "the stomach apparently stops digesting alcohol at all," according to the researchers.[44] *Glamour* warned readers that "the damaging effects of alcohol on the liver and other organs begin sooner and progress more rapidly in women than in men—placing women who drink heavily at far greater risk than men."[45] Although the stated goal of this article was to empower young women to make educated choices about drinking, its content and tone evoke the persistent theme that while alcoholism might be less common among women than among men, it is a more severe condition.

Scientific reports of sex differences in addiction have only increased during the 2000s. The now-familiar charge that women progress more quickly than men through the stages of addiction has recurred, with the qualification that this finding refers to a subset of women who are "vulnerable to addiction."[46] Animal research replicates this dynamic; female rats acquire drug taking more quickly than males and progress to addictive-like behavior more rapidly.[47] Since addiction is defined by the National Institute on Drug Abuse today as a "chronic relapsing brain disease,"[48] these reports about the biological bases of sex differences carry considerable scientific and cultural authority.[49] The salience of sex differences is reinforced by public health guidelines that also vary by gender: The National Institute for Alcohol Abuse and Alcoholism measures "moderate" drinking and "binge" drinking differently for women and men.[50]

Making sense of these findings is challenging; identifying difference is not an inherently feminist act, and assertions of biological sex differences have been used many times to deny social and political equality. As the drug scholar Nancy Campbell points out, the "differences that matter" in addiction may not be biological at all but, rather, unequal power relations and responsibilities in social terms.[51] So there is reason to be cautious. Still, today's scientific methods and the motivations of most researchers are quite different than those of a century ago; ideally current findings will be interrogated more thoroughly and applied in a more nuanced way, with greater awareness of their political and cultural implications.

The history presented in this book shows that alcoholic women have suffered from comparisons with alcoholic men on the one hand and nonalcoholic women on the other. As scientists, clinicians, advocates, and the general public increasingly emphasize differences between male and female alcoholics, some voices have returned to a focus on what women have in common whether they are alcoholic or not. In 2013, the journalist Gabrielle Glaser published *Her Best-Kept Secret: Why Women Drink—and How They Can Regain Control*. Glaser begins the book by announcing that she is not an alcoholic; it is an effective rhetorical device, riffing on the now-familiar AA opening in which one declares that he or she is an alcoholic. But Glaser also points out that most writing by women about alcohol is based on personal experience, taking the form of what she calls "addiction chronicles."[52] By contrast, Glaser's book is primarily a work of reporting. Still, she muses at some length about her own wine-drinking habits, evoking the evangelical self-scrutiny of the antebellum United States as well as the numerous quizzes and exercises produced in the twentieth century by public health advocates, along the lines of "How Do You Know If You have a Drinking Problem?"

Like Marian Sandmaier's pioneering work on female alcoholics thirty years ago, Glaser analyzes the drinking habits of middle-class American women in light of their everyday pressures. Both Sandmaier and Glaser identify uneven rates of social change as stressors for women—as more women work outside the home in ever-more demanding careers, they still carry considerable domestic responsibilities. The costs involved in juggling all this take a toll even on privileged women, and according to Glaser, more and more women turn to alcohol as a result. She explains, "For many women, the unfulfilling, stressful tasks of running a household, mixed with the regret of lost opportunities and the loneliness of social isolation, add up to a 750-milliliter reason to drink."[53] In some ways, her account sounds like it could have been written in the 1960s about "the housewife with the secret sickness." But there is an important difference: Glaser claims common ground here even though she declares she is not an alcoholic. In this way, she contradicts the modern alcoholism paradigm, which posited a fundamental difference between alcoholics and everyone else. Instead, she asserts that the circumstances of all women's lives merit serious evaluation. It is too soon to tell whether feminist analyses such as Glaser's will lead to a new understanding of drinking problems in women. For now, though, her words are an important reminder that we do not need to be bound by the rigid, either-or categories of the past.

Acknowledgments

This project began under the tutelage of Estelle Freedman, and I recall her guidance and support with gratitude. Like all historians, I depend on the efforts of archivists to serve as stewards of the past. I especially appreciate the extraordinary generosity of William L. White, who has not only written a masterful history of addiction treatment but has shared his work and the marvelous collection of materials he has amassed at the Illinois Addiction Studies Archive. I also thank the staff at the Special Collections Research Center, Syracuse University Libraries; the General Service Office Archives of Alcoholics Anonymous; the John Hay Library of Brown University; the Schlesinger Library; and the A. T. Still Memorial Library and National Center for Osteopathic History. I would also like to thank the *Journal of Historical Biography*, the *Alcoholism Treatment Quarterly*, the University of Massachusetts Press, and McGill-Queen's University Press for permission to revise and print text that first appeared in their publications.

Alcohol and drug scholars constitute a genuine community featuring a rare combination of seriousness of purpose and a lively sense of humor. I have benefited from many rich discussions over the years and would especially like to thank Sarah W. Tracy, Caroline Acker, David Herzberg, Alexine Fleck, and Ingrid Walker. Lori Rotskoff served as an important interlocutor and friend. I owe a particular debt to Trysh Travis, whose invitation to serve as a contributing editor to *Points: The Blog of the Alcohol and Drugs History Society* prompted me to think and write about alcohol and gender in new ways. Nancy D. Campbell has served as a valued mentor and fellow traveler in the wilds of interdisciplinarity. I value ongoing conversations with Trysh and Nancy very much.

I finished this book while at the University of Michigan, and I am thankful for the institutional and financial support of the History Department, the Residential College, the Institute for Research on Women and Gender (IRWG), and the University of Michigan Substance Abuse Research Center (UMSARC). Through IRWG and UMSARC, I met a creative and committed group of scholars, including Carol Boyd, Amy Krentzman, Ernest Kurtz, and John Traynor. My ongoing collaboration with Jill Becker and Beth Glover Reed, first fostered through UMSARC and IRWG, has been unlike anything I ever experienced. I am so glad to have this opportunity to continue to learn in unexpected and fascinating (if occasionally frustrating) ways and grateful beyond measure for their personal and professional support.

I have been fortunate to find a stellar group of historians of medicine and of women and gender at the University of Michigan. I would especially like to thank the participants in my manuscript workshop, which was expertly orchestrated by Geoff Eley. In particular, the careful reading and encouragement offered by Joel Howell, Alexandra Stern, Barron Lerner, and Janet Golden represented a privilege, indeed. Martin Pernick and Regina Morantz-Sanchez read the complete manuscript more than once; I will always remember how each of them showed me that I had something worthwhile to say even when I did not always believe it myself.

Others at Michigan and beyond have been enormously helpful as well. Judy Houck's insightful reading of the manuscript at a much earlier stage has continued to pay dividends. David Young's metaphors about horse racing and lawn care came at just the right time. Matt Lassiter has pushed me repeatedly to develop a stronger voice, and I appreciate his encouragement. Charlie Bright is a model of the engaged historian and teacher, and I am grateful for his wise counsel on all matters.

Rutgers University Press has demonstrated consummate professionalism, efficiency, and kindness toward an anxious author. The comments of the anonymous readers helped improve the book. Janet Golden and Rima D. Apple, series editors, have been most helpful. Peter Mickulas has been unfailingly generous and supportive all the way through this process.

I owe a special thank-you to my family and dear friends. Laura Ettinger and Alexandra Lord provide an intellectual affinity, sisterly camaraderie, and emotional support that have become foundational in my life. Carol Didget Pomfret, as she well knows, is the sister I never had. There was Doug, who made this book real in so many ways. My parents and brother have provided encouragement, love, and practical support for my entire life. Their curiosity about what I do means a great deal to me. My children, Jeremy and Sawyer, joined me when this project was already under way. Now, guys, we can begin a new chapter!

Notes

Introduction

1. Floyd Miller, "What the Alcoholic Owes to Marty Mann," *Reader's Digest* 82 (January 1963): 173–180. The discussion in the following three paragraphs is based on this article.
2. Mann's experiences in early AA are discussed more fully in chapter 3. My thinking about Mann's public health career has been informed by the work of Barron H. Lerner, *When Illness Goes Public: Celebrity Patients and How We Look at Medicine* (Baltimore: Johns Hopkins University Press, 2006).
3. Miller, "What the Alcoholic Owes to Marty Mann," 180.
4. Bruce Dorsey, *Reforming Men and Women: Gender in the Antebellum City* (Ithaca, NY: Cornell University Press, 2002); Elaine Frantz Parsons, *Manhood Lost: Fallen Drunkards and Redeeming Women in the Nineteenth-Century United States* (Baltimore: Johns Hopkins University Press, 2003); and Lori Rotskoff, *Love on the Rocks: Men, Women, and Alcohol in Post–World War II America* (Chapel Hill: University of North Carolina Press, 2002).
5. Shelley F. Greenfield, Sumita G. Manwani, and Jessica E. Nargiso, "Epidemiology of Substance Use Disorders in Women," *Obstetrics and Gynecology Clinics of North America* 30, no. 3 (September 2003): 413.
6. National Institute on Alcohol Abuse and Alcoholism, National Institutes of Health, U.S. Department of Health and Human Services, "Alcohol: A Women's Health Issue," NIH Publication no. 03 4956, revised (Washington, DC: National Institute on Alcohol Abuse and Alcoholism, 2008), and "Women and Alcohol," fact sheet, December 2015, http://pubs.niaaa.nih.gov/publications/womensfact/womensFact.pdf; Centers for Disease Control and Prevention, "Fact Sheets—Excessive Alcohol Use and Risks to Women's Health," March 7, 2016, www.cdc.gov/alcohol/fact-sheets/womens-health.htm, and "Alcohol and Public Health—Frequently Asked Questions," August 2, 2016, www.cdc.gov/alcohol/faqs.htm, specifically "What does moderate drinking mean?" and "What do you mean by heavy drinking?"
7. Gabrielle Glaser, *Her Best-Kept Secret: Why Women Drink—and How They Can Regain Control* (New York: Simon & Schuster, 2013); and Ann Downsett Johnson, *Drink: The Intimate Relationship between Women and Alcohol* (New York: HarperWave, 2013). As we will see in the epilogue, these works evoked earlier efforts by feminist journalists and social scientists to call attention to women's problem drinking.
8. Stephanie Wilder-Taylor, *Sippy Cups Are Not for Chardonnay: And Other Things I Had to Learn as a New Mom* (New York: Gallery Books, 2006); Rachael Brownell, *Mommy Doesn't Drink Here Anymore: Getting through the First Year of Sobriety* (San Francisco: Conari Press, 2009); and Brenda Wilhelmsom, *Diary of an Alcoholic Housewife* (Center City, MN: Hazelden, 2011).
9. J. B. Becker, A. N. Perry, and C. Westenbroek, "Sex Differences in the Neural Mechanisms Mediating Addiction: A New Synthesis and Hypothesis," *Biology of Sex Differences* 3 (2012): 14.

10. Ruth Bordin, *Woman and Temperance: The Quest for Power and Liberty, 1873–1900* (Philadelphia: Temple University Press, 1981).
11. Sarah Stage, *Female Complaints: Lydia Pinkham and the Business of Women's Medicine* (New York: W. W. Norton, 1979).
12. David T. Courtwright, *Forces of Habit: Drugs and the Making of the Modern World* (Cambridge, MA: Harvard University Press, 2001).
13. See, e.g., Sarah Whitney Tracy and Caroline Acker, eds., *Altering American Consciousness: The History of Alcohol and Drug Use in the United States, 1800–2000* (Amherst: University of Massachusetts Press, 2004). Recent work also focuses on pharmaceuticals: see David Herzberg, *Happy Pills in America: From Miltown to Prozac* (Baltimore: Johns Hopkins University Press, 2009); and Andrea Tone, *The Age of Anxiety: A History of America's Turbulent Affair with Tranquilizers* (New York: Basic Books, 2009). See also Ronald Roizen, "The American Discovery of Alcoholism, 1933–1939" (Ph.D. diss., University of California, Berkeley, 1991); Bruce Holley Johnson, "The Alcoholism Movement in America: A Study in Cultural Innovation" (Ph.D. diss., University of Illinois, 1973); A. E. Wilkerson, Jr., "A History of the Concept of Alcoholism as a Disease" (D.S.W. diss., University of Pennsylvania, 1966); and Genevieve M. Ames, "American Beliefs about Alcoholism: Historical Perspectives on the Medical-Moral Controversy," in *The American Experience with Alcohol: Contrasting Cultural Perspectives*, ed. Linda A. Bennett and Genevieve M. Ames (New York: Plenum Press, 1985), 23–39. W. J. Rorabaugh, *The Alcoholic Republic: An American Tradition* (New York: Oxford University Press, 1979), covers the early history of the United States.
14. John C. Burnham, *Bad Habits: Drinking, Smoking, Taking Drugs, Gambling, Sexual Misbehavior, and Swearing in American History* (New York: New York University Press, 1993).
15. Stage, *Female Complaints*; David F. Musto, *The American Disease: Origins of Narcotic Control* (New York: Oxford University Press, 1987); Mark E. Lender and James K. Martin, *Drinking in America: A History* (New York: Free Press, 1987); and H. Wayne Morgan, *Drugs in America: A Social History, 1880–1980* (Syracuse, NY: Syracuse University Press, 1981).
16. David T. Courtwright, *Dark Paradise: Opiate Addiction in America before 1940* (Cambridge, MA: Harvard University Press, 1982), and "The Female Opiate Addict in Nineteenth-Century America," *Essays in Arts and Sciences* 10, no. 2 (March 1982): 161–171; and Caroline J. Acker, *Creating the American Junkie: Addiction Research in the Classic Era of Narcotic Control* (Baltimore: Johns Hopkins University Press, 2002).
17. Acker, *Creating the American Junkie*; Nancy D. Campbell, *Using Women: Gender, Drug Policy, and Social Justice* (New York: Routledge, 2000); and Nancy D. Campbell and Elizabeth Ettore, *Gendering Addiction: The Politics of Drug Treatment in a Neurochemical World* (Basingstoke: Palgrave Macmillan, 2011).
18. Lynn Dumenil, *The Modern Temper: American Culture and Society in the 1920s* (New York: Hill & Wang, 1995).
19. David E. Kyvig, *Repealing National Prohibition* (Chicago: University of Chicago Press, 1979, rev. ed., 2000). The work of Catherine Gilbert Murdock is important in understanding drinking customs before and during Prohibition, although she devotes only limited attention to inebriety or problem drinking. See her "Domesticating Drink: Women and Alcohol in Prohibition America" (Ph.D. diss., University of Pennsylvania, 1995), later published as *Domesticating Drink: Women, Men, and*

Alcohol in America, 1870–1940 (Baltimore: Johns Hopkins University Press, 1998). Similarly, Kenneth Rose's analysis of women's involvement in the repeal campaign covers the rhetoric of the Woman's Organization for National Prohibition Reform but spends little time on women's drinking itself. See Kenneth D. Rose, *American Women and the Repeal of Prohibition* (New York: New York University Press, 1996).

20. Roizen, "The American Discovery of Alcoholism"; Courtwright, *Forces of Habit* and *Dark Paradise*; Musto, *The American Disease*; and Acker, *Creating the American Junkie*.
21. Carol Groneman, *Nymphomania: A History* (New York: W. W. Norton, 2000); Dumenil, *The Modern Temper*; Lizabeth Cohen, *A Consumer's Republic: The Politics of Mass Consumption in Postwar America* (New York: Alfred A. Knopf, 2003); and John D'Emilio and Estelle B. Freedman, *Intimate Matters: A History of Sexuality in America* (New York: Harper & Row, 1988).
22. See, e.g., "Women Are Drinking Too Much," *Facts*; "Women Who Drink," *Sunday Mirror*; undated pamphlet and clipping in Oversize Package no. 3 in Marty Mann Papers, Special Collections Research Center, Syracuse University Libraries (hereafter MMP). This theme continues to the present; see, e.g., the National Center on Addiction and Substance Abuse at Columbia University, *Women under the Influence* (Baltimore: Johns Hopkins University Press, 2006).
23. Joan Kelly, "Did Women Have a Renaissance?" in her *Women, History, and Theory* (1977; reprint, Chicago: University of Chicago Press, 1984).
24. Allan M. Brandt, *The Cigarette Century: The Rise, Fall, and Deadly Persistence of the Product That Defined America* (New York: Basic Books, 2007).
25. Letter, "Massachusetts—Readers' Digest," box 4, MMP.
26. The literature on medicalization is large. See, e.g., Charles E. Rosenberg, "Framing Disease: Illness, Society, and History," in *Framing Disease: Studies in Cultural History*, ed. Charles E. Rosenberg and Janet Golden (New Brunswick, NJ: Rutgers University Press, 1992), xiii–xxiv; Robert A. Nye, "The Evolution of the Concept of Medicalization in the Late Twentieth Century," *Journal of History of the Behavioral Sciences* 39, no. 2 (Spring 2003): 115–129; and Paul Starr, *The Social Transformation of American Medicine* (New York: Basic Books, 1982). On medicalization of alcoholism specifically, see Sarah Whitney Tracy, *Alcoholism in America from Reconstruction to Prohibition* (Baltimore: Johns Hopkins University Press, 2005).
27. See Peter Conrad, *The Medicalization of Society: On the Transformation of Human Conditions into Treatable Disorders* (Baltimore: Johns Hopkins University Press, 2007); and Judith Houck, *Hot and Bothered: Women, Medicine, and Menopause in Modern America* (Cambridge, MA: Harvard University Press, 2006), 12–13, on the dynamic process and blunt instrument.
28. Laura D. Hirshbein, *American Melancholy: Constructions of Depression in the Twentieth Century* (New Brunswick, NJ: Rutgers University Press, 2009), 6.
29. Harry Gene Levine, "The Discovery of Addiction: Changing Conceptions of Habitual Drunkenness in America," *Journal of Studies on Alcohol* 39 (1978): 143–174; and Mark Edward Lender, "Jellinek's Typology of Alcoholism: Some Historical Antecedents," *Journal of Studies on Alcohol* 40 (1979): 361–373. William L. White analyzes the disease concept and also provides a very thorough account of alcoholism treatment in American history in his *Slaying the Dragon: The History of Addiction Treatment and Recovery in America* (Bloomington, IL: Chestnut Hill Health Systems, 1998; 2nd ed., 2014).

30. The venereal diseases may offer the closest parallel, in that those who suffer from the condition are blamed for bringing on their fate through their conduct. See, e.g., Allan M. Brandt, *No Magic Bullet: A Social History of Venereal Disease in the United States since 1880* (New York: Oxford University Press, 1985); and Elizabeth Fee, "Venereal Disease: The Wages of Sin?" in *Passion and Power: Sexuality in History*, ed. Kathy Peiss and Christina Simmons (Philadelphia: Temple University Press, 1989), 178–198.
31. See Starr, *The Social Transformation of American Medicine*; and Joanne Meyerowitz, *How Sex Changed: A History of Transsexuality in the United States* (Cambridge, MA: Harvard University Press, 2002).
32. Rima D. Apple, *Perfect Motherhood: Science and Childrearing in America* (New Brunswick, NJ: Rutgers University Press, 2006).
33. Acker, *Creating the American Junkie*.
34. See esp. Campbell, *Using Women*.
35. This type of addiction resurfaced in the "Valium Panic of the 1970s." See Herzberg, *Happy Pills in America*; and Tone, *The Age of Anxiety*. For female inebriety in the earlier period, see Cheryl Krasnick Warsh, "'Oh Lord, Pour a Cordial in Her Wounded Heart': The Drinking Woman in Victorian and Edwardian Canada," in *Drink in Canada*, ed. Cheryl Krasnick Warsh (Montreal: McGill-Queen's University Press, 1993), 70–91; Mark Edward Lender, "Women Alcoholics: Prevalence Estimates and Their Problems as Reflected in Turn-of-the-Century Institutional Data," *International Journal of the Addictions* 16, no. 3 (1981): 443–448, and "A Special Stigma: Women and Alcoholism in the Late 19th and Early 20th Centuries," in *Alcohol Interventions: Historical and Sociocultural Approaches*, ed. David L. Strug, S. Priyadarsini, and Merton M. Hyman (New York: Hayworth Press, 1986), 41–57. In his *Substance and Shadow: Women and Addiction in the United States* (Cambridge, MA: Harvard University Press, 1996), Stephen R. Kandall (with the assistance of Jennifer Petrillo) surveys women's addiction from the nineteenth century to the present, but he excludes alcohol from his study, focusing instead on opiates and narcotics.
36. See, e.g., E. M. Jellinek, "Recent Trends in Alcoholism and in Alcohol Consumption," *Quarterly Journal of Studies on Alcohol* 8 (1947): 1–43; Norman Jolliffe, "The Alcoholic Admissions to Bellevue Hospital," *Science* 83, no. 2152 (March 27, 1936): 306–309; Frederick Lemere, Paul O'Hallaren, and Milton A. Maxwell, "Sex Ratio of Alcoholic Patients Treated over a 20-Year Period," *Quarterly Journal of Studies on Alcohol* 17 (1956): 437–442; J. V. Lowrie and F. G. Ebaugh, "A Post-Repeal Study of 300 Chronic Alcoholics," *American Journal of Medical Science* 203 (1942): 120–124; and B. Malzberg, "First Admissions with Alcoholic Psychoses in New York State," *Quarterly Journal of Studies on Alcohol* 10 (1949): 461–470.
37. "National Report on Lady Booze Hounds a Cause of Concern," *Mitchell (South Dakota) Republic*, February 26 [no year specified], in Oversize Package no. 1; "Women Are Drinking Too Much," *Facts*; and "Women Who Drink," *Sunday Mirror*, in Oversize Package no. 3, MMP.
38. Tracy, *Alcoholism in America*, demonstrates this point cogently.
39. Bert Hansen, "American Physicians' 'Discovery' of Homosexuals, 1880–1900: A New Diagnosis in a Changing Society," in Rosenberg and Golden, *Framing Disease*, 104–133; and Barbara Sicherman, "The Uses of a Diagnosis: Doctors, Patients, and Neurasthenia," *Journal of the History of Medicine and Allied Sciences* 32, no. 1 (1977): 33–54.

40. Janet Golden, *Message in a Bottle: The Making of Fetal Alcohol Syndrome* (Cambridge, MA: Harvard University Press, 2005), analyzes medicalization and demedicalization in the case of Fetal Alcohol Syndrome.
41. Tracy, *Alcoholism in America*, esp. xiv–xvii. Trysh Travis, *The Language of the Heart: A Cultural History of the Recovery Movement from Alcoholics Anonymous to Oprah Winfrey* (Chapel Hill: University of North Carolina Press, 2009), explores "recovery" as a social and cultural phenomenon in twentieth-century America.
42. Barbara Ehrenreich and Deirdre English, *For Her Own Good: 150 Years of the Experts' Advice to Women* (New York: Anchor Books, 1978); Ann Douglas Wood, "The 'Fashionable Diseases': Women's Complaints and Their Treatments in Nineteenth-Century America," 222–238, with response by Regina Markell Morantz, "The Perils of Feminist History," 239–245, in *Women and Health in America: Historical Readings*, ed. Judith Walzer Leavitt (Madison: University of Wisconsin Press, 1984).
43. Elizabeth Lunbeck, *The Psychiatric Persuasion: Knowledge, Gender and Power in Modern America* (Princeton, NJ: Princeton University Press, 1994); Linda Gordon, *Heroes of Their Own Lives: The Politics and History of Family Violence* (New York: Penguin Books, 1988); and Judith Walzer Leavitt, *Brought to Bed: Childbearing in America, 1750–1950* (New York: Oxford University Press, 1986).
44. Barron H. Lerner, *The Breast Cancer Wars: Faith, Hope, and the Pursuit of a Cure in Twentieth-Century America* (New York: Oxford University Press, 2001); Houck, *Hot and Bothered*; and Wendy Kline, *Bodies of Knowledge: Sexuality, Reproduction, and Women's Health in the Second Wave* (Chicago: University of Chicago Press, 2010).
45. Leavitt, *Brought to Bed*, provides a detailed and cogent analysis of the campaign for Twilight Sleep.
46. Houck, *Hot and Bothered*, 11.
47. Laura Schmidt and Constance Weisner, "The Emergence of Problem-Drinking Women as a Special Population in Need of Treatment," in *Recent Developments in Alcoholism*, vol. 12, *Women and Alcohol*, ed. Mark Galanter (New York: Plenum Press, 1995), 309–334.
48. Kline, *Bodies of Knowledge*, 1–2.
49. My analysis here has benefited from discussion with Trysh Travis as well as from her book, *Language of the Heart*.
50. Nancy Lurie, "The World's Longest Ongoing Protest Demonstration: North American Indian Drinking Patterns," *Pacific Historical Review* 40 (1971): 311–332.
51. For an insightful and carefully nuanced view of the reading of women's illness as "resistance," see Carroll Smith-Rosenberg, "The Hysterical Woman: Sex Roles and Role Conflict in Nineteenth-Century America," in her *Disorderly Conduct: Visions of Gender in Victorian America* (New York: Oxford University Press, 1985), 197–216. For an example of the "alcoholism-as-feminist-strategy" view, see Melinda Kanner, "Drinking Themselves to Life, or the Body in the Bottle," in *Reading the Social Body*, ed. Catherine B. Burroughs and Jeffrey David Ehrenreich (Iowa City: University of Iowa Press, 1993), 156–184. In *The Invisible Alcoholics*, Sandmaier calls alcohol a "cheap substitute" for equality (64).
52. Joan Jacobs Brumberg, *Fasting Girls: The Emergence of Anorexia Nervosa as a Modern Disease* (Cambridge, MA: Harvard University Press, 1988). Leavitt, *Brought to Bed*, is another classic example. See also Leavitt, *Women and Health in America*; and Rima D. Apple, ed., *Women, Health, and Medicine in America: A Historical*

Handbook (New York: Garland Publishers, 1990). Groneman, *Nymphomania*, offers suggestive parallels with alcoholism, particularly in a shift from biological to psychological models and with a similar concern about how much is too much.

53. H. I. Kushner, "Taking Biology Seriously: The Next Task for Historians of Addiction?" *Bulletin of the History of Medicine* 80 (2006): 115–143.

54. Golden, *Message in a Bottle*; Moira Plant, *Women, Drinking, and Pregnancy* (London: Tavistock Publications, 1985). In her study of women and drugs, Nancy Campbell argues that drugs are granted an omnipotence that fundamentally alters the addict. Those who wanted to prohibit alcohol believed the same of it, but that association faded after Repeal—except, again, in the case of women. See Campbell, *Using Women*, 7.

55. See John W. Crowley, *The White Logic: Alcoholism and Gender in American Modernist Fiction* (Amherst: University of Massachusetts Press, 1994); and Bruce Holley Johnson, "The Alcoholism Movement in America," esp. the appendix, for discussion of terminology.

1. The Female Inebriate in the Temperance Paradigm

1. This case was reported by Dr. McCowen, "Clinical Cases in Private Practice," *Quarterly Journal of Inebriety (QJI)* 10 (1888): 233–234. Discussion in these two paragraphs is based on this article.

2. Leonard Blumberg, "The American Association for the Study and Cure of Inebriety," *Alcoholism: Clinical and Experimental Research* 2, no. 3 (July 1978): 235–240; Edward M. Brown, "'What Shall We Do with the Inebriate?': Asylum Treatment and the Disease Concept of Alcoholism in the Late Nineteenth Century," *Journal of the History of the Behavioral Sciences* 21 (January 1985): 48–59; Mark Edward Lender, "Jellinek's Typology of Alcoholism: Some Historical Antecedents," *Journal of Studies on Alcohol* 40, no. 5 (1979): 361–373; A. E. Wilkerson, Jr., "A History of the Concept of Alcoholism as a Disease" (D.S.W. diss., University of Pennsylvania, 1966); and A. Jaffe, "Reform in American Medical Science: The Inebriety Movement and the Origins of the Psychological Disease Theory of Addiction, 1870–1920," *British Journal of Addiction* 73 (1978): 139–147. In her *Alcoholism in America from Reconstruction to Prohibition* (Baltimore: Johns Hopkins University Press, 2005), Sarah W. Tracy explores the complex relationships between physicians and other advocates of a medicalized views of problem drinking, including judges, legislators, and inebriates themselves. She also examines tensions between inebriate specialists and temperance advocates.

3. The literature on the temperance movement is extensive. For classic early studies, see Jack S. Blocker, *American Temperance Movements: Cycles of Reform* (Boston: Twayne, 1989); Harry Gene Levine, "Demon of the Middle Class: Self-Control, Liquor, and the Ideology of Temperance in the Nineteenth-Century America" (Ph.D. diss., University of California at Berkeley, 1978); Ruth Bordin, *Woman and Temperance: The Quest for Power and Liberty, 1873–1900* (Philadelphia: Temple University Press, 1981), and *Frances Willard: A Biography* (Chapel Hill: University of North Carolina Press, 1986); Janet Zollinger Giele, *Two Paths to Women's Equality: Temperance, Suffrage, and the Origins of Modern Feminism* (New York: Twayne, 1995); Richard F. Hamm, *Shaping the Eighteenth Amendment: Temperance Reform, Legal Culture, and the Polity, 1880–1920* (Chapel Hill: University of North Carolina Press, 1995); and Paul E. Johnson, *A Shopkeeper's Millennium: Society and Revivals in Rochester, New York, 1815–1837* (New York: Hill & Wang, 1978).

4. Elaine Frantz Parsons, *Manhood Lost: Fallen Drunkards and Redeeming Women in the Nineteenth-Century United States* (Baltimore: Johns Hopkins University Press, 2003); Eion F. Cannon, *The Saloon and the Mission: Addiction, Conversion, and the Politics of Redemption in American Culture* (Amherst: University of Massachusetts Press, 2013); Bruce Dorsey, *Reforming Men and Women: Gender in the Antebellum City* (Ithaca, NY: Cornell University Press, 2002); Matthew W. Osborn, *Rum Maniacs: Alcoholic Insanity in the Early American Republic* (Chicago: University of Chicago Press, 2014); Rodney Hessinger, *Seduced, Abandoned, and Reborn: Visions of Youth in Middle-Class America, 1780–1850* (Philadelphia: University of Pennsylvania Press, 2005); and Scott C. Martin, *Devil of the Domestic Sphere: Temperance, Gender, and Middle-Class Ideology, 1800–1860* (DeKalb: Northern Illinois University Press, 2008).
5. Martin, *Devil of the Domestic Sphere*, 32.
6. Ibid., 35–37.
7. Carroll Smith-Rosenberg, "Puberty to Menopause: The Cycle of Femininity in Nineteenth-Century America," in her *Disorderly Conduct: Visions of Gender in Victorian America* (New York: Oxford University Press, 1985); Adele E. Clark, "Women's Health: Life-Cycle Issues," in *Women, Health, and Medicine in America: A Historical Handbook*, ed. Rima D. Apple (New York: Garland Publishers, 1990); Carroll Smith-Rosenberg and Charles Rosenberg, "The Female Animal: Medical and Biological Views of Woman and Her Role in Nineteenth-Century America," in *Women and Health in America: Historical Readings*, ed. Judith Walzer Leavitt (Madison: University of Wisconsin Press, 1984), 12–27.
8. Judith Walzer Leavitt, *Brought to Bed: Childbearing in America, 1750–1950* (New York: Oxford University Press, 1986). Mrs. C.'s case also shows important transitions and fluidity in medical practice. She delivered her baby at home, as was standard at that time, but the use of forceps suggests she was attended by a male physician rather than a female midwife. Yet the prescription for wine recalled an older form of "dosing," almost a folk custom.
9. Martin, *Devil of the Domestic Sphere*.
10. The following discussion draws on the *Quarterly Journal of Inebriety*, the publication of the American Association for the Study and Cure of Inebriety. An American group, these doctors shared many ties with their British colleagues, whose writings appeared often in the *Journal*.
11. Chapter 2 examines women's public drinking.
12. Lawrence D. Longo, "The Rise and Fall of Battey's Operation: A Fashion in Surgery," in Leavitt, *Women and Health in America*, 270–284.
13. See sources cited in note 7 above.
14. McCowen, "Clinical Cases in Private Practice," *QJI* 10 (1888): 234.
15. George M. Beard, "Neurasthenia as a Cause of Inebriety," *QJI* 3 (1879): 200; "Some Remarks on the Morphine Habit," *QJI* 18 (1896): 241.
16. McCowen, "Clinical Cases in Private Practice," *QJI* 10 (1888): 233.
17. "Cursed by Her Appetite," *QJI* 7 (1885): 182.
18. "The Causes of Inebriety among Women," *QJI* 20 (1898): 430.
19. "Observations on Inebriety," *QJI* 9 (1887): 154.
20. McCowen, "Clinical Cases in Private Practice," *QJI* 10 (1888): 232.
21. "Inebriety from Tea," *QJI* 8 (1886): 187–188. See also "Coffee Inebriety," *QJI* 10 (1888): 370–372. Technological developments such as the telephone ensured additional privacy for women who wished to order alcohol from druggists. See Perry R.

Duis, *The Saloon: Public Drinking in Chicago and Boston, 1880–1920* (Urbana: University of Illinois Press, 1983), 220, 223.
22. Sarah Stage, *Female Complaints: Lydia Pinkham and the Business of Women's Medicine* (New York: W. W. Norton, 1979).
23. Ibid., 167.
24. Catherine Gilbert Murdock's Ph.D. dissertation is an insightful examination of the ways in which women's drinking habits helped to transform Americans' relationship with alcohol; see "Domesticating Drink: Women and Alcohol in Prohibition America" (Ph.D. diss., University of Pennsylvania, 1995), 120–121, 124–125. This study was later published as *Domesticating Drink: Women, Men, and Alcohol in America, 1870–1940* (Baltimore: Johns Hopkins University Press, 1998). Page references in this chapter are to the dissertation. Also see David T. Courtwright, "The Female Opiate Addict in Nineteenth-Century America," *Essay in Arts and Sciences* 10, no. 2 (March 1982): 161–171; and H. Wayne Morgan, *Drugs in America: A Social History, 1880–1980* (Syracuse, NY: Syracuse University Press, 1981). Some experts maintained that women might use opium as a general tonic rather than alcohol. See "Inebriety in Women," *QJI* 6 (1884): 247; and T. D. Crothers, "Is Alcoholism Increasing among American Women?" *North American Review* 155 (December 1892): 735.
25. Crothers, "Is Alcoholism Increasing among American Women?," 734–735; no author, no title, *QJI* 6 (1884): 119; and "Clinical Notes of Cases of Opium Inebriety," *QJI* 20 (1898): 189–191.
26. "The Transmissibility of Morphine," *QJI* 22 (1900): 349; "Beware of Chlorodyne," *QJI* 19 (1897): 197; Norman Kerr, "Inebriety, a Disease Allied to Insanity," *QJI* 6 (1884): 228, 232; "Morphinism in Women," *QJI* 20 (1898): 202–208; and T. D. Crothers, "Some Injuries from the Use of Opium in Infancy," *QJI* 22 (1900): 303, and "Is Alcoholism Increasing among American Women?," 734, 736.
27. Agnes Sparks, "Alcoholism in Women—Its Cause, Consequence, and Cure," *QJI* 20 (1898): 31–32. William L. White describes her as "one of the earliest women working within addiction medicine" in his *Slaying the Dragon: The History of Addiction Treatment and Recovery in America* (Bloomington, IL: Chestnut Hill Health Systems, 1998), 44.
28. The term "race" in this context did not mean the human race, but only people of white, northern European descent.
29. See Carl Degler, *In Search of Human Nature: The Decline and Revival of Darwinism in American Social Thought* (New York: Oxford University Press, 1991).
30. Although this discussion evokes the warning labels about drinking during pregnancy with which we are familiar today, the historian Janet Golden persuasively argues that these nineteenth-century concerns, including the clinical findings that informed them, should not be regarded as simply an earlier form of Fetal Alcohol Syndrome, which was named as such in the 1970s. Any diagnosis is specific to its own historical context, and Fetal Alcohol Syndrome could only emerge in the wake of ideas about fetuses prompted by late twentieth-century developments such as the thalidomide episode of the 1960s and the Supreme Court's *Roe v. Wade* decision in 1973. See Janet Golden, *Message in a Bottle: The Making of Fetal Alcohol Syndrome* (Cambridge, MA: Harvard University Press, 2005), esp. ch. 2.
31. "Alcoholic Heredity," *QJI* 10 (1888): 102.
32. Although much of this writing was produced by European authors, particularly British, the articles appeared in American journals and helped shape the American view of female inebriety. Similar concerns were expressed in Britain; see David W.

Gutzke, "'The Cry of the Children': The Edwardian Medical Campaign against Maternal Drinking," *British Journal of Addiction* 79 (1984): 71–84.
33. "Observations on Inebriety," *QJI* 9 (1887): 154.
34. "Inebriety as a Cause of Infant Mortality," *QJI* 2 (1877–1878): 124; "Alcohol on the Offspring," *QJI* 2 (1877–1878): 190; "English Experiences in Treating Inebriates at Home," *QJI* 18 (1896): 261; and R. Demme, "The Influence of Alcohol upon the Organism of the Child," *Wood's Medical and Surgical Monographs* 12 (1891): 225.
35. Demme, "The Influence of Alcohol upon the Organism of the Child," 225.
36. "Observations on Inebriety," *QJI* 9 (1887): 74; Stephen Lett, "Why Do Men Drink?" *QJI* 19 (1897): 266; and "Alcoholic Heredity," *QJI* 10 (1888): 101.
37. H. L. Staples, "Alcoholism," *QJI* 22 (1900): 413.
38. Gertrude Atherton, *Daughter of the Vine* (London: John Lane / The Bodley Head, 1899).
39. "Cirrhosis from Inebriety," *QJI* 3 (1879): 107; "Heredity in Alcoholism," *QJI* 2 (1877–1878): 178; "Alcoholic Heredity," *QJI* 10 (1888): 101–106; and Lett, "Why Do Men Drink?" *QJI* 19 (1897): 266.
40. "Alcohol on the Offspring," *QJI* 2 (1877–78), 190; "Inebriety in Women," *QJI* 6 (1884): 250; and "Alcoholic Heredity," *QJI* 10 (1888): 103.
41. "Heredity in Alcoholism," *QJI* 2 (1877–1878): 178–179.
42. "Alcohol on the Offspring," *QJI* 2 (1877–78): 190.
43. "Notes, etc.," *QJI* 1 (1877): 120. In this attitude, physicians resembled temperance advocates, but most doctors in the American Association for the Study and Cure of Inebriety were not prohibitionists. See also W. C. Sullivan, "A Note on the Influence of Maternal Inebriety on the Offspring," *QJI* 21 (1899): 325.
44. "Heredity in Alcoholism," *QJI* 2 (1877–1878): 178; and E. S. Talbot, "Degeneracies the Result of Alcohol and Other Narcotics," *QJI* 34 (1913): 173. See also "A Note on the Influence of Maternal Inebriety on the Offspring," *QJI* 20 (1898): 331–332; and "Female Inebriety," *QJI* 20 (1898): 103.
45. "Alcohol in Pre-natal Life," *QJI* 22 (1900): 334; "Cirrhosis from Inebriety," *QJI* 3 (1879): 107; and "Inebriety in Women," *QJI* 6 (1884): 250. Some physicians maintained that alcohol, by damaging the reproductive organs and germ cells so severely that embryos did not survive, in fact had a eugenic effect. See, e.g., E. S. Talbot, "Alcohol in Its Relation to Degeneracy," *Journal of the American Medical Association* 48 (1907): 399–401. For more on constitutional weakness, see, e.g., H. Emerson, "Alcohol: A Public Health Problem," *American Journal of Public Health* 7 (1917): 558.
46. Lucy M. Hall, "Prison Experiences with Inebriates," *QJI* 10 (1888): 112.
47. "The Transmissibility of Morphine," *QJI* 22 (1900): 347, 349, 353; and "Alcohol in Pre-natal Life," *QJI* 22 (1900): 334–335.
48. "Alcohol on Nursing Children," *QJI* 2 (1877–1878): 123; "Influence of Alcohol in Nursing," *QJI* 9 (1887): 118–119; "Observations on Inebriety," *QJI* 9 (1887): 151; "Alcohol and Infant Convulsions," *QJI* 20 (1898): 347; and "Convulsions in a Child due to Intemperance in the Nurse," *QJI* 21 (1899): 372.
49. "Alcohol to Nursing Mothers," *QJI* 2 (1877–1878): 96.
50. Demme, "The Influence of Alcohol upon the Organism of the Child," 220. See also "Alcohol in Infancy and Childhood," *QJI* 22 (1900): 354; and "Inebriety a Cause of Infant Mortality," *QJI* 2 (1877–1878): 124.
51. Crothers, "Some Injuries," *QJI* 22 (1900): 303. It is worth noting that Crothers expressed surprise that her inebriety was not the result of "pain or sickness."

52. "Beginning of Inebriety," *QJI* 20 (1898): 178.
53. Crothers, "Some Injuries," *QJI* 22 (1900): 304. See also "Inebriety in Children," *QJI* 8 (1886): 38–39; and Charles L. Dana, "Alcoholism in New York and the Classification of Inebriates," *American Journal of Insanity* 50 (1893): 30.
54. "A Note on the Influence of Maternal Inebriety on the Offspring," *QJI* 20 (1898): 335–336; "Inebriety a Cause of Infant Mortality," *QJI* 2 (1877–1878): 124; and Henry William Blair, *The Temperance Movement; or, The Conflict between Man and Alcohol* (Boston: William E. Smythe Co., 1888), 166.
55. "Observations on Inebriety," *QJI* 9 (1887): 151.
56. "Some Clinical Aspects of Inebriety," *QJI* 20 (1898): 173–174.
57. Stephen Crane, "Maggie: A Girl of the Streets," in *Maggie and Other Stories by Stephen Crane* (New York: Pocket Books, 1960), quoted at 8, 10.
58. Caroline Lee Hentz, "The Victim of Excitement," in her *Love after Marriage, and Other Stories of the Heart* (Philadelphia: T. B. Peterson & Bros., 1870), quoted at 57.
59. Many historians of women have written on the central position of motherhood in the nineteenth-century construction of femininity. Classic studies include Barbara Welter, "The Cult of True Womanhood, 1820–1860," *American Quarterly* 18 (Summer 1966): 151–174; Nancy F. Cott, *The Bonds of Womanhood: 'Woman's Sphere' in New England, 1780–1835* (New Haven, CT: Yale University Press, 1977); and Mary P. Ryan, Cradle of the Middle Class: The Family in Oneida County, New York, 1790–1865 (Cambridge: Cambridge University Press, 1981).
60. John W. Crowley, ed., *Drunkard's Progress: Narratives of Addiction, Despair, and Recovery* (Baltimore: Johns Hopkins University Press, 1999).
61. Katherine A. Chavigny, "Reforming Drunkards in Nineteenth-Century America: Religion, Medicine, Therapy," in *Altering American Consciousness: The History of Alcohol and Drug Use in the United States, 1800–2000*, ed. Sarah W. Tracy and Caroline Acker (Amherst: University of Massachusetts Press, 2004), 108–123; and White, *Slaying the Dragon*.
62. Crowley, *Drunkard's Progress*, 10.
63. Ruth M. Alexander, "'We are Engaged as a Band of Sisters': Class and Domesticity in the Washingtonian Temperance Movement, 1840–1850," *Journal of American History* 75, no. 3 (December 1988): 763–785.
64. Crowley, *Drunkard's Progress*, "my health," quoted at 72, and "with the first stimulant," quoted at 74.
65. Ibid., "far too loudly," quoted at 77.
66. Ibid., 13.
67. Atherton, *Daughter of the Vine*, explanation of withdrawal on 291.
68. No author, no title, *QJI* 8 (1886): 3; "Notes on Alcoholic Paralysis," *QJI* 8 (1886): 97.
69. "Inebriety in Women," *QJI* 6 (1884): 248.
70. "English Experiences in Treating Inebriates at Home," *QJI* 18 (1896): 261–262.
71. "Morphinism in Women," *QJI* 20 (1898): 203; and Dr. Thomeuf, "Alcoholism in Women," in *Wood's Medical and Surgical Monographs* 7 (1890): 351.
72. Sparks, "Alcoholism in Women," *QJI* 20 (1898): 32.
73. Crothers, "Is Alcoholism Increasing among American Women?" 734.
74. "The Danger of Alcohol Administered in Uterine Disease," *QJI* 1 (1876–77): 239–240.
75. "Extracts from Foreign Correspondence," *QJI* 1 (1877): 92; "Abstracts and Reviews," *QJI* 2 (1877): 38; and Sparks, "Alcoholism in Women," *QJI* 20 (1898): 33.
76. Isaiah DeZouche, "Duty of the State with Regard to Inebriates," *QJI* 10 (1888): 127; "Cursed by Her Appetite," *QJI* 7 (1885): 182–183; and J. J. Pitcairn, "The Prison

Treatment of Inebriates," *QJI* 19 (1897): 146. They also reported some of the things family members did to female inebriates in an attempt to break their habit and/or punish them. One father, for example, hung his inebriate daughter up by her wrists until she fainted.
77. Tracy, *Alcoholism in America*, 94.
78. Sparks, "Alcoholism in Women," *QJI* 20 (1898): 129.
79. Mark Edward Lender, "Women Alcoholics: Prevalence Estimates and Their Problems as Reflected in Turn-of-the-Century Institutional Data," *International Journal of the Addictions* 16, no. 3 (1981): 443–448. See also Cheryl Krasnick Warsh, "'Oh Lord, Pour a Cordial in Her Wounded Heart': The Drinking Woman in Victorian and Edwardian Canada," in *Drink in Canada*, ed. Cheryl Krasnick Warsh (Montreal: McGill-Queen's University Press, 1993): 70–91; and Mark Edward Lender, "A Special Stigma: Women and Alcoholism in the Late 19th and Early 20th Centuries," in *Alcohol Interventions: Historical and Sociocultural Approaches*, ed. David L. Strug, S. Priyadarsini, and Merton M. Hyman (New York: Hayworth Press, 1986), 41–57.
80. Tracy, *Alcoholism in America*, 159.
81. Ibid., 192.
82. Jim Baumohl, "Inebriate Institutions in North America, 1840–1920," *British Journal of Addiction* 85 (1990): 1187–1204; Sarah Whitney Tracy, "The Foxborough Experiment: Medicalizing Inebriety at the Massachusetts Hospital for Dipsomaniacs and Inebriates" (Ph.D. diss., University of Pennsylvania, 1992); and Brown, "What Shall We Do with the Inebriate?"
83. Tracy, *Alcoholism in America*, 51.
84. See White, *Slaying the Dragon*, 50–63, and advertisements from the Keeley archives. The characterization of Dwight as a "therapeutic community" is from William L. White (personal communication, June 2, 2010).
85. Tracy, *Alcoholism in America*, 116. This practice foreshadowed the early years of Alcoholics Anonymous, where female alcoholics were relegated to the care of non-alcoholic wives, as discussed in chapter 3.
86. Tracy, *Alcoholism in America*, 103.
87. Thomeuf, "Alcoholism in Women," 352; and "London's Women Drunkards," *Outlook* 69 (October 12, 1901): 344.
88. "Dipsomania: Its Medical and Legal Aspects," *QJI* 3 (1879): 218; George H. McMichael, "Alcoholism as a Disease," QJI 19 (1897): 256; H. L. Staples, "Alcoholism," *QJI* 22 (1900): 413.
89. "A Note on the Influence of Maternal Inebriety on the Offspring," *QJI* 20 (1898): 332.
90. Sparks, "Alcoholism in Women," *QJI* 20 (1898): 36. See also Staples, "Alcoholism," *QJI* 22 (1900): 415.
91. Stage, *Female Complaints*, 161–171.
92. David F. Musto, "The Harrison Act," in his *The American Disease: Origins of Narcotic Control* (New York: Oxford University Press, 1987), 54–68.

2. "Lit Ladies": Women's Drinking during the Progressive Era and Prohibition

1. "Mrs. Gould's Life at Home, Drunken Orgy," *Los Angeles Times*, June 17, 1909.
2. The question of their engagement drew press coverage from 1895 to 1898, including discussion of whether they would elope, the financial implications of such a marriage for Gould given his family's disapproval, and the couple's joint travel and

public displays of affection. See, e.g., "Will Gould Wed Miss Clemmons?" *Milwaukee Journal*, January 5, 1898.
3. "Pint a Lady's Limit," *Washington Post*, October 30, 1908.
4. "Prince Enraged Gould, She Says," *New York Times*, June 2, 1909.
5. "The Wrong Dearie," *Washington Post*, June 19, 1909; and "Will Not Call for Mr. Gould," *Los Angeles Times*, June 22, 1909.
6. Mrs. C. is discussed in chapter 1.
7. Elaine F. Parsons, *Manhood Lost: Fallen Drunkards and Redeeming Women in the Nineteenth-Century United States* (Baltimore: Johns Hopkins University Press, 2003). Also see my notes to the Introduction and Chapter 1 for additional information on the historiography of the temperance movement.
8. Madelon Powers, *Faces along the Bar: Lore and Order in the Workingman's Saloon, 1870–1920* (Chicago: University of Chicago Press, 1998), 35; Roy Rosenzweig, *Eight Hours for What We Will: Workers and Leisure in an Industrial City, 1870–1920* (Cambridge: Cambridge University Press, 1983), 42–44.
9. Perry R. Duis, *The Saloon: Public Drinking in Chicago and Boston, 1880–1920* (Urbana: University of Illinois Press, 1983), 106. See also Catherine G. Murdock, *Domesticating Drink: Women, Men, and Alcohol in America* (Baltimore: Johns Hopkins University Press, 1998), 159.
10. Duis, *The Saloon*, 96.
11. Stephen Crane, "Maggie: A Girl of the Streets," in *Maggie and Other Stories by Stephen Crane* (New York: Pocket Books, 1960).
12. Duis, *The Saloon*, 3, 96, and 106; Crane, "Maggie," 9; and Murdock, *Domesticating Drink*, 170–171.
13. Powers, *Faces along the Bar*, 32.
14. Ibid., 32–33; and Duis, *The Saloon*, 186. Temperance advocates criticized the practice of offering free food to lure more people into the saloon, where the salty meal prompted them to drink even more.
15. Oliver Allstrom, "Ladies' Entrance" (1910), reprinted in Leon Fink, ed., *Major Problems in the Gilded Age and Progressive Era* (Lexington, MA: D. C. Heath, 1993), 188–189.
16. Duis, *The Saloon*, 196. See also Joanne J. Meyerowitz, *Women Adrift: Independent Wage Earners in Chicago, 1880–1930* (Chicago: University of Chicago Press, 1988); Kathy Peiss, *Cheap Amusements: Working Women and Leisure in Turn-of-the-Century New York* (Philadelphia: Temple University Press, 1986); and Mary E. Odem, *Delinquent Daughters: Protecting and Policing Adolescent Female Sexuality in the United States, 1885–1920* (Chapel Hill: University of North Carolina Press, 1995).
17. Vice Commission of Chicago, *The Social Evil in Chicago* (Chicago: Gunthorp-Warren Printing Co., 1911), quoted in Walter Clarke, "Prostitution and Alcohol," *Social Hygiene* 3 (1917): 84n3.
18. Kathy Peiss, "'Charity Girls' and City Pleasures: Historical Notes on Working-Class Sexuality, 1880–1920," in *Passion and Power: Sexuality in History*, ed. Kathy Peiss and Christina Simmons (Philadelphia: Temple University Press, 1989), 57–69.
19. Crane, "Maggie," 61, 63, 64–65.
20. Gladys Mary Hall, *Prostitution in the Modern World: A Survey and a Challenge* (New York: Emerson Books, 1936), 90.
21. Clarke, "Prostitution and Alcohol," 82.
22. Ibid., 82; and W. W. Sanger, *History of Prostitution* (New York: Medical Publishing Co., 1910), 541–542. See also Vice Commission of Chicago, "The Social Evil and

the Saloon," chapter 2 in *The Social Evil in Chicago* (Chicago: Gunthorp-Warren Printing Co., 1911), 119–140, for a discussion of "How Women Enter Lives of Prostitution through the Saloon," 127–129.
23. Mary Murphy, "Bootlegging Mothers and Drinking Daughters: Gender and Prohibition in Butte, Montana," *American Quarterly* 46, no. 2 (1994): 181. The Vice Commission of Chicago, *The Social Evil in Chicago*, 34, reports findings from a 1911 survey of Chicago saloons: "929 unescorted women in these [445] saloons, who by their actions and conversation were believed to be prostitutes."
24. Clarke, "Prostitution and Alcohol," 84, 85.
25. One reformer referred to "liquor and lust" and the "brothel and the saloon" as the "devil's Siamese twins." See Clifford G. Roe, *The Great War on White Slavery* (1911), 319 (in the Bishop-Kirk Collection).
26. Murphy, "Bootlegging Mothers and Drinking Daughters," 181–182.
27. V. V. Anderson and C. M. Leonard, "Drunkenness as Seen among Women in Court," *Mental Hygiene* 3 (1919): 266, 268.
28. Frances A. Kellor, "Criminality among Women," *Arena* 23 (May 1900): 516.
29. Ibid., 521.
30. Anderson and Leonard, "Drunkenness as Seen among Women," 268–269.
31. Clarke, "Prostitution and Alcohol," 83. See also Kellor, "Criminality among Women," 524.
32. Similar ideas animated reform work with, and medical treatment of, young, working-class women whose primary problem was being "oversexed" or nymphomaniacs. See Carol Groneman, *Nymphomania: A History* (New York: W. W. Norton, 2000), 53.
33. Lynn Dumenil, "The New Woman," chapter 3 in *The Modern Temper: American Culture and Society in the 1920s* (New York: Hill & Wang, 1995), 98–144.
34. Murdock, *Domesticating Drink*, 157–158.
35. Ibid., 108, 123, 140–141. Murdock even argues that "Women's moderate, at-home drinking formed the formation of alcohol-consumption patterns in the twentieth century" (123), although she notes that alcohol did not define sociability in the middle-class home as it did in the saloon.
36. Discussed in chapter 1.
37. Gertrude Atherton, *Daughter of the Vine* (London: John Lane / The Bodley Head, 1899), 37.
38. "Woman and Drink," *Current Literature* 34, no. 2 (February 1903): 226.
39. David E. Kyvig, *Repealing National Prohibition* (Chicago: University of Chicago Press, 1979; rev. ed., 2000); Murdock, *Domesticating Drink*; Michael A. Lerner, *Dry Manhattan: Prohibition in New York City* (Cambridge, MA: Harvard University Press, 2007); and Mark Edward Lender and James Kirby Martin, *Drinking in America: A History* (New York: Free Press, 1987), chapter 3. See also Paul Aaron and David Musto, "Temperance and Prohibition in America: A Historical Overview," in *Alcohol and Public Policy: Beyond the Shadow of Prohibition*, ed. M. H. Moore and D. R. Gerstein (Washington, DC: National Academy Press, 1981). Debates about the effectiveness or failure of Prohibition have been ongoing for decades. See, e.g., Sean Dennis Cashman, *Prohibition: The Lie of the Land* (New York: Free Press, 1981); or Andrew Sinclair, *Prohibition: The Era of Excess* (Boston: Little, Brown, 1962). While they did not always specify the criteria used to evaluate the Prohibition experiment, many writers took repeal to be sufficient proof of defeat. The historian John C. Burnham questioned this apparent consensus in a now-classic

article, "New Perspectives on the Prohibition 'Experiment' of the 1920s," *Journal of Social History* 2, no. 1 (1968): 51–68, and in his *Bad Habits: Drinking, Smoking, Taking Drugs, Gambling, Sexual Misbehavior, and Swearing in American History* (New York: New York University Press, 1993).

40. "Women Bootleggers a Problem," *Literary Digest*, February 5, 1927, 46; Ernest W. Mendeville, "What Happened to Sally?" *Outlook* 139, no. 10 (March 11, 1925): 374–376; and "Lady Bootlegger," *Scribner's Magazine* 92, no. 4 (October 1932): 229–231. For an account of the colorful figure of "Texas" Guinan, known as "Queen of the Night Clubs," see Stanley Walker, *The Night Club Era* (New York: Frederick A. Stokes Co., 1933), 240–245. Lender and Martin, *Drinking in America*, 140, describe one West Virginia grandmother who ran a still; and Murphy analyzes "Bootlegging Mothers." Catherine G. Murdock, "Domesticating Drink: Women and Alcohol in Prohibition America" (Ph.D. diss., University of Pennsylvania, 1995), discusses moonshining, 186–188, 194. On Irish widows in the nineteenth century, see Roy Rosenzweig, Eight Hours for What We Will: Workers and Leisure in an Industrial City, 1870–1920 (Cambridge: Cambridge University Press, 1983), 42–44.
41. Joshua Zeitz, *Flapper: A Madcap Story of Sex, Style, Celebrity, and the Women Who Made America Modern* (New York: Crown Publishers, 2006).
42. This is what sexual reformers had hoped for during the nineteenth century as well, that women would establish a single standard that men would learn to follow.
43. Kay Kennedy, "Sisters of the Hollow Leg," *Outlook and Independent* 155 (May 21, 1930): 93.
44. Marty Mann, "Alcoholics Anonymous Official Tells of Life Plagued by Liquor," *Washington (DC) Times Herald*, May 22, 1945. Other profiles included accounts of her early drinking, such as S. J. Woolf, "The Sick Person We Call an Alcoholic," *New York Times Magazine*, April 21, 1946, Marty Mann Papers, Special Collections Research Center, Syracuse University Libraries (hereafter MMP).
45. Woolf, "The Sick Person We Call an Alcoholic," MMP.
46. Newspaper clipping from *Wilmington (DE) Daily Journal*, February 22 (no year); "Nancy Craig Program—WJZ," MMP. For more on courtship rituals during this period, see Beth Bailey, *From Front Porch to Back Seat: Courtship in Twentieth-Century America* (Baltimore: Johns Hopkins University Press, 1988). The dances and parties Mann described were clearly shaped by the conventions of her socioeconomic class.
47. Eudora R. Richardson, "Drinking Mothers," *Outlook and Independent* 158 (June 10, 1931): 174.
48. Ibid.; Kennedy, "Sisters of the Hollow Leg," 92; and Margaret Culkin Banning, "Lit Ladies," *Harper's*, January 1930, 163. On cigarettes, see Cassandra Tate, "Milady's Cigarette," chapter 4 in *Cigarette Wars: The Triumph of the "Little White Slaver"* (New York: Oxford University Press, 1999), 93–118. See also Alan M. Brandt, *The Cigarette Century: The Rise, Fall, and Deadly Persistence of the Product That Defined America* (New York: Basic Books, 2007). Commentator Frederick Lewis Allen included strong language in this list. See Burnham, *Bad Habits*, 25.
49. Murphy, "Bootlegging Mothers and Drinking Daughters," 181, 187–188.
50. Paula S. Fass, *The Damned and the Beautiful: American Youth in the 1920s* (Oxford: Oxford University Press, 1977), 321.
51. Joan Jacobs Brumberg, *The Body Project: An Intimate History of American Girls* (New York: Random House, 1997), 154–155.

52. William K. Anderson, "Shall I Send My Daughter to Europe?" *Christian Century* 48 (June 10, 1931): 774.
53. Cigarettes present an interesting comparison. Because cigarettes were legal during the 1920s, they could be advertised heavily. These ads as well as movies show that cigarettes, like alcohol, were linked with female sexuality and modernity. But they were not perceived to have quite the same disinhibiting effect as alcohol. See Tate, "Milady's Cigarette."
54. Zeitz makes this point clearly in *Flapper*.
55. Anderson, "Shall I Send My Daughter to Europe?," 774.
56. Ione Nicoll, "Should Women Vote Wet?" *North American Review* 229 (May 1930): 562, 564.
57. "On Girls Learning to Drink," *Literary Digest*, January 7, 1933, 20. Kenneth D. Rose, *American Women and the Repeal of Prohibition* (New York: New York University Press, 1996), provides a thorough analysis of the ways in which the WONPR used "home protection" rhetoric to further their campaign for repeal.
58. Ron Roizen, "The American Discovery of Alcoholism, 1933–1939" (Ph.D. diss., University of California at Berkeley, 1991).
59. See, e.g., Daniel Okrent, *Last Call: The Rise and Fall of Prohibition* (New York: Scribner, 2010); and Lerner, *Dry Manhattan*.
60. Allan M. Brandt, *No Magic Bullet: A Social History of Venereal Disease in the United States since 1880* (New York: Oxford University Press, 1985), 40–41, 46, 161.
61. Burnham maintains, in fact, that the significant decline in alcohol-related admissions is "the most convincing evidence of the success of prohibition" ("New Perspectives," 60).
62. George G. Sears, "Hospital Administration under the Eighteenth Amendment," *Boston Medical and Surgical Journal* 189, no. 12 (September 20, 1923): 399, on delirium tremens becoming extinct; Hugh B. Gray, "The Experience of the Washingtonian Home," *New England Journal of Medicine* 200, no. 18 (May 2, 1929): 936–937, on a charity home closing its doors.
63. Lender and Martin, *Drinking in America*, 160; Leonard Blumberg, "The American Association for the Study and Cure of Inebriety," *Alcoholism: Clinical and Experimental Research* 2, no. 3 (July 1978): 239–240; A. Jaffe, "Reform in American Medical Science: The Inebriety Movement and the Origins of the Psychological Disease Theory of Addiction, 1870–1920," *British Journal of Addiction* 73 (1978): 139–147; and Jim Baumohl, "Inebriate Institutions in North America, 1840–1920," *British Journal of Addiction* 85 (1990): 1187–1204.
64. Norman Jolliffe, "The Alcoholic Admissions to Bellevue Hospital," *Science* 83, no. 2152 (March 27, 1936): 308–309. See also Sears, "Hospital Administration"; Gray, "The Experience of the Washingtonian Home"; Horatio M. Pollock and Edith M. Furbush, "Prohibition and Alcoholic Mental Disease," *Mental Hygiene* 8 (1924): 548–570; and Horatio M. Pollock and Frederick W. Brown, "Recent Statistics of Alcoholic Mental Disease," *Mental Hygiene* 13 (1929): 591–614.
65. Gray, "The Experience of the Washingtonian Home," 36.
66. Sears, "Hospital Administration," 398. Similarly, one Chicago physician reported a case under the colorful title "Three Months Amnesia following Moonshine Whiskey Debauch," addressing the extent to which moonshine whiskey caused different kinds of hallucinations and delirium. See B. Lemchen, "Three Months Amnesia

Following Moonshine Whiskey Debauch," *Illinois Medical Journal* 48 (September 1925): 246–248.
67. Burnham makes this point convincingly in his 1968 essay, "New Perspectives."
68. Gray, "The Experience of the Washingtonian Home," 936–937.
69. Pollock and Furbush, "Prohibition and Alcoholic Mental Disease," 548–570; and Pollock and Brown, "Recent Statistics," 613. Clark Warburton reported similar findings in *The Economic Results of Prohibition* (New York: Columbia University Press, 1932). He concluded that "the frequency of cases of alcoholism, cirrhosis of the liver, nephritis, and alcoholic insanity decreased to a marked degree" during wartime prohibition and the early years of national prohibition. He noted that, although such rates then began to increase, they remained below prewar rates (216–217).
70. Jolliffe, "The Alcoholic Admissions," 306–309. Of course, the relative absence of men due to military service in 1918–1919 may also have contributed to a proportional increase in female patients, although Joliffe does not address this possibility.
71. Sears, "Hospital Administration," 398.
72. Pollock and Furbush, "Prohibition and Alcoholic Mental Disease," 556–558.
73. Pollock and Brown, "Recent Statistics," 609–613.
74. Nicoll, "Should Women Vote Wet?," 563–564.
75. Sears, "Hospital Administration," 398.
76. "Effect of Prohibition on Alcoholism," *Literary Digest*, July 14, 1923, 21.
77. Nicoll, "Should Women Vote Wet?," 563.
78. Pauline Morton Sabin, "Women's Revolt against Prohibition," *Review of Reviews* 80, no. 478 (November 1929): 88.
79. Lerner, *Dry Manhattan*, 96.
80. Sarah Stage, *Female Complaints: Lydia Pinkham and the Business of Women's Medicine* (New York: W. W. Norton, 1979), 196, 198.
81. Karl Abraham, "The Psychological Relations between Sexuality and Alcoholism," *International Journal of Psycho-analysis* 8 (1926): 2–10. The discussion in this and the following four paragraphs is based on this article, from which quotations are drawn.
82. Susan Cahn, *Coming on Strong: Gender and Sexuality in Twentieth-Century Women's Sport* (Cambridge, MA: Harvard University Press, 1994).
83. Murdock, *Domesticating Drink*.
84. Kennedy, "Sisters of the Hollow Leg," 92.
85. Ibid.
86. Edna Yost, "Carry Nation Wets," *Outlook and Independent*, September 25, 1929, 146–147, 159. This article built on the long association of temperance workers with extremism. Even though the pressure now involved drinking rather than abstention, the figure of Carry Nation provided a useful shorthand for any excesses regarding drinking choices.
87. Banning, "Lit Ladies," 162.
88. Biographical Note for Margaret Culkin Banning, at the Margaret Culkin Banning Papers, Archives and Special Collections, Vassar College Libraries, http://specialcollections.vassar.edu/findingaids/banning_margaret_culkin.html.
89. Banning, "Lit Ladies," 162–163, for reasons for drinking, quotation on 166–167. Banning and others discussed women's vanity as a reason for drinking, as women sought to appear youthful and charming but should avoid the risks of intoxication, including the toll it could take on their appearance. See Kennedy, "Sisters of the Hollow Leg," 117, 119. See also "Alcohol: Beauty Blaster," *Everybody's Magazine*

35 (December 1916): 763–764. For more on the importance of appearance for girls and women, see Brumberg, *The Body Project*; and Kathy Peiss, *Hope in a Jar: The Making of America's Beauty Culture* (New York: Metropolitan Books, 1998).
90. Banning, "Lit Ladies," 163.
91. Ibid., 161–166.
92. Kennedy, "Sisters of the Hollow Leg," 92.
93. Richardson, "Drinking Mothers," 174.
94. Ibid., 174–175.
95. Ibid., 175.
96. Ibid., 174–175.
97. Ibid.
98. "This Moderate Drinking," *Harper's Monthly Magazine*, March 1931, 427.
99. Banning, "Lit Ladies," 169.
100. Richardson, "Drinking Mothers," 191.
101. Banning, "Lit Ladies," 168.
102. Kyvig, *Repealing National Prohibition*, 104.
103. Ibid., 22, 24; Lender and Martin, *Drinking in America*, 144–145. See also Jack S. Blocker, "Did Prohibition Really Work? Alcohol Prohibition as Public Health Innovation," *American Journal of Public Health* 96 (February 2006): 233–243. For an overview of changing assessments of Prohibition over time, see Ian Tyrrell, "The U.S. Prohibition Experiment: Myths, History and Implications," *Addiction* 92 (November 1997): 1405–1409.
104. Kyvig, *Repealing National Prohibition*. See also Jack S. Blocker, *American Temperance Movements: Cycles of Reform* (Boston: Twayne, 1989).
105. Burnham, *Bad Habits*, 34–38.
106. Richardson, "Drinking Mothers," 174.
107. "Women Become People" (Editorial), *Outlook and Independent*, April 21, 1931, 586–587.
108. Murdock, *Domesticating Drink*, 202, 248, 257.

3. "More to Overcome than the Men": Women in Alcoholics Anonymous

1. The contours and details of Mann's life come from her speeches, press coverage of her public health campaign, her Alcoholics Anonymous narrative, and the biography by Sally Brown and David R. Brown, *Mrs. Marty Mann: The First Lady of Alcoholics Anonymous* (Center City, MN: Hazelden/Pittman Archives Press, 2001). Brown and Brown recount Mann's introduction to AA and her first AA meeting in chapters 12 and 13.
2. Alcoholics Anonymous, *Alcoholics Anonymous: The Story of How Many Thousands of Men and Women Have Recovered from Alcoholism* ("The Big Book"), rev. ed. (New York: Alcoholics Anonymous World Services, 1955), 228.
3. Sidney Fields, "The Birth of the National Committee for Education on Alcoholism, Part 1: The Search," *Guideposts* (n.d.). See also other clippings such as "Poison for Ladies"; and S. J. Woolf, "The Sick Person We Call an Alcoholic," *New York Times Magazine*, April 21, 1946, Marty Mann Papers, Special Collections Research Center, Syracuse University Libraries (hereafter MMP).
4. Marty Mann, "Mrs. Mann Tells about Final Victory over Alcoholism," MMP.
5. The account in the following three paragraphs is drawn from Alcoholics Anonymous, "The Big Book," 1955 ed.; Ernest Kurtz, *Not-God: A History of Alcoholics Anonymous* (Center City, MN: Hazelden Educational Services, 1979); William L.

White, *Slaying the Dragon: The History of Addiction Treatment and Recovery in America* (Bloomington, IL: Chestnut Hill Health Systems, 1998); Lillian Mae Hallberg, "Rhetorical Dimensions of Institutional Language: A Case Study of Women Alcoholics" (Ph.D. diss., University of Iowa, 1988); and Nan Robertson, *Getting Better: Inside Alcoholics Anonymous* (New York: William Morrow, 1988). Following AA tradition, only first names will be used here for AA members, with the exception of the cofounders, Bill Wilson and Dr. Bob Smith, and also with Marty Mann, who broke her own anonymity.

For additional discussion of male alcoholics in AA, and the development of Al-Anon, see Lori Rotskoff, *Love on the Rocks: Men, Women, and Alcohol in Post–World War II America* (Chapel Hill: University of North Carolina Press, 2002). For the spread of the AA philosophy through American culture, including print culture, see Trysh Travis, *The Language of the Heart: A Cultural History of the Recovery Movement from Alcoholics Anonymous to Oprah Winfrey* (Chapel Hill: University of North Carolina Press, 2009).

6. Travis, *The Language of the Heart*, 63.
7. Rotskoff, *Love on the Rocks*, 112–113.
8. See, e.g., Rotskoff, *Love on the Rocks*; and Travis, *The Language of the Heart*.
9. Travis, *The Language of the Heart*, 5.
10. Rotskoff, *Love on the Rocks*.
11. In later decades there has been substantial critique of the Twelve Steps from a feminist perspective, arguing that the "surrender" that is considered fundamental to the AA program is particularly destructive for women. This chapter, however, focuses more on the social practices of AA in its early years.
12. "Women in AA: First Groups," Alcoholics Anonymous Archives, New York, New York (hereafter AA Archives-NYC).
13. *Dr. Bob and the Good Oldtimers* (New York: Alcoholics Anonymous World Services, 1980), 246.
14. Ibid., 242.
15. Mary C. Darrah, *Sister Ignatia: Angel of Alcoholics Anonymous* (Chicago: Loyola University Press, 1992), 124.
16. *Dr. Bob and the Good Oldtimers*, 235.
17. *Lois Remembers: Memoirs of the Co-Founder of Al-Anon and the Wife of the Co-Founder of Alcoholics Anonymous* (New York: Al-Anon Family Group Headquarters, 1979), 91–100; Darrah, *Sister Ignatia*, 114–118.
18. *Dr. Bob and the Good Oldtimers*, 241.
19. Ibid., 244.
20. Ibid.
21. Ibid., 247.
22. *Cleveland Press* clipping, July 29, 1950, in Scrapbook (1950–1952), AA Archives-NYC.
23. Alcoholics Anonymous, "The Big Book," 1955 ed., 490–491.
24. "California—Readers Digest," box 5, MMP.
25. See the "To Wives" chapter in Alcoholics Anonymous, "The Big Book," 1955 (note that the chapter was not entitled "To Spouses"); for discussion of the authorship of that chapter, see Darrah, *Sister Ignatia*, 122.
26. Alcoholics Anonymous, "The Big Book," 1955 ed., 269, 273.
27. Woolf, "The Sick Person We Call an Alcoholic," MMP.

28. Eleanor Roberts, "Women Drunkards, Pitiful Creatures, Get Helping Hand," [Boston, no newspaper name], in Scrapbook (1939–1942), AA Archives-NYC.
29. Ibid.
30. "Atlantic City Speech," box 1, MMP.
31. See, e.g., the plea by Joe, who founded a group in the Bronx in 1944. "'More women,' says Joe. 'We need more women at our meetings.'" *Grapevine* 1, no. 5 (October 1944), MMP.
32. For discussion of the relative comfort women found in cities as opposed to small towns or rural areas and the 25–40 percent figure for some large cities, see "Women in A.A. 1st Groups—Corr." See also "Thoughts re: Bill and Women Members," handwritten note in folder "Women in AA: General," on women in the South facing particularly acute issues of shame and stigma. See also J. D. Owens, "Women Drunks Win Sympathy," *Detroit Times*, September 30, 1953, in folder "Women in AA: General." On women outnumbering men, see "Women Alcoholics Outnumber Men," *Argus Press* (Owosso, Michigan), January 11, 1950, in Scrapbook (1950–1952). See also "Old Topers Ask Ladies to Join Them on Wagon," *Chicago Tribune*, June 9, 1943, in Scrapbook (1943) on Chicago; "Women in AA: 1st Groups—Corr," on New York in early 1940s; an undated clipping states that New York City alone had sixty women in AA (see Josephine Horen, "More Women Joining Group to Cure Selves of Drinking," *White Plains (New York) Reporter Dispatch* (n.d.), in Scrapbook (1943)). All of the foregoing sources are from AA Archives-NYC. "War's Strains Seen as Peril to Alcoholics," *Jacksonville (Florida) Times-Union*, March 25, 1945, MMP, quotes Mann as saying that more than one third of AA members in New York were women.
33. Alcoholics Anonymous, "The Big Book," 1955 ed., 330–331.
34. Ibid., 519–520.
35. Ibid., 492–493.
36. Ibid., 415. She does not identify Mann by full name but we can be reasonably certain it was she, given Mann's prominence in the New York fellowship. Her observation that Mann was "neither a bloated wreck nor a reformer" likely pleased Mann, who sought to maintain a sophisticated image as part of her public health campaign.
37. "Mrs. Mann (Personal Letters), 1946–47," box 1; "Mrs. Mann (Personal Letters), February 1949–1950," box 2; "MM-Personal Letters, 1958–1960," box 2, MMP.
38. "Mrs. Mann (Personal Letters), 1946–47," box 1, MMP.
39. "Mrs. Mann (Personal Letters), February 1949 to 1950," box 2, MMP.
40. Lillian Roth, *I'll Cry Tomorrow* (New York: Frederick Fell Publishers, 1954), 198.
41. Ibid., 218, 214, 222.
42. Ibid., 233–235.
43. "Thoughts re: Bill and Women Members," handwritten notes, no author, n.d., in folder "Women in AA: General." The May 1945 issue of the *Grapevine* (vol. 1) included several articles about women in the fellowship; see the folder "Women in AA: General." Also see the *Cleveland Press* clipping, July 29, 1950, in Scrapbook (1950–1952), all in AA Archives-NYC.
44. New Jersey police chief: see Josephine Horen, "More Women Joining Group to Cure Selves of Drinking," *White Plains (New York) Reporter Dispatch* (n.d.), in Scrapbook (1943), AA Archives-NYC. Harvard psychiatrist: see "What about Women Alcoholics?" (p. 43), in folder "Women in AA: General," AA Archives-NYC.
45. "Women in AA: First Groups," AA Archives-NYC.

46. "Women's Group of San Diego—1945," typed pages with cover note dated April 27, 1948, in folder "Women in AA—1st Groups Corr," AA Archives-NYC.
47. "MM—Personal Letters—1961–1964," box 2, MMP.
48. "Women in AA: First Groups," AA Archives-NYC.
49. Other scholars have examined this tension; see esp. Travis, *The Language of the Heart*.
50. Charles E. Schamel, "The Washington Group: Foundations, 1936–1941" (Washington, DC: Washington Area Intergroup Association, Intergroup Archives Project, rev. exp. ed., 1995), 54; held in AA Archives-NYC.
51. *Dr. Bob and the Good Oldtimers*, 247–248.
52. Reference to the "Negro problem" in a group in correspondence, but no details are provided, not even the location of the group ("Women in AA: 1st Groups—Corr."); numeric estimate is in a clipping on the 1950 Cleveland convention, Scrapbook (1950–52), AA Archives-NYC.
53. Alcoholics Anonymous, "The Big Book," 1955 ed.; see also Kurtz, *Not-God*.
54. Darrah, *Sister Ignatia*, 83.
55. Charles C. Hewitt, "A Personality Study of Alcohol Addiction," *Quarterly Journal of Studies on Alcohol* 4, no. 3 (December 1943): 376.
56. "'New Horizons in the Prevention of Alcoholism.' Address given by Mrs. Mann at Boston, on October 4, 1950," MMP. Mann notes in this speech that the attitude had changed over the previous ten years, with the new goal being to bring the "crisis" to the man, rather than waiting for the man to hit the crisis.
57. Alcoholics Anonymous, "The Big Book," 1955 ed., 266.
58. Ibid., 413. Such an overt reference in the narratives to the physical danger and vulnerability that alcoholic women were exposed to was rare.
59. Ibid., 378, 518.
60. "Old Topers Ask Ladies to Join Them on Wagon," *Chicago Tribune*, June 9, 1943, in Scrapbook (1943), AA Archives-NYC.
61. Chas. Neville, "Now 'Alcoholics Anonymous' Tackles the Lady Souse Problem," newspaper article, November 6, [1943?], in Scrapbook (1943), AA Archives-NYC.
62. "A.A.'s Country-Wide News Circuit," *Grapevine* 1, no. 12 (May 1945): 7, in folder "Women in AA: General," AA Archives-NYC.
63. This account is drawn from Schamel, "The Washington Group." See also "Women in AA: 1st Groups—Corr," AA Archives-NYC.
64. "Monument to AA," photocopied clipping, no newspaper title or date, in folder "Women in AA: General," AA Archives-NYC. See also *Dr. Bob and the Good Oldtimers*, 244, for memories of how Ethel sponsored many women. See also Darrah, *Sister Ignatia*, 124–125.
65. See Brown and Brown, *Mrs. Marty Mann*.
66. *Pass It On: The Story of Bill Wilson and How the AA Message Reached the World* (New York: Alcoholics Anonymous World Services, 1984), 310–311, in AA Archives-NYC. For more on these episodes, see Brown and Brown, *Mrs. Marty Mann*, esp. chapter 18, "Rocking the Boat." See also Bruce Holley Johnson, "The Alcoholism Movement in America: A Study in Cultural Innovation" (Ph.D. diss., University of Illinois, 1973).
67. *Alcoholics Anonymous Comes of Age: A Brief History of Alcoholics Anonymous* (New York: Alcoholics Anonymous World Services, 1957), 199.
68. *Dr. Bob and the Good Oldtimers*, 241.
69. Travis, *The Language of the Heart*, 102.

4. Defining a Disease: Gender, Stigma, and the Modern Alcoholism Movement

1. "Lady Lushes on the Loose!" *New York Daily Mirror Sunday Magazine*, December 20, 1944, Marty Mann Papers, Special Collections Research Center, Syracuse University Libraries (hereafter MMP).
2. "Women Nowadays Called 'Hard' Drinkers," *New York Herald-Tribune*, January 5, 1947; "A Growing Liability: The Woman 'Bar Fly,'" *New York Daily Mirror*, January 5, 1948, MMP.
3. Noel F. Busch, "Lady Tipplers," *Life* 22 (April 14, 1947): 85; "Mrs. Drunkard," *Newsweek* 31 (March 8, 1948): Clippings, MMP.
4. H. I. Phillips, "The Sun Dial," *New York Sun*, January 27, 1947, MMP.
5. Ron Roizen, "The American Discovery of Alcoholism, 1933–1939" (Ph.D. diss., University of California, Berkeley, 1991); Barron H. Lerner, *One for the Road: Drunk Driving since 1900* (Baltimore: Johns Hopkins University Press, 2011).
6. Although the NCEA is today known as the National Council on Alcoholism and Drug Dependence, it did not change its name and mission until 1990. See National Council on Alcoholism and Drug Dependence, "A Symbol of Help and Hope" (New York: National Council on Alcoholism and Drug Dependence, n.d.), ncadd.org/images/stories/PDF/history_charts_60_years_1944_2004.pdf. See also William L. White, *Slaying the Dragon: The History of Addiction Treatment and Recovery in America* (Bloomington, IL: Chestnut Hill Health Systems, 1998), 197. Transsexuals and homosexuals also created taxonomies for the same reasons during the mid-twentieth century; see Joanne Meyerowitz, *How Sex Changed: A History of Transsexuality in the United States* (Cambridge, MA: Harvard University Press, 2002), 176–185.
7. Sally Brown and David R. Brown, *Mrs. Marty Mann: The First Lady of Alcoholics Anonymous* (Center City, MN: Hazelden / Pittman Archives Press, 2001), 246.
8. David E. Kyvig, *Repealing National Prohibition* (Chicago: University of Chicago Press, 1979; rev. ed., 2000), 186–187 and throughout.
9. Catherine G. Murdock, *Domesticating Drink: Women, Men, and Alcohol in America, 1870–1940* (Baltimore: Johns Hopkins University Press, 1998).
10. Kyvig, *Repealing National Prohibition*, 28.
11. W. J. Rorabaugh, "Drinking in the 'Thin Man' Films, 1934–1947," *Social History of Alcohol and Drugs* 18 (2003): 51–68.
12. Norman H. Clark, *The Dry Years: Prohibition and Social Change in Washington*, rev. ed. (Seattle: University of Washington Press, 1988), 268 and 270.
13. Meyerowitz, *How Sex Changed*, 65.
14. See, e.g., Busch, "Lady Tipplers"; "Mrs. Drunkard"; "Dressing for the Cocktail Lounge," *Christian Century* 54 (January 20, 1937): 75–77.
15. Jack S. Blocker, "Did Prohibition Really Work? Alcohol Prohibition as a Public Health Innovation," *American Journal of Public Health* 96 (February 2006): 240–241; J. W. Riley, Jr., C. F. Marden, and M. Lifshitz, "The Motivational Pattern of Drinking," *Quarterly Journal of Studies on Alcohol* 9 (1948–1949): 353–362; C. A. Hecht, R. J. Grine, and S. E. Rothrock, "The Drinking and Dating Habits of 336 College Women in a Coeducational Institution," *Quarterly Journal of Studies on Alcohol* 9 (1948–1949): 252. See also John C. Burnham, *Bad Habits: Drinking, Smoking, Taking Drugs, Gambling, Sexual Misbehavior, and Swearing in American History* (New York: New York University Press, 1993), Chapter 3, "Drinking," 50–85; and Mark Edward Lender and James Kirby Martin, *Drinking in America: A History* (New York: Free Press, 1987).

16. Merton M. Hyman et al., *Drinkers, Drinking, and Alcohol-Related Mortality and Hospitalizations* (New Brunswick, NJ: Center of Alcohol Studies, Rutgers University, 1980); Lori Rotskoff, *Love on the Rocks: Men, Women, and Alcohol in Post–World War II America* (Chapel Hill: University of North Carolina Press, 2002), 52–53.
17. Rotskoff, *Love on the Rocks*, 52.
18. Pamela E. Pennock, *Advertising Sin and Sickness: The Politics of Alcohol and Tobacco Marketing, 1950–1990* (DeKalb: Northern Illinois University Press, 2007), 45.
19. Hecht, Grine, and Rothrock, "The Drinking and Dating Habits of 336 College Women," 252.
20. Phillips, "The Sun Dial"; "Lady Lushes on the Loose!"
21. "Why Some Women Should Not Drink," *Cosmopolitan*, n.d., n.p.; "Women Are Drinking Too Much," *Facts*, n.d., n.p., MMP.
22. Rotskoff, *Love on the Rocks*, 85.
23. Ibid., 54–56.
24. "Women Who Drink," *Sunday Mirror*, n.d., MMP.
25. Christine Jorgensen offers intriguing parallels. Both she and Mann claimed that science had liberated them, and while both cultivated some aspects of conventional femininity, especially in appearance and demeanor, they also demonstrated assertiveness and authority. See Meyerowitz, *How Sex Changed*.
26. This paragraph and the following two paragraphs are drawn from materials related to the history and bylaws of the National Committee for Education on Alcoholism, MMP; as well as "Committee for Education on Alcoholism Historic Event, Says Dwight Anderson," *Grapevine* 1, no. 5 (October 1944), MMP; Bruce Holley Johnson, "The Alcoholism Movement in America: A Study in Cultural Innovation" (Ph.D. diss., University of Illinois, 1973), 249, 266–275; and Brown and Brown, *Mrs. Marty Mann*, 155, 158. See also Ernest Kurtz, *Not-God: A History of Alcoholics Anonymous* (Center City, MN: Hazelden Educational Services, 1979), 117–119.
27. White, *Slaying the Dragon*, chapters 19–20.
28. Brown and Brown, *Mrs. Marty Mann*, 155–156, describe how Mann reworked earlier formulations by Dwight Anderson.
29. Mann to Howard Haggard, August 10, 1948, quoted in Johnson, "The Alcoholism Movement in America," 291. Trysh Travis explains how the "disease model" of alcoholism functioned as a metaphor in her *Language of the Heart: A Cultural History of the Recovery Movement from Alcoholics Anonymous to Oprah Winfrey* (Chapel Hill: University of North Carolina Press, 2009), chapter 1. She couples her analysis of the cultural influence of this metaphor with a consideration of the "material conditions and the communications structures" through which it gained and exercised power (58).
30. "Transcript of Keynote Address," MMP. For more on tuberculosis during the early twentieth century, see Sheila M. Rothman, *Living in the Shadow of Death: Tuberculosis and the Social Experience of Illness in American History* (Baltimore: Johns Hopkins University Press, 1994), esp. pt. 4.
31. "Memo on: National Committee for Education on Alcoholism," MMP.
32. S. J. Woolf, "The Sick Person We Call an Alcoholic," *New York Times Magazine*, April 21, 1946, MMP.
33. Typed fragment, folder "NCA—Historical," box 3; "Memo on: NCEA," folder "NCA—Historical," box 3, MMP.

34. Kenneth D. Rose, *American Women and the Repeal of Prohibition* (New York: New York University Press, 1996); and Murdock, "Domesticating Drink."
35. "Adelaide Hawley Program—WEAF (June 5, 1945)," MMP.
36. Ernest H. Cherrington, *Standard Encyclopedia of the Alcohol Problem* (Westerville, OH: American Issue Publishing Co., 1928), 4:1850–1852; D. Leigh Colvin, *Prohibition in the United States* (New York: George H. Doran Co., 1926), 321–322; and Herbert Ashbury, *The Great Illusion: An Informal History of Prohibition* (New York: Greenwood Press, 1968), 117–120. Many writers who regard Prohibition as a failure, even a tragic mistake, depict Nation with condescending language, for example: "Motivated by prurience and sexual nausea, she was part fraud, part fanatic, but not a total fool." See Sean Dennis Cashman, *Prohibition: The Lie of the Land* (New York: Free Press, 1981), ix.
37. Dorothy Jones, "500,000 U.S. Women Victims of Alcoholism, Speaker Says," *Detroit News*, November 25, 1946; and "Women Drinkers," *Erie (Pennsylvania) Times*, December 2 [no year], MMP.
38. Woolf, "The Sick Person We Call an Alcoholic."
39. Ibid.
40. My thinking here is influenced by Regina Morantz-Sanchez in her *Conduct Unbecoming a Woman: Medicine on Trial in Turn-of-the-Century Brooklyn* (New York: Oxford University Press, 1999) and how Dr. Mary Dixon-Jones used various professional scripts to define herself as a female physician and surgeon.
41. Brown and Brown, *Mrs. Marty Mann*, 179–182. See also Kurtz, *Not-God*; and Johnson, "The Alcoholism Movement in America."
42. Brown and Brown, *Mrs. Marty Mann*, 243–245.
43. See, e.g., Edith S. Lisansky, "Alcoholism in Women: Social and Psychological Concomitants," *Quarterly Journal of Studies on Alcohol* 18 (1957): 588–623.
44. Wallace Mason Yater, *Fundamentals of Internal Medicine* (New York: D. Appleton-Century Co., 1944), 609–612. The section was little changed in subsequent editions, suggesting that Mann's public health message did not immediately influence these domains.
45. See Kaye Middleton Fillmore, "The Epidemiology of Alcohol Use and Abuse among Women: A History of Science Approach," *Bulletin of the Society of Psychologists in Addictive Behaviors* 3, no. 3 (1982): 130–136.
46. E. M. Jellinek, "Phases in the Drinking History of Alcoholics," *Quarterly Journal of Studies on Alcohol* 7 (1946): 1–88, esp. 1–3. I discuss the psychiatric approach in chapter 5.
47. Ibid., 6–7.
48. Ironically, despite becoming known as the father of the modern disease model, Jellinek himself came to dislike a simple equation of alcoholism and disease, arguing later in his career that many subtypes of alcoholism existed. Nonetheless, his early concepts had considerable staying power in both scholarly literature and public understanding. Some of his other writings include Howard W. Haggard and E. M. Jellinek, *Alcohol Explored* (New York: Doubleday, Doran, and Co., 1942); and E. M. Jellinek, "Phases of Alcohol Addiction," *Quarterly Journal of Studies on Alcohol* 13 (1952): 673–684.
49. Jellinek, "Phases in the Drinking History of Alcoholics," 6.
50. Jellinek, in ibid., analyzed ninety-eight of the surveys; in addition to women's responses, he excluded seventeen that featured insufficient information—not listing age in relation to questions for example—and twenty-eight that represented the

average responses of an AA group rather than individual data. It is possible that some of these respondents were women as well.

51. E. M. Jellinek, "Recent Trends in Alcoholism and in Alcohol Consumption," *Quarterly Journal of Studies on Alcohol* 8 (1947): 1–43; N. Jolliffe, "The Alcoholic Admissions to Bellevue Hospital," *Science* 83 (March 27, 1936): 306–309; F. Lemere, P. O'Hallaren, and M. A. Maxwell, "Sex Ratio of Alcoholic Patients Treated over a 20-Year Period," *Quarterly Journal of Studies on Alcohol* 17 (1956): 437–442; J. V. Lowrie and F. G. Ebaugh, "A Post-Repeal Study of 300 Chronic Alcoholics," *American Journal of Medical Science* 203 (1942): 120–124; and B. Malzberg, "First Admissions with Alcoholic Psychoses in New York State," *Quarterly Journal of Studies on Alcohol* 10 (1949): 461–470.
52. Jellinek, "Phases in the Drinking History of Alcoholics," 79.
53. Twila Florence Fort, "A Preliminary Study of Social Factors in the Alcoholism of Women" (M.A. thesis, Texas Christian University, 1949), 1, 4. The discussion in the following four paragraphs is based on the Fort thesis.
54. See ibid., 10, for focus of Fort's study.
55. Ibid., 28.
56. Ibid., 26–27.
57. Ibid., 37.
58. Ibid., 5, 26.
59. Brown and Brown, *Mrs. Marty Mann*, 220.
60. Marty Mann, *Marty Mann's New Primer on Alcoholism* (1950; rev. ed., New York: Rinehart, 1958), 215.
61. Ibid., 10–11.
62. Ibid., 215.
63. Travis, *Language of the Heart*, 63.
64. Robin Room, "Alcoholism and Alcoholics Anonymous in U.S. Films, 1945–1962: The Party Ends for the 'Wet Generations,'" *Journal of Studies on Alcohol* 50 (1989): 368–383. See also Rotskoff, *Love on the Rocks*, for analysis of films of this era.
65. Brown and Brown, *Mrs. Marty Mann*, 177; Johnson, "The Alcoholism Movement in America," 282–283.
66. In her essay "Beyond the Feminine Mystique," Joanne Meyerowitz shows that stories in women's magazines celebrated the accomplishments of high-achieving career women like Mann. That Mann had herself overcome alcoholism would have reinforced the inspirational message that Meyerowitz identified here. See Joanne Meyerowitz, "Beyond the Feminine Mystique: A Reassessment of Postwar Mass Culture, 1946–1958," in *Not June Cleaver: Women and Gender in Postwar America, 1945–1960*, ed. Joanne Meyerowitz (Philadelphia: Temple University Press, 1994), 229–262.

5. "A Special Masculine Neurosis": Psychiatrists Look at Alcoholism

1. Douglas Noble, "Psychodynamics of Alcoholism in a Woman," *Psychiatry* 12 (1949): 413–425. The discussion in the following five paragraphs is based on this article, and the quotations are drawn from it.
2. The collection edited by Joanne Meyerowitz, *Not June Cleaver: Women and Gender in Postwar America, 1945–1960* (Philadelphia: Temple University Press, 1994), makes this point convincingly.
3. Ellen Herman, *The Romance of American Psychology: Political Culture in the Age of Experts* (Berkeley: University of California Press, 1995); and Andrea Tone, *The*

Age of Anxiety: A History of America's Turbulent Affair with Tranquilizers (New York: Basic Books, 2009). See also Elizabeth Lunbeck, *The Psychiatric Persuasion: Knowledge, Gender, and Power in Modern America* (Princeton, NJ: Princeton University Press, 1994). On psychoanalysis, see Nathan G. Hale, Jr., *The Rise and Crisis of Psychoanalysis in the United States: Freud and the Americans, 1917–1985* (New York: Oxford University Press, 1995); and Mari Jo Buhle, *Feminism and Its Discontents: A Century of Struggle with Psychoanalysis* (Cambridge, MA: Harvard University Press, 1998).

4. Kenneth J. Tillotson and Robert Fleming, "Personality and Sociological Factors in the Prognosis and Treatment of Chronic Alcoholism," *New England Journal of Medicine* 217, no. 16 (October 14, 1937): 611.
5. American Psychiatric Association Committee on Nomenclature and Statistics, *Diagnostic and Statistical Manual: Mental Disorders* (Washington, DC: American Psychiatric Association, 1952), with alcoholism as personality disorder described on 39. The first edition is now referred to as *DSM-I*.
6. Marty Mann Papers, Special Collections Research Center, Syracuse University Libraries (hereafter MMP).
7. Lori Rotskoff, *Love on the Rocks: Men, Women and Alcohol in Post–World War II America* (Chapel Hill: University of North Carolina Press, 2002), analyzes the ways in which psychiatrists and psychiatric social workers understood men's alcoholism and recovery as part of a "gender crisis" and the need to return to conventional roles in marriage after World War II.
8. R. S. Banay, "Cultural Influences in Alcoholism," *Journal of Nervous and Mental Disease* 102 (1945): 265–275; A. Meyerson, "Alcohol: A Study of Social Ambivalence," *Quarterly Journal of Studies on Alcohol* 1 (1940–1941): 13–20; and J. P. Shalloo, "Some Cultural Factors in the Etiology of Alcoholism," *Quarterly Journal of Studies on Alcohol* 2 (1941–1942): 464–478.
9. Banay, "Cultural Influences in Alcoholism," 269.
10. Simon Weijl, "Theoretical and Practical Aspects of Psychoanalytic Therapy of Problem Drinkers," *Quarterly Journal of Studies on Alcohol* 5 (1944–1945): 206–208.
11. J. H. Wall, "A Study of Alcoholism in Men," *American Journal of Psychiatry* 92 (1936): 1391.
12. R. P. Knight, "The Psychoanalytic Treatment in a Sanatorium of Chronic Addiction to Alcohol," *Journal of the American Medical Association* 111 (October 15, 1938): 1444.
13. R. P. Knight, "The Psychodynamics of Chronic Alcoholism," *Journal of Nervous and Mental Diseases* 86 (November 1937): 544; Harold W. Lovell, *Hope and Help for the Alcoholic* (Garden City, NY: Doubleday, 1951), 76; Knight, "The Psychoanalytic Treatment in a Sanatorium," 1444. See also M. M. Miller, "Treatment of Chronic Alcoholism by Hypnotic Aversion," *Journal of the American Medical Association* 171, no. 11 (November 14, 1959): 167.
14. J. Levine, "The Sexual Adjustment of Alcoholics," *Quarterly Journal of Studies on Alcohol* 16 (1955): 679.
15. Banay, "Cultural Influences in Alcoholism," 273.
16. See Karl Abraham, "The Psychological Relations between Sexuality and Alcoholism," *International Journal of Psycho-analysis* 8 (1926): 2–10.
17. Knight, "The Psychodynamics of Chronic Alcoholism," 545.
18. Weijl, "Theoretical and Practical Aspects of Psychoanalytic Therapy of Problem Drinkers," 202.

19. See John D'Emilio, "The Homosexual Menace: The Politics of Sexuality in Cold War America," in *Passion and Power: Sexuality in History*, ed. Kathy Peiss and Christina Simmons (Philadelphia: Temple University Press, 1989), 226–240.
20. Edward A. Strecker, *Their Mothers' Sons: The Psychiatrist Examines an American Problem* (Philadelphia: Lippincott, 1951), esp. chap. "Mom in a Bottle"; quoted on 14, 122, 125.
21. Charles H. Durfee, "Some Practical Observations on the Treatment of Problem Drinkers," *Quarterly Journal of Studies on Alcohol* 7, no. 2 (September 1946): 234.
22. Few alcoholic patients were psychoanalyzed because of the length and cost of psychoanalytic treatment, but many psychiatrists, even those who had not received psychoanalytic training, were clearly influenced by psychoanalytic theory. See, for example, Knight, "The Psychoanalytic Treatment in a Sanatorium," 1443–1448. Mann's correspondence also reflects the influence of psychoanalytic language and concepts, and several of her correspondents spent time at the Menninger Clinic, where Knight worked.
23. Durfee, "Some Practical Observations."
24. Weijl, "Theoretical and Practical Aspects," 210–211.
25. Wall, "A Study of Alcoholism in Men," 1400.
26. D. J. Myerson, "An Active Therapeutic Method of Interrupting the Dependence Relationships of Certain Male Alcoholics," *Quarterly Journal of Studies on Alcohol* 14 (1953): 423–424.
27. Strecker, *Their Mothers' Sons*, 125.
28. Obituary for Benjamin Karpman, M.D. (1886–1962), *American Journal of Psychiatry* 119 (May 1, 1963): 1119–1120.
29. Benjamin Karpman, *The Alcoholic Woman: Case Studies in the Psychodynamics of Alcoholism* (Washington, DC: Linacre Press, 1948), x.
30. Ibid., vii.
31. Ibid., 187, 217, 233.
32. Rosenbaum calls the mothers of the alcoholic women in her study "ungiving" and the fathers "ineffectual"; see B. Rosenbaum, "Married Women Alcoholics at the Washingtonian Hospital," *Quarterly Journal of Studies on Alcohol* 19 (1958): 85–86. Dorothy Jean Deex, "A Study of the Housewife Role among Alcoholic Women In-Patients at the Washingtonian Hospital" (M.S. thesis, Boston University School of Social Work, 1954), cites a "lack of preparation" for the role of homemaker, 18. See also Twila Florence Fort, "A Preliminary Study of Social Factors in the Alcoholism of Women" (M.A. thesis, Texas Christian University, 1949), 169.
33. Karpman, *The Alcoholic Woman*, details in "The Case of Miss Elizabeth Chesser," 3–65; and F. J. Curran, "Personality Studies in Alcoholic Women," *Journal of Nervous and Mental Disease* 86 (1937): 656–664.
34. This tension was not unique to psychiatric discussions of alcoholism. Doctors who treated "nymphomania," psychologists and physicians who cared for transsexual patients, and other mental health professionals who dealt with family conflict all contributed to a potential questioning of conventional gender roles and behaviors. Psychology could be "politically flexible," but it retained a focus on individual adjustment through therapy. See, for example, Carol Groneman, *Nymphomania: A History* (New York: W. W. Norton, 2000), 81, on how doctors insisted that their female patients must accept femininity. See also Herman, *The Romance of American Psychology*; and Joanne Meyerowitz, *How Sex Changed: A History of Transsexuality in the United States* (Cambridge, MA: Harvard University Press, 2002).

35. Curran, "Personality Studies," 649; R. J. Van Amberg, "A Study of 50 Women Patients Hospitalized for Alcohol Addiction," *Diseases of the Nervous System* 3–4 (1943): 250; James H. Wall, "A Study of Alcoholism in Women," *American Journal of Psychiatry* 93 (1937): 944; and H. Wortis and L. R. Sillman, eds., "Case Histories of Compulsive Drinkers," *Quarterly Journal of Studies on Alcohol* 6 (1945–46): 320–321. On the pattern of masculinity, see L. Sillman, "Chronic Alcoholism," *Journal of Nervous and Mental Diseases* 107 (1948): 140–141.
36. Joanne Meyerowitz shows how doctors' focus on unconventional childhood behavior reflected an active attempt by scientists and medical professionals to understand biological sex differences and gender formation in the middle decades of the twentieth century (*How Sex Changed*, 98–99). Medical discourse on infertile women echoed this theme, similarly emphasizing the nonconforming childhood behavior of women who sought treatment for infertility. See Elaine Tyler May, *Barren in the Promised Land: Childless Americans and the Pursuit of Happiness* (New York: Basic Books, 1995), 174.
37. Edith S. Lisansky, "Alcoholism in Women: Social and Psychological Concomitants," *Quarterly Journal of Studies on Alcohol* 18 (1957): 614. See also Wall, "A Study of Alcoholism in Women." Men's reasons for drinking often included vague moods, such as boredom, irritability, or shyness.
38. Joseph Hirsh, *The Problem Drinker* (New York: Duell, Sloan, & Pearce, 1949), 50.
39. Sarah Stage, *Female Complaints: Lydia Pinkham and the Business of Women's Medicine* (New York: W. W. Norton, 1979), 244.
40. As in the nineteenth century, some women were not drinking liquor, as such; they were using remedies that had high alcohol content. See Hirsh, *The Problem Drinker*, 50, who warns against this practice. See also C. Landis and J. F. Cushman, eds., "Case Studies of Compulsive Drinkers," *Quarterly Journal of Studies on Alcohol* 6 (1945–1946): 167; N. D. C. Lewis, "Personality Factors in Alcoholic Addiction," *Quarterly Journal of Studies on Alcohol* 1 (1940–1941): 41; Van Amberg, "A Study of 50 Women Patients," 249; Durfee, "Some Practical Observations," 237–238; Fort, "A Preliminary Study," 121, 152; and Rosenbaum, "Married Women Alcoholics," 88.
41. Wall, "A Study of Alcoholism in Women," 944.
42. Lisansky, "Alcoholism in Women," 591.
43. Some of the most prominent researchers on alcohol questions, including E. M. Jellinek, dismissed the idea that alcohol damaged germ cells or produced deformities in children. See Moira Plant, *Women, Drinking, and Pregnancy* (London: Tavistock Publications, 1985), 14–15.
44. Anne Roe, "The Adult Adjustment of Children of Alcoholics Raised in Foster Homes," *Quarterly Journal of Studies on Alcohol* 5 (1944): 378–393.
45. "Questions and Answers," *Hygeia* 14 (March 1936): 285. See also T. Swann Harding, "Alcohol, Health, Longevity, and Offspring," *American Journal of Pharmacy* 111 (1939): 351–358; and Paul Popenoe, "Heredity and Environment as Related to Alcoholism," *Eugenical News* (1946–1947): 35–38.
46. "Queries and Minor Notes: Effect of Single Large Alcohol Intake on Fetus," *Journal of the American Medical Association* 120 (1942): 88; "Queries and Minor Notes: Effect of Alcoholism at Time of Conception," *Journal of the American Medical Association* 132 (1946): 419; "Queries and Minor Notes: Smoking and Drinking during Pregnancy," *Journal of the American Medical Association* 154 (1954): 186; "Queries and Minor Notes: Alcoholism and Heredity," *Journal of the American*

Medical Association 136 (1948): 849; and "Notes and Queries: Alcohol and Pregnancy," *Practitioner* 160 (1948): 73. See also Hirsh, *The Problem Drinker*, 50–51, who maintains that alcohol consumed by the mother is not harmful to the fetus or to the nursing infant. For detailed discussion of developments in science that affected these issues, see Philip J. Pauly, "How Did the Effects of Alcohol on Reproduction Become Scientifically Uninteresting?" *Journal of the History of Biology* 29 (1996): 1–28.

47. Cited in May, *Barren in the Promised Land*, 161; see also 141–142. May, 194, also notes that the assumption that women were "naturally fulfilled in motherhood" was so strong that "anxiety or ambivalence surrounding pregnancy was actually considered a pathological condition."
48. Rebecca Plant, *Mom: The Transformation of American Motherhood in Modern America* (Chicago: University of Chicago Press, 2010).
49. H. H. Hart, "Personality Factors in Alcoholism," *Archives of Neurology and Psychiatry* 24 (1930): 130; Rosenbaum, "Married Women Alcoholics," 86; I. Wolf, "Alcoholism and Marriage," *Quarterly Journal of Studies on Alcohol* 19 (1958): 511–513; and Wortis and Sillman, "Case Histories," 310. On hostility toward children, see Deex, "A Study of the Housewife Role," 55.
50. Wall, "A Study of Alcoholism in Women," 948.
51. Karpman, *The Alcoholic Woman*, 231.
52. Fort, "A Preliminary Study," 176.
53. Brett Harvey, *The Fifties: A Women's Oral History* (New York: HarperCollins, 1993), 125–126.
54. Wall, "A Study of Alcoholism in Women," 947.
55. Karpman, *The Alcoholic Woman*, 231. See Lunbeck, *The Psychiatric Persuasion*, 72–74, for a discussion of psychiatrists' "faintly feminist" but inconsistent perspective on issues of gender and sexuality.
56. Wall, "A Study of Alcoholism in Women," 947. Reflecting different orientations in their training, and perhaps the fact that they were more likely to be women themselves, social workers were more likely to address family issues, although not necessarily social constraints, in treatment. Their approach is discussed further in chapter 6.
57. See Elaine Tyler May, *Homeward Bound: American Families in the Cold War Era* (New York: Basic Books, 1988), on the sexualized wife and mother and sexual containment. See John D'Emilio and Estelle B. Freedman, *Intimate Matters: A History of Sexuality in America* (New York: Harper & Row, 1988), 241, on "sexual liberalism." Also see Lunbeck, *The Psychiatric Persuasion*, 308; and Groneman, *Nymphomania*.
58. Karpman, *The Alcoholic Woman*, 16, 117, 147.
59. Fort, "A Preliminary Study," 91.
60. Karpman, *The Alcoholic Woman*, 227. Karpman was not alone in holding this view; other experts claimed that women had an "unconscious desire" to be raped; see Rotskoff, *Love on the Rocks*, 156.
61. Shalloo, "Some Cultural Factors," 472.
62. Fort, "A Preliminary Study," 224; also see 82, 130.
63. Ibid., 269; and Landis and Cushman, "Case Studies," 166–167.
64. Fort, "A Preliminary Study," 289–290.
65. Ibid., 226, 175.
66. Rosenbaum, "Married Women Alcoholics," 86; and Wolf, "Alcoholism and Marriage," 511–513. Also see Fort, "A Preliminary Study," 19, 25, and, on marriage

being an independent and dependent variable in alcoholism, for examples, see 193, 197, 242, 280. See also Deex, "A Study of the Housewife Role," 76, 80; and Karpman, *The Alcoholic Woman*, 125–126.

67. In *Nymphomania*, Groneman describes this apparent paradox as well. See esp. 39–45.
68. Banay, "Cultural Influences in Alcoholism," 267. A similar case was reported by Hart, "Personality Factors," 127. See also Curran, "Personality Studies," 649–650; Levine, "The Sexual Adjustment of Alcoholics," 676–677; Wall, "A Study of Alcoholism in Women," 944–945; Van Amberg, "A Study of 50 Women Patients," 250; Wortis and Sillman, "Case Histories," 322; and Tillotson and Fleming, "Personality and Sociologic Factors," 613.
69. Roth and Burt later divorced, but at the time of her memoir and the film based on it, the marriage was portrayed as affectionate and successful. See Lillian Roth, *I'll Cry Tomorrow* (New York: Frederick Fell Publishers, 1954).
70. Curran, "Personality Studies," 665; and Levine, "The Sexual Adjustment of Alcoholics," 677.
71. Elizabeth Lapovsky Kennedy and Madeline Davis, "The Reproduction of Butch-Fem Roles: A Social Constructionist Approach," in Peiss and Simmons, *Passion and Power*, 241–256. See also Lillian Faderman, *Odd Girls and Twilight Lovers: A History of Lesbian Life in Twentieth-Century America* (New York: Columbia University Press, 1991).
72. See, for example, George Chauncey, *Gay New York: Gender, Urban Culture, and the Making of the Gay Male World, 1890–1940* (New York: Basic Books, 1994).
73. Compare Hart, "Personality Factors," 120, versus Wall, "A Study of Alcoholism in Women," 952.
74. Karpman, *The Alcoholic Woman*, 128, 137, 141.
75. Ibid., 140.
76. N.R. to Mann, n.d., folder "Mrs. Mann (Personal Letters) Jan. 1948–Dec. 1948," box 1, MMP.
77. Sally Brown and David R. Brown, *Mrs. Marty Mann: The First Lady of Alcoholics Anonymous* (Center City, MN: Hazelden/Pittman Archives Press, 2001), esp. chap. 15, "Priscilla."
78. Ron Roizen, personal communication, May 12, 1996.
79. Curran, "Personality Studies," 665. See also William C. Garvin, "Post Prohibition Alcoholic Psychoses in New York State," *American Journal of Psychiatry* 9 (January 1930): 747.
80. Curran, "Personality Studies," 647, 649, for "conscious knowledge." Also see L. L. Orestein and W. Goldfarb, "A Note on the Incidence of Syphilis in Alcoholics," *Quarterly Journal of Studies on Alcohol* 1 (1940–1941): 442–443.

6. "The Doctor Didn't Want to Take an Alcoholic":
The Challenge of Medicalization at Midcentury

1. Wilma Wilson, *They Call Them Camisoles* (Los Angeles: Lymanhouse, 1940). For a contemporary review, see "Woman Who Overindulged Tells Inside Story of 'Cure,'" *Los Angeles Times*, February 16, 1941.
2. See Wilson, *Camisoles*, 129 (for jury trial), 237 (for recoiled in horror).
3. See ibid., 76 (for commitments not in vain), 89 (for too depraved).
4. "Soldier Held in Beach Death," *Los Angeles Times*, June 6, 1943; "Accused's Garb Version Differ at Soldier Trial," *Los Angeles Times*, June 17, 1943; and "Court-Martial Weighs Death," *Los Angeles Times*, June 16, 1943.

5. Alcoholics Anonymous, *Alcoholics Anonymous: The Story of How Many Thousands of Men and Women Have Recovered from Alcoholism*, new and rev. ed. (New York: Alcoholics Anonymous World Services, 1955), 267–268 (hereafter "The Big Book").
6. Ibid., 345–346. It is unclear who had her committed.
7. Ibid., 407.
8. C. N. Davis, "The Alcoholic Problem as the Doctor Views It," *Pennsylvania Medical Journal* 49 (June 1946): 1020, 1024.
9. Alcoholics Anonymous, "The Big Book," 535.
10. "New York—*Readers' Digest*," box 4, Marty Mann Papers, Special Collections Research Center, Syracuse University Libraries (hereafter MMP).
11. On the changing meaning of hospitals over time, see Charles Rosenberg, *The Care of Strangers: The Rise of America's Hospital System* (New York: Basic Books, 1992).
12. Merrill Moore and M. Geneva Gray, "Alcoholism at the Boston City Hospital," *New England Journal of Medicine* 221, no. 2 (July 13, 1939): 47–48.
13. Council on Medical Education and Hospitals, "Hospital Facilities for Alcoholic Patients," *Journal of the American Medical Association* 141 (1949): 620.
14. Ibid., 620–621. The total number of hospitals in the survey was 6,276, with 1,718 accepting alcoholic patients. See Mary C. Darrah, *Sister Ignatia: Angel of Alcoholics Anonymous* (Chicago: Loyola University Press, 1992), 78, on hospitalization.
15. Darrah, *Sister Ignatia*, 83; see also 87–88.
16. M. A. Block, "Alcoholism: The Physician's Duty," *GP* 6, no. 3 (1952): 56.
17. Martha Brunner-Orne, "Treatment and Rehabilitation of Alcohol Addicts in a General Hospital Setting," *Journal of the American Medical Woman's Association* 10 (1955): 195.
18. Marty Mann, *Primer on Alcoholism* (New York: Rinehart & Co., 1950), 111–112.
19. William L. White, *Slaying the Dragon: The History of Addiction Treatment and Recovery in America* (Bloomington, IL: Chestnut Hill Health Systems, 1998), 188. See also Bruce H. Johnson, "The Alcoholism Movement in America: A Study in Cultural Innovation" (Ph.D. diss., University of Illinois, 1973); and A. E. Wilkerson, Jr., "A History of the Concept of Alcoholism as a Disease" (D.S.W. diss., University of Pennsylvania, 1966).
20. Floyd Miller, "What the Alcoholic Owes to Marty Mann," *Reader's Digest* 82 (January 1963): 173–180.
21. "Kansas—*Readers' Digest*," box 4, MMP.
22. Michael M. Miller, "Treatment of Chronic Alcoholism by Hypnotic Aversion," *Journal of the American Medical Association* 171, no. 11 (November 14, 1959): 165.
23. The Washingtonian example is in Dorothy Jean Deex, "A Study of the Housewife Role among Alcoholic Women In-Patients at the Washingtonian Hospital" (M.S. thesis, Boston University School of Social Work, 1954), 79. The binge episode is in Twila Florence Fort, "A Preliminary Study of Social Factors in the Alcoholism of Women" (M.A. thesis, Texas Christian University, 1949), 163.
24. Moore and Gray, "Alcoholism at the Boston City Hospital," 49.
25. Marty Mann, *Marty Mann's New Primer on Alcoholism* (New York: Rinehart & Co., 1958), 213.
26. Paul E. Feldman and Elias Cohen, "A Statistical Study of the Admission of Alcoholic Patients to a Large Mental Hospital," *American Journal of Psychiatry* 111 (1955): 677–679. Feldman and Cohen also reported that, while fewer female than male alcoholics were admitted overall, the alcoholic women were much more

likely to suffer from psychoses. The New York data are in Robert J. Van Amberg, "A Study of 50 Women Patients Hospitalized for Alcohol Addiction," *Diseases of the Nervous System* 3–4 (August 1943): 248. Many psychiatrists expressed concern that it was very difficult to convince patients to stay in the hospital long enough. See, for example, Robert P. Knight, "The Psychoanalytic Treatment in a Sanatorium of Chronic Addiction to Alcohol," *Journal of the American Medical Association* 111, no. 6 (October 15, 1938): 1446.

27. F. J. Curran, "Personality Studies in Alcoholic Women," *Journal of Nervous and Mental Disease* 86 (1937): 645; and Kenneth J. Tillotson and Robert Fleming, "Personality and Sociologic Factors in the Prognosis and Treatment of Chronic Alcoholism," *New England Journal of Medicine* 217, no. 16 (October 14, 1937): 611.

28. Among male patients, alcoholics represented 1.8 percent of all outpatients and 33.6 percent of all inpatients, while for women the corresponding figures were 0.2 percent and 13.5 percent. See Moore and Gray, "Alcoholism at the Boston City Hospital," 46, 48–49.

29. "The Alcoholic in the General Hospital," folder "Mrs. Mann's Manuscripts, 1948–," box 1, MMP.

30. Lillian Roth, *I'll Cry Tomorrow* (New York: Frederick Fell Publishers, 1954), 131–132. Colitis is mentioned on 163.

31. Ibid., 183–189, 191.

32. Ibid., 131–132, 208. In another example, Wall recommended that "warm wet packs and prolonged baths" were superior to sedatives in producing relaxation, but he did not indicate that sedatives could be themselves addictive. See James H. Wall, "A Study of Alcoholism in Men," *American Journal of Psychiatry* 92 (May 1936): 1399.

33. Stephen R. Kandall, *Substance and Shadow: Women and Addiction in the United States* (Cambridge, MA: Harvard University Press, 1996), 138–141. See also Andrea Tone, *The Age of Anxiety: A History of America's Turbulent Affair with Tranquilizers* (New York: Basic Books, 2009); and David Herzberg, *Happy Pills in America: From Miltown to Prozac* (Baltimore: Johns Hopkins University Press, 2009).

34. Harold I. Goldman, "Treatment of Postalcoholic Syndrome with Triflupromazine Hydrochloride," *Journal of the American Medical Association* 171, no. 11 (November 14, 1959): 1502–1503, and "Outpatient Treatment of Postalcoholic Syndrome," *Journal of the American Medical Association* 167 (August 23, 1958): 2069–2071.

35. Douglas Noble, "Psychodynamics of Alcoholism in a Woman," *Psychiatry* 12 (1949): 418, 420.

36. "New Jersey—*Readers' Digest*," box 4, MMP.

37. Herzberg, *Happy Pills*, esp. 83–84, 86, 91–101; and Tone, *The Age of Anxiety*, 142–143, 146.

38. Tone, *The Age of Anxiety*, xii, 80.

39. Other "modern" and "scientific" treatments for alcoholism during this period included antihistamines and the injection of adrenal cortex extract. See Morton M. Stern, "Antihistamine Treatment of Alcoholism," *Journal of Nervous and Mental Diseases* 122 (1955): 198–199; Howard W. Lovell, *Hope and Help for the Alcoholic* (New York: Doubleday, 1956), 168–169; and Mann, *Primer on Alcoholism*, 113.

40. Mann, *Primer on Alcoholism*, 123.

41. Frederick Lemere and Walter L. Votegin et al., "The Conditioned Reflex Treatment of Chronic Alcoholism," *Journal of the American Medical Association* 120, no. 4 (1942): 269–270.

42. C. C. Turner, "The Conditioned Reflex in the Treatment of Alcoholism—Case Reports," *Memphis Medical Journal* 17 (December 1942): 223–224.
43. James H. Wall, "A Study of Alcoholism in Women," *American Journal of Psychiatry* 93 (1937): 950.
44. Miriam Van Waters Papers, Schlesinger Library, Radcliffe College, box 21, file 239 (hereafter MVW Papers). On the increasing commitments of alcoholic women during the 1940s, see Estelle B. Freedman, *Maternal Justice: Miriam Van Waters and the Female Reform Tradition* (Chicago: University of Chicago Press, 1996), 259.
45. Alcoholics Anonymous, "The Big Book," 264.
46. "New York—*Readers' Digest*," box 4, MMP.
47. "New York City—*Readers' Digest*," box 4, MMP.
48. Sheldon Glueck and Eleanor T. Glueck, *Five Hundred Delinquent Women* (New York: Alfred A. Knopf, 1934), 57–59.
49. "Altrusa Project," MVW Papers, box 22, file 247.
50. "New Jersey—*Readers' Digest*," box 4, MMP.
51. "California—*Readers' Digest*," box 4, MMP.
52. Alcoholics Anonymous, "The Big Book," 558.
53. "Fasso Frees Woman to Accept Aid of 'Alcoholics Anonymous,'" *New Rochelle (New York) Standard-Star*, October 14, 1943. See also the Scrapbook (1943), Alcoholics Anonymous Archives—New York City.
54. MVW Papers, box 22, file 249, and box 31, file 397.
55. MVW Papers, box 22, file 247.
56. "Altrusa Project," MVW Papers, box 22, file 247; "People Seen While in Custody at R.W.," MVW Papers, box 22, file 249. See also Freedman, *Maternal Justice*.
57. "Report," MVW Papers, box 22, file 247.
58. Mann, *Marty Mann's New Primer on Alcoholism*, 34.
59. Wilson, *They Call Them Camisoles*, 138.
60. This sentiment started to percolate through alcoholism literature during this mid-century moment. See, for example, Edith S. Lisansky, "Alcoholism in Women: Social and Psychological Concomitants," *Quarterly Journal of Studies on Alcohol* 18 (1957): 588–623; and Charles H. Durfee, "Some Practical Observations on the Treatment of Problem Drinkers," *Quarterly Journal of Studies on Alcohol* 7, no. 2 (September 1946): 228–239.
61. Joanne Meyerowitz, "Beyond the Feminine Mystique," in her *Not June Cleaver: Women and Gender in Postwar America, 1945–1960* (Philadelphia: Temple University Press, 1994), 229–262.
62. Dorothy Jean Deex, "A Study of the Housewife Role among Alcoholic Women In-Patients at the Washingtonian Hospital" (M.S. thesis, Boston University School of Social Work, 1954). This and the following six paragraphs are based on this thesis. Specifics here are on 1–2, 9–11, 22, 24. Deex does not say how many male patients were admitted during the same period. All the women in the sample were white; she notes that there were no black women (or, presumably, women from other racial backgrounds) treated as inpatients during this period. See 62.
63. Ibid., 29.
64. Ibid., 50.
65. Ibid., 13.
66. Ibid., 5 (two groups), 34 ("day to day reality" quotation), 57 (other factors), 45–46 (implications for treatment), 52–53 (better prognosis).

67. Ibid., 9. Although she expressed considerable caution about not extrapolating inappropriately from the very small sample size, Deex reported that the vast majority of women who underwent role shift (eight out of nine women) experienced "beneficial results."
68. Ibid., 73–74.
69. Ibid., 76–78.
70. Ibid., 85–87.
71. Ibid., 102.
72. Ibid., 63–64 (for Mrs. A.), 79 (for Mrs. H.).
73. Ibid., 103.
74. Ibid., 18. Deex also indicates hierarchy and specialization between doctors (psychiatrists in this case) and social workers, 13. For the professionalization of social work, see Elizabeth Lunbeck, *The Psychiatric Persuasion: Knowledge, Gender, and Power in Modern America* (Princeton, NJ: Princeton University Press, 1994).
75. Lori Rotskoff, *Love on the Rocks: Men, Women, and Alcohol in Post–World War II America* (Chapel Hill: University of North Carolina Press, 2002), chap. 4, "The Dilemma of the Alcoholic Marriage." Rotskoff also notes that very little research was conducted on the husbands of alcoholic women in the midcentury period (153).

Epilogue

1. Lisa Belkin, "How Could a Mother Drive Drunk?" Motherlode: Adventures in Parenting column, *New York Times*, August 5, 2009.
2. Lisa W. Foderaro and Liz Robbins, "Grief Grips Long Island Community at Funeral for 5 Crash Victims," *New York Times*, July 31, 2009.
3. Al Baker and Lisa W. Foderaro, "Tests Show Driver Was Drunk in Parkway Crash That Killed 8," *New York Times*, August 5, 2009.
4. Ibid.
5. Ibid.
6. Belkin, "How Could a Mother Drive Drunk?"
7. Floyd Miller, "What the Alcoholic Owes to Marty Mann," *Reader's Digest* 82 (January 1963): 173–180.
8. See, for example, Vera L. Lindbeck, "The Woman Alcoholic: A Review of the Literature," *International Journal of the Addictions* 7, no. 3 (1972): 567–580; and Marc Shuckit, "The Alcoholic Woman: A Literature Review," *Psychiatry in Medicine* 3 (1972): 37–43. Feminist social scientists also looked to the past, although their historical analysis was not fully developed. See Edith S. Lisansky Gomberg, "Historical and Political Perspectives: Women and Drug Use," *Journal of Social Issues* 38 (1982): 9–23; and Kaye Middleton Fillmore, "The Epidemiology of Alcohol Use and Abuse among Women: A History of Science Approach," *Bulletin of the Society of Psychologists in Addictive Behaviors* 3, no. 3 (1984): 130–136, and "Issues in the Changing Drinking Patterns among Women in the Last Century," *Women and Alcohol: Health-Related Issues*, Research Monograph no. 16 (Washington, DC: National Institute on Alcohol Abuse and Alcoholism, 1986).
9. Research on female alcoholics did increase. Examples include Sharon C. Wilsnack and Linda J. Beckman, eds., *Alcohol Problems in Women: Antecedents, Consequences, and Intervention* (New York: Guilford Press, 1984); Peter G. Fellios, "Alcoholism in Women: Causes, Treatment, and Prevention," in *Alcoholism and*

Substance Abuse in Special Populations, ed. Gary W. Lawson and Ann W. Lawson (Rockville, MD: Aspen Publishers, 1989); Edith Lynn Hornik, *The Drinking Woman* (New York: Association Press, 1977); Marian Sandmaier, *The Invisible Alcoholics: Wine and Alcohol Abuse in America* (New York: McGraw-Hill, 1980); and Barry A. Kinsey, *The Female Alcoholic: A Social Psychological Study* (Springfield, IL: Charles C. Thomas Publisher, 1966). Much of this research included considerably more attention to differences among women in terms of race, class, and sexual orientation than did earlier discussions. See also Laura Schmidt and Constance Weisner, "The Emergence of Problem-Drinking Women as a Special Population in Need of Treatment," in *Recent Developments in Alcoholism*, vol. 12: *Women and Alcohol*, ed. Mark Galanter (New York: Plenum Press, 1995), 309–334. For further analysis of these developments, see Trysh Travis, *The Language of the Heart: A Cultural History of the Recovery Movement from Alcoholics Anonymous to Oprah Winfrey* (Chapel Hill: University of North Carolina Press, 2009).

10. Nancy Olson, *With a Lot of Help from Our Friends: The Politics of Alcoholism* (New York: Writers Club Press, 2003), esp. chap. 31; and Sally Brown and David R. Brown, *Mrs. Marty Mann: The First Lady of Alcoholics Anonymous* (Center City, MN: Hazelden/Pittman Archives Press, 2001), 304.

11. Of course, this was also a circular process, in that social views of alcohol as distinct from other drugs led to this institutional division. Morris Chafetz, the first director of the NIAAA, advocated strongly for the normalization of social drinking and for humane care for alcoholics. In much of his writing, he followed the pattern of the modern alcoholism movement in that he included occasional examples of women drinkers and female alcoholics without analysis or reflection. See Morris E. Chafetz and Harold W. DeMone, Jr., *Alcoholism and Society* (New York: Oxford University Press, 1962); and Morris E. Chafetz, *Liquor: The Servant of Man* (Boston: Little, Brown, 1965).

12. Travis, *The Language of the Heart*; Nancy D. Campbell, *Using Women: Gender, Drug Policy, and Social Justice* (New York: Routledge, 2000); and Nancy Campbell and Elizabeth Ettore, *Gendering Addiction: The Politics of Drug Treatment in a Neurochemical World* (Basingstoke: Palgrave Macmillan, 2011).

13. Jean Kirkpatrick, *Turnabout: New Help for the Woman Alcoholic* (Fort Lee, NJ: Barricade Books, 1977).

14. Ford published two memoirs, and a number of biographies have been written. See, for example, John Robert Greene, *Betty Ford: Candor and Courage in the White House* (Lawrence: University Press of Kansas, 2004).

15. Sally Quinn, "Betty Ford: Speaking Out without Speaking Up," *Washington Post*, September 18, 1974. See also Eleanor Randolph, "Betty Ford Is a Breath of Fresh Air with Candor," *Chicago Tribune*, September 9, 1974.

16. Greene, *Betty Ford*, 103.

17. The television show *Intervention* began on the A&E Network in 2005. Each episode focuses on a particular addict, for whom family members and friends, along with a specialist, stage an intervention. The website for the program records how many of the individuals who have appeared on the show over the years are currently sober. See "About," *Intervention*, A&E Network, n.d., www.aetv.com/intervention/about.

18. See, for example, "Betty Ford: True to Form," *Washington Post*, April 25, 1978.

19. Jennings Parrott, "Newsmakers," *Los Angeles Times*, April 25, 1978.

20. "An Insidious Thing," *Chicago Tribune*, April 12, 1978. See also Victor Cohn, "Women's Drug Dependency Called an Epidemic," *Washington Post*, April 12, 1978.

21. Betty Ford, *Betty: A Glad Awakening*, with Chris Chase (New York: Jove Books, 1988), 60.
22. "Betty Ford Being Treated for 'Addiction to Alcohol,'" *Chicago Tribune*, April 22, 1978.
23. "Mrs. Ford's Illness Described," *New York Times*, April 16, 1978.
24. Ford, *Betty*, 110, 132.
25. Although twelve-step programs were apparently important in Ford's own recovery and are utilized at the Betty Ford Center, the tradition of anonymity means that that component was not as prominent in press coverage.
26. See, for example, Ford, *Betty*, chap. 10.
27. Vera Glaser, "Reluctant 'Passenger,'" *Chicago Tribune*, November 3, 1973.
28. Marjorie Hunter, "Betty Ford's Renaissance: The Best Time of Her Life," *New York Times*, November 10, 1978.
29. David Herzberg, *Happy Pills in America: From Miltown to Prozac* (Baltimore: Johns Hopkins University Press, 2009); and Andrea Tone, *The Age of Anxiety: A History of America's Turbulent Affair with Tranquilizers* (New York: Basic Books, 2009).
30. Sandmaier, *The Invisible Alcoholics*, xviii.
31. Lori Rotskoff, *Love on the Rocks: Men, Women and Alcohol in Post–World War II America* (Chapel Hill: University of North Carolina Press, 2002).
32. Janet Golden, *Message in a Bottle: The Making of Fetal Alcohol Syndrome* (Cambridge, MA: Harvard University Press, 2005).
33. Campbell, *Using Women*.
34. "Babies and Drinking: A Chance to Stop Fetal Alcohol Exposure," *Minneapolis Star Tribune*, April 8, 1999, metro ed.
35. Kim Ode, "Drinking and Pregnancy Still Shouldn't Mix," *Minneapolis Star Tribune*, August 15, 1998, metro ed.
36. "Mothers' Vices during Pregnancy: Drinking on Rise despite Risks to Fetus," *Cleveland Plain-Dealer*, February 16, 1998. While explaining that "heavy" drinking—more than two drinks per day—can cause FAS and that "moderate" consumption—one to two drinks per day—can cause the milder form of the syndrome known as Fetal Alcohol Effect (FAE), this article and many others emphasized that pregnant women should not drink at all. This article also quoted an assistant professor of obstetrics and gynecology from Columbia University who explained that women should gradually wean themselves from alcohol in the months before they try to become pregnant.
37. Golden, *Message in a Bottle*, provides an insightful analysis of this demedicalization process.
38. See also Barron H. Lerner, *One for the Road: Drunk Driving since 1900* (Baltimore: Johns Hopkins University Press, 2011), which includes a detailed analysis of MADD and the intriguing trajectories of Lightner and other mothers involved in such advocacy.
39. "Fraternity at UCLA Suspended over Party," *Los Angeles Times*, August 21, 1996, home ed.
40. Marian Sandmaier, "The Wrong Idea about Date Rape," *St. Louis Post-Dispatch*, July 29, 1994.
41. Jon Krakauer, *Missoula: Rape and the Justice System in a College Town* (New York: Doubleday, 2015).
42. "Gender Gap in Drug Abuse Said to Close," *New York Times*, June 6, 1996.
43. "Women and Drugs," *Wall Street Journal*, June 6, 1996.

44. Gina Kolata, "Why a Drink for a Woman Acts Like Two for a Man," *New York Times*, January 11, 1990.
45. Peter Jaret, "Young Women and Alcohol," *Glamour*, April 1995, 262–265, 292–295.
46. K. T. Brady and C. L. Randall, "Gender Differences in Substance Use Disorders," *Psychiatric Clinics of North America* 22 (1999): 241–252.
47. J. B. Becker and M. Hu, "Sex Differences in Drug Abuse," *Frontiers in Neuroendocrinology* 29 (2008): 36–47; and J. B. Becker, A. N. Perry, and C. Westenbroek, "Sex Differences in the Neural Mechanisms Mediating Addiction: A New Synthesis and Hypothesis," *Biology of Sex Differences* 3 (2012): 14.
48. National Institute on Drug Abuse, "The Science of Drug Abuse and Addiction: The Basics," *Media Guide*, October 26, 2016, www.drugabuse.gov/publications/media-guide/science-drug-abuse-addiction.
49. See, for example, Campbell and Ettore, *Gendering Addiction*.
50. National Institute on Alcohol Abuse and Alcoholism, "Drinking Levels Defined," n.d., www.niaaa.nih.gov/alcohol-your-health/overview-alcohol-consumption/moderate-binge-drinking.
51. Campbell, *Using Women*, 13.
52. Gabrielle Glaser, *Her Best-Kept Secret: Why Women Drink—and How They Can Regain Control* (New York: Simon & Schuster), 1.
53. Ibid., 55.

Bibliography

Archival Sources and Manuscript Collections

Alcoholics Anonymous Archives, New York, NY.
Bishop-Kirk Collection, John Hay Library, Brown University, Providence, RI.
Illinois Addiction Studies Archive, Bloomington, IL.
Keeley Collection, Abraham Lincoln Presidential Library, Springfield, IL.
Margaret Culkin Banning Papers, Archives and Special Collections, Vassar College Libraries, Poughkeepsie, NY.
Marty Mann Papers, Department of Special Collections, Syracuse University Library, Syracuse, NY.
Department of Special Collections, A. T. Still Memorial Library and National Center for Osteopathic History, Kirksville College of Osteopathic Medicine, Kirksville, MO.
Miriam Van Waters Papers, Schlesinger Library, Radcliffe College, Cambridge, MA.

Primary Sources

Abraham, Karl. "The Psychological Relations between Sexuality and Alcoholism." *International Journal of Psycho-analysis* 8 (1926): 2–10.
"Alcohol: Beauty Blaster." *Everybody's Magazine* 35 (December 1916): 763–764.
Alcoholics Anonymous. *Alcoholics Anonymous: The Story of How Many Thousands of Men and Women Have Recovered from Alcoholism* ["The Big Book"]. New and rev. ed. New York: Alcoholics Anonymous World Services, 1955. Originally published as Alcoholics Anonymous, *Alcoholics Anonymous: The Story of How Many More than One Hundred Men Have Recovered from Alcoholism* (New York: World Publishing, 1939).
Alcoholics Anonymous. *Alcoholics Anonymous Comes of Age: A Brief History of Alcoholics Anonymous*. New York: Alcoholics Anonymous World Services, 1957.
"Alcoholism and Prohibition." *Literary Digest* (February 28, 1925): 24.
Allstrom, Oliver. "Ladies' Entrance" (1910). Reprinted in *Major Problems in the Gilded Age and Progressive Era*, edited by Leon Fink, 188–189. Lexington, MA: D. C. Heath, 1993.
Anderson, V. V., and C. M. Leonard. "Drunkenness as Seen among Women in Court." *Mental Hygiene* 3 (1919): 266–274.
Anderson, William K. "Shall I Send My Daughter to Europe?" *Christian Century* 48 (June 10, 1931): 773–775.
Arlitt, A. H., and W. G. Well. "The Effect of Alcohol on Reproductive Tissues." *Journal of Experimental Medicine* 26 (1917): 769–778.
Atherton, Gertrude. *Daughter of the Vine*. London: John Lane / Bodley Head, 1899.
"Babies and Drinking: A Chance to Stop Fetal Alcohol Exposure." *Minneapolis Star Tribune* (April 8, 1999), metro ed.
Banay, R. S. "Cultural Influences in Alcoholism." *Journal of Nervous and Mental Disease* 102 (1945): 265–275.
Banning, Margaret Culkin. "Lit Ladies." *Harper's* (January 1930): 161–169.
Becker, J. B., and M. Hu. "Sex Differences in Drug Abuse." *Frontiers in Neuroendocrinology* 29 (2008): 36–47.

Becker, J. B., A. N. Perry, and C. Westenbroek. "Sex Differences in the Neural Mechanisms Mediating Addiction: A New Synthesis and Hypothesis." *Biology of Sex Differences* 3 (2012): 1–35.

Blair, Henry William. *The Temperance Movement; or, The Conflict between Man and Alcohol*. Boston: William E. Smythe Co., 1888.

Block, M. A. "Alcoholism: The Physician's Duty." *GP* 6, no. 3 (1952): 53–58.

Brady, K. T., and C. L. Randall. "Gender Differences in Substance Use Disorders." *Psychiatric Clinics of North America* 22 (1999): 241–252.

Brownell, Rachael. *Mommy Doesn't Drink Here Anymore: Getting through the First Year of Sobriety*. San Francisco: Conari Press, 2009.

Brunner-Orne, Martha. "Treatment and Rehabilitation of Alcohol Addicts in a General Hospital Setting." *Journal of the American Medical Woman's Association* 10 (1955): 193–195.

Busch, Noel F. "Lady Tipplers." *Life* 22 (April 14, 1947): 85.

Chafetz, Morris E. *Liquor: The Servant of Man*. Boston: Little, Brown, & Co., 1965.

Chafetz, Morris E., and Harold W. DeMone, Jr. *Alcoholism and Society*. New York: Oxford University Press, 1962.

Cherrington, Ernest H. *Standard Encyclopedia of the Alcohol Problem*. Vol. 4. Westerville, OH: American Issue Publishing Co., 1928.

Clarke, Walter. "Prostitution and Alcohol." *Social Hygiene* 3 (1917): 75–90.

Colvin, D. Leigh. *Prohibition in the United States*. New York: George H. Doran Co., 1926.

Council on Medical Education and Hospitals. "Hospital Facilities for Alcoholic Patients." *Journal of the American Medical Association* 141 (1949): 620–621.

Crane, Stephen. "Maggie: A Girl of the Streets." In *Maggie and Other Stories by Stephen Crane*. New York: Pocket Books, 1960.

Crothers, T. D. "Is Alcoholism Increasing among American Women?" *North American Review* 155 (December 1892): 731–736.

Curran, F. J. "Personality Studies in Alcoholic Women." *Journal of Nervous and Mental Disease* 86 (1937): 645–667.

Davis, C. N. "The Alcoholic Problem as the Doctor Views It." *Pennsylvania Medical Journal* 49 (June 1946): 1018–1026.

Deex, Dorothy Jean. "A Study of the Housewife Role among Alcoholic Women In-Patients at the Washingtonian Hospital." M.S. thesis, Boston University School of Social Work, 1954.

Demme, R. "The Influence of Alcohol upon the Organism of the Child." *Wood's Medical and Surgical Monographs* 12 (1891): 207–233.

"Dressing for the Cocktail Lounge." *Christian Century* 54 (January 20, 1937): 75–77.

Dufur, J. Ivan. "Nervous Pathology of the Drug Habit." *Journal of the American Osteopathic Association* 16, no. 2 (1916): 742–745.

Durfee, Charles H. "Some Practical Observations on the Treatment of Problem Drinkers." *Quarterly Journal of Studies on Alcohol* 7, no. 2 (September 1946): 228–239.

"Effect of Prohibition on Alcoholism." *Literary Digest* (July 14, 1923): 21.

E.H.J.S. "Alcohol and Eugenics." *Nature* 85, no. 2154 (February 9, 1911): 479–480.

Emerson, H. "Alcohol: A Public Health Problem." *American Journal of Public Health* 7 (1917): 555–559.

Feldman, Paul E., and Elias Cohen. "A Statistical Study of the Admission of Alcoholic Patients to a Large Mental Hospital." *American Journal of Psychiatry* 111 (1955): 677–679.

Fellios, Peter G. "Alcoholism in Women: Causes, Treatment, and Prevention." In *Alcoholism and Substance Abuse in Special Populations*, edited by Gary W. Lawson and Ann W. Lawson, 11–34. Rockville, MD: Aspen Publishers, 1989.
First Steps. New York: Al-anon Family Group Headquarters, 1986.
Fiske, David. "'Psychotic Reaction' to Tetraethylthiuram Disulfide (Antabuse) Therapy." *Journal of the American Medical Association* 150, no. 11 (November 15, 1952): 1110–1111.
Fleming, Robert, and Kenneth J. Tillotson. "Further Studies on the Personality and Sociologic Factors in the Prognosis and Treatment of Chronic Alcoholism." *New England Journal of Medicine* 221, no. 19 (November 9, 1939): 741–745.
Ford, Betty. *Betty: A Glad Awakening*. With Chris Chase. New York: Jove Books, 1988.
———. *The Times of My Life*. New York: Harper & Row, 1978.
Fort, Twila Florence. "A Preliminary Study of Social Factors in the Alcoholism of Women." M.A. thesis, Texas Christian University, 1949.
"Fraternity at UCLA Suspended over Party." *Los Angeles Times* (August 21, 1996), home ed.
Garvin, William C. "Post Prohibition Alcoholic Psychoses in New York State." *American Journal of Psychiatry* (January 1930): 739–754.
"Gender Gap in Drug Abuse Said to Close." *New York Times* (June 6, 1996).
Glueck, Sheldon, and Eleanor T. Glueck. *Five Hundred Delinquent Women*. New York: Alfred A. Knopf, 1934.
Goldman, Harold I. "Outpatient Treatment of Postalcoholic Syndrome." *Journal of the American Medical Association* 167 (August 23, 1958): 2069–2071.
———. "Treatment of Postalcoholic Syndrome with Triflupromazine Hydrochloride." *Journal of the American Medical Association* 171, no. 11 (November 14, 1959): 1502–1503.
Gray, Hugh B. "The Experience of the Washingtonian Home." *New England Journal of Medicine* 200, no. 18 (May 2, 1929): 936–937.
Greenfield, Shelly F., Sumita G. Manwani, and Jessica E. Nargiso. "Epidemiology of Substance Use Disorders in Women." *Obstetrics and Gynecology Clinics of North America* 30, no. 3 (September 2003): 413–446.
Haggard, Howard W., and E. M. Jellinek. *Alcohol Explored*. New York: Doubleday, Doran, & Co., 1942.
Hall, Gladys Mary. *Prostitution in the Modern World: A Survey and a Challenge*. New York: Emerson Books, 1936.
Harding, T. Swann. "Alcohol, Health, Longevity, and Offspring." *American Journal of Pharmacy* 111 (1939): 351–358.
Hart, H. H. "Personality Factors in Alcoholism." *Archives of Neurology and Psychiatry* 24 (1930): 116–134.
Hecht, C. A., R. J. Grine, and S. E. Rothrock. "The Drinking and Dating Habits of 336 College Women in a Coeducational Institution." *Quarterly Journal of Studies on Alcohol* 9 (1948–1949): 252–258.
Hentz, Caroline Lee. "The Victim of Excitement." In *Love after Marriage, and Other Stories of the Heart*. Philadelphia: T. B. Peterson & Bros., 1870.
Hewitt, Charles C. "A Personality Study of Alcohol Addiction." *Quarterly Journal of Studies on Alcohol* 4, no. 3 (December 1943): 368–386.
Hirsh, Joseph. *The Problem Drinker*. New York: Duell, Sloan, & Pearce, 1949.
Jaret, Peter. "Young Women and Alcohol." *Glamour* (April 1995): 262–265, 292–295.

Jellinek, E. M. "Phases in the Drinking History of Alcoholics." *Quarterly Journal of Studies on Alcohol* 7 (1946): 1–88.

———. "Phases of Alcohol Addiction." *Quarterly Journal of Studies on Alcohol* 13 (1952): 673–684.

———. "Recent Trends in Alcoholism and in Alcohol Consumption." *Quarterly Journal of Studies on Alcohol* 8 (1947): 1–43.

Jolliffe, Norman. "The Alcoholic Admissions to Bellevue Hospital." *Science* 83, no. 2152 (March 27, 1936): 306–309.

Karpman, Benjamin. *The Alcoholic Woman: Case Studies in the Psychodynamics of Alcoholism.* Washington, DC: Linacre Press, 1948.

"Karpman, Benjamin, M.D. (1886–1962)." *American Journal of Psychiatry* 119 (May 1, 1963): 1119–1120.

Kellor, Frances A. "Criminality among Women." *Arena* 23 (May 1900): 516–524.

Kennedy, Kay. "Sisters of the Hollow Leg." *Outlook and Independent* 155 (May 21, 1930): 92–93, 117, 119.

Kerner, O. J. B. "Initiating Psychotherapy with Alcoholic Patients." *Quarterly Journal of Studies on Alcohol* 17 (1956): 479–484.

Kinsey, Barry A. *The Female Alcoholic: A Social Psychological Study.* Springfield, IL: Charles C. Thomas, 1966.

Kirkpatrick, Jean. *Turnabout: New Help for the Woman Alcoholic.* Fort Lee, NJ: Barricade Books, 1977.

Knapp, Caroline. *Drinking: A Love Story.* New York: Delta, 1996.

Knight, Robert P. "The Psychoanalytic Treatment in a Sanatorium of Chronic Addiction to Alcohol." *Journal of the American Medical Association* 111, no. 6 (October 15, 1938): 1443–1448.

———. "The Psychodynamics of Chronic Alcoholism." *Journal of Nervous and Mental Diseases* 86 (November 1937): 538–548.

Kolata, Gina. "Why a Drink for a Woman Acts Like Two for a Man." *New York Times* (January 11, 1990).

"Lady Bootlegger." *Scribner's Magazine* 92, no. 4 (October 1932): 229–231.

Landis, C., and J. F. Cushman, eds. "Case Studies of Compulsive Drinkers." *Quarterly Journal of Studies on Alcohol* 6 (1945–1946): 164–168.

Lemchen, B. "Three Months Amnesia following Moonshine Whiskey Debauch." *Illinois Medical Journal* 48 (September 1925): 246–248.

Lemere, Frederick, Paul O'Hallaren, and Milton A. Maxwell. "Sex Ratio of Alcoholic Patients Treated over a 20-Year Period." *Quarterly Journal of Studies on Alcohol* 17 (1956): 437–442.

Lemere, Frederick, Walter L. Voegtlin, William R. Broz, Paul O'Hollaren, and Warren E. Tupper. "The Conditioned Reflex Treatment of Chronic Alcoholism." *Journal of the American Medical Association* 120, no. 4 (1942): 269–270.

Levine, J. "The Sexual Adjustment of Alcoholics." *Quarterly Journal of Studies on Alcohol* 16 (1955): 675–680.

Lewis, N. D. C. "Personality Factors in Alcoholic Addiction." *Quarterly Journal of Studies on Alcohol* 1 (1940–1941): 21–44.

Lindbeck, Vera L. "The Woman Alcoholic: A Review of the Literature." *International Journal of the Addictions* 7, no. 3 (1972): 567–580.

Lisansky, Edith S. "Alcoholism in Women: Social and Psychological Concomitants." *Quarterly Journal of Studies on Alcohol* 18 (1957): 588–623.

Lois Remembers: Memoirs of the Co-founder of Al-Anon and Wife of the Co-founder of Alcoholics Anonymous. New York: Al-Anon Family Group Headquarters, 1979.

"The Long Lives of Women." *Literary Digest* (May 27, 1916): 1529.

Lovell, Howard W. *Hope and Help for the Alcoholic.* New York: Doubleday, 1956.

Lowrie, J. V., and F. G. Ebaugh. "A Post-Repeal Study of 300 Chronic Alcoholics." *American Journal of Medical Science* 203 (1942): 120–124.

Lundberg, Ferdinand, and Marynia F. Farnham. *Modern Woman: The Lost Sex.* New York: Harper & Bros., 1947.

MacNicholl, T. A. "Alcohol Use and the Disabilities of School Children." *Journal of the American Medical Association* 48 (1907): 396–399.

Malzberg, B. "First Admissions with Alcoholic Psychoses in New York State." *Quarterly Journal of Studies on Alcohol* 10 (1949): 461–470.

Mann, Marty. *Marty Mann's New Primer on Alcoholism.* New York: Rinehart & Co., 1958. Originally published as Marty Mann, *Primer on Alcoholism* (New York: Rinehart & Co., 1950).

Maus, L. M. "Alcohol and Racial Degeneracy." *Medical Record* 85 (1914): 102–105.

McCowen, Dr. "Clinical Cases in Private Practice." *Quarterly Journal of Inebriety* 10 (1888): 233–234.

Mendeville, Ernest W. "What Happened to Sally?" *Outlook* 139, no. 10 (March 11, 1925): 374–376.

Meyerson, A. "Alcohol: A Study of Social Ambivalence." *Quarterly Journal of Studies on Alcohol* 1 (1940–1941): 13–20.

Miller, Floyd. "What the Alcoholic Owes to Marty Mann." *Reader's Digest* 82 (January 1963): 173–180.

Miller, Michael M. "Treatment of Chronic Alcoholism by Hypnotic Aversion." *Journal of the American Medical Association* 171, no. 11 (November 14, 1959): 164–167.

Moore, Merrill, and M. Geneva Gray. "Alcoholism at the Boston City Hospital." *New England Journal of Medicine* 221, no. 2 (July 13, 1939): 45–61.

"Mothers' Vices during Pregnancy: Drinking on Rise Despite Risks to Fetus." *Cleveland Plain-Dealer* (February 16, 1998).

"Mrs. Drunkard." *Newsweek* 31 (March 8, 1948): 22–23.

Myerson, D. J. "An Active Therapeutic Method of Interrupting the Dependence Relationships of Certain Male Alcoholics." *Quarterly Journal of Studies on Alcohol* 14 (1953): 419–426.

National Institute on Alcohol Abuse and Alcoholism, National Institutes of Health, U.S. Department of Health and Human Services. "Alcohol: A Women's Health Issue." NIH Publication no. 03 4956, revised. Washington, DC: National Institute on Alcohol Abuse and Alcoholism, 2008.

Nicoll, Ione. "Should Women Vote Wet?" *North American Review* 229 (May 1930): 561–565.

Noble, Douglas. "Psychodynamics of Alcoholism in a Woman." *Psychiatry* 12 (1949): 413–425.

"Notes and Queries: Alcohol and Pregnancy." *Practitioner* 160 (1948): 73.

Ode, Kim. "Drinking and Pregnancy Still Shouldn't Mix." *Minneapolis Star Tribune* (August 15, 1998), metro ed.

Olson, Nancy. *With a Lot of Help from Our Friends: The Politics of Alcoholism.* New York: Writers Club Press, 2003.

"On Girls Learning to Drink." *Literary Digest* (January 7, 1933): 20.

Orestein, L. L., and W. Goldfarb. "A Note on the Incidence of Syphilis in Alcoholics." *Quarterly Journal of Studies on Alcohol* 1 (1940–1941): 442–443.
Pfeffer, A. Z., Philip Friedland, and S. Bernard Wortis. "Group Psychotherapy with Alcoholics: A Preliminary Report." *Quarterly Journal of Studies on Alcohol* 10, no. 2 (September 1949): 198–216.
Pollock, Horatio M., and Frederick W. Brown. "Recent Statistics of Alcoholic Mental Disease." *Mental Hygiene* 13 (1929): 591–614.
Pollock, Horatio M., and Edith M. Furbush. "Prohibition and Alcoholic Mental Disease." *Mental Hygiene* 8 (1924): 548–570.
Popenoe, Paul. "Heredity and Environment as Related to Alcoholism." *Eugenical News* (1946–1947): 35–38.
"Queries and Minor Notes: Alcoholism and Heredity." *Journal of the American Medical Association* 136 (1948): 849.
"Queries and Minor Notes: Effect of Alcoholism at Time of Conception." *Journal of the American Medical Association* 132 (1946): 419.
"Queries and Minor Notes: Effect of Single Large Alcohol Intake on Fetus." *Journal of the American Medical Association* 120 (1942): 88.
"Queries and Minor Notes: Smoking and Drinking during Pregnancy." *Journal of the American Medical Association* 154 (1954): 186.
"Questions and Answers." *Hygeia* 14 (March 1936): 285.
Revelle, G. G. *Alcoholic Wife*. Boston: Beacon Press, 1960.
Richardson, Eudora R. "Drinking Mothers." *Outlook and Independent* 158 (June 10, 1931): 174–175, 191.
Riley, J. W., Jr., C. F. Marden, and M. Lifshitz, "The Motivational Pattern of Drinking." *Quarterly Journal of Studies on Alcohol* 9 (1948–1949): 353–362.
Roe, Anne. "The Adult Adjustment of Children of Alcoholics Raised in Foster Homes." *Quarterly Journal of Studies on Alcohol* 5 (1944): 378–393.
Rosenbaum, B. "Married Women Alcoholics at the Washingtonian Hospital." *Quarterly Journal of Studies on Alcohol* 19 (1958): 79–89.
Roth, Lillian. *I'll Cry Tomorrow*. New York: Frederick Fell Publishers, 1954.
Rotman, D. B. "Alcoholism: A Social Disease." *Journal of the American Medical Association* 127 (1945): 564–567.
Sabin, Pauline Morton. "Women's Revolt against Prohibition." *Review of Reviews* 80, no. 478 (November 1929): 88.
Sandmaier, Marian. "The Wrong Idea about Date Rape." *St. Louis Post-Dispatch* (July 29, 1994).
Sanger, W. W. *History of Prostitution*. New York: Medical Publishing Co., 1910.
Sears, George G. "Hospital Administration under the Eighteenth Amendment." *Boston Medical and Surgical Journal* 189, no. 12 (September 20, 1923): 397–399.
Shalloo, J. P. "Some Cultural Factors in the Etiology of Alcoholism." *Quarterly Journal of Studies on Alcohol* 2 (1941–1942): 464–478.
Shuckit, Marc. "The Alcoholic Woman: A Literature Review." *Psychiatry in Medicine* 3 (1972): 37–43.
Sillman, L. "Chronic Alcoholism." *Journal of Nervous and Mental Disease* 107 (1948): 127–149.
Stern, Morton M. "Antihistamine Treatment of Alcoholism." *Journal of Nervous and Mental Diseases* 122 (1955): 198–199.
Stockard, C. R. "The Influence of Alcoholism on the Offspring." *Proceedings of the Society for Experimental Biology and Medicine* (1911–1912): 71–72.

Strecker, Edward A. *Their Mothers' Sons: The Psychiatrist Examines an American Problem.* Philadelphia: J. P. Lippincott, 1951.
Talbot, E. S. "Alcohol in Its Relation to Degeneracy." *Journal of the American Medical Association* 48 (1907): 399–401.
"This Moderate Drinking." *Harper's Monthly Magazine* (March 1931): 419–427.
Thomeuf, Dr. "Alcoholism in Women." In *Wood's Medical and Surgical Monographs* 7 (1890): 343–355.
Tillotson, Kenneth J., and Robert Fleming. "Personality and Sociological Factors in the Prognosis and Treatment of Chronic Alcoholism." *New England Journal of Medicine* 217, no. 16 (October 14, 1937): 611–615.
Turner, C. C. "The Conditioned Reflex in the Treatment of Alcoholism—Case Reports." *Memphis Medical Journal* 17 (December 1942): 223–224.
Van Amberg, Robert J. "A Study of 50 Women Patients Hospitalized for Alcohol Addiction." *Diseases of the Nervous System* 3–4 (August 1943): 246–251.
Vice Commission of Chicago. *The Social Evil in Chicago.* Chicago: Gunthorp-Warren Printing Co., 1911.
Walker, Stanley. *The Night Club Era.* New York: Frederick A. Stokes Co., 1933.
Wall, James H. "A Study of Alcoholism in Men." *American Journal of Psychiatry* 92 (May 1936): 1389–1401.
———. "A Study of Alcoholism in Women." *American Journal of Psychiatry* 93 (1937): 943–955.
Warburton, Clark. *The Economic Results of Prohibition.* New York: Columbia University Press, 1932.
Weijl, Simon. "Theoretical and Practical Aspects of Psychoanalytic Therapy of Problem Drinkers." *Quarterly Journal of Studies on Alcohol* 5, no. 2 (September 1944): 200–211.
Wilder-Taylor, Stephanie. *Sippy Cups Are Not for Chardonnay: And Other Things I Had to Learn as a New Mom.* New York: Gallery Books, 2006.
Wilhelmson, Brenda. *Diary of an Alcoholic Housewife.* Center City, MN: Hazelden, 2011.
Wilson, Samuel Paynter. *Chicago by Gaslight.* Chicago: n.p., 1910.
Wilson, Wilma. *They Call Them Camisoles.* Los Angeles: Lymanhouse, 1940.
Wing, Nell. *Grateful to Have Been There: My Forty-Two Years with Bill and Lois and the Evolution of Alcoholics Anonymous.* Park Ridge, IL: Parkside Publishing, 1992.
Wolf, I. "Alcoholism and Marriage." *Quarterly Journal of Studies on Alcohol* 19 (1958): 511–513.
"Woman and Drink." *Current Literature* 34, no. 2 (February 1903): 226.
"Women and Drugs." *Wall Street Journal* (June 6, 1996).
"Women Become People." *Outlook and Independent* (April 21, 1931): 586–587.
"Women Bootleggers a Problem." *Literary Digest* (February 5, 1927): 46.
Woods, M. "Relation of Alcoholism to Epilepsy." *Journal of the American Medical Association* 48, no. 6 (1907): 469–471.
Wortis, H., and L. R. Sillman, eds. "Case Histories of Compulsive Drinkers." *Quarterly Journal of Studies on Alcohol* 6 (1945–1946): 320–325.
Yater, Wallace Mason. *Fundamentals of Internal Medicine,* 609–612. New York: D. Appleton-Century Co., 1944.
Yost, Edna. "Carry Nation Wets." *Outlook and Independent* (September 25, 1929): 146–147, 159.

Secondary Sources

Aaron, Paul, and David Musto. "Temperance and Prohibition in America: A Historical Overview." In *Alcohol and Public Policy: Beyond the Shadow of Prohibition*, edited by M. H. Moore and D. R. Gerstein. Washington, DC: National Academy Press, 1981.

Acker, Caroline J. *Creating the American Junkie: Addiction Research in the Classic Era of Narcotic Control*. Baltimore: Johns Hopkins University Press, 2002.

Alexander, Ruth M. "'We Are Engaged as a Band of Sisters': Class and Domesticity in the Washingtonian Temperance Movement, 1840–1850." *Journal of American History* 75, no. 3 (December 1988): 763–785.

Ames, Genevieve M. "American Beliefs about Alcoholism: Historical Perspectives on the Medical-Moral Controversy." In *The American Experience with Alcohol: Contrasting Cultural Perspectives*, edited by Linda A. Bennett and Genevieve M. Ames, 23–39. New York: Plenum Press, 1985.

Apple, Rima D. *Perfect Motherhood: Science and Childrearing in America*. New Brunswick, NJ: Rutgers University Press, 2006.

———. *Vitamania: Vitamins in American Culture*. New Brunswick, NJ: Rutgers University Press, 1996.

———, ed. *Women, Health, and Medicine in America: A Historical Handbook*. New York: Garland Publishers, 1990.

Ashbury, Herbert. *The Great Illusion: An Informal History of Prohibition*. New York: Greenwood Press, 1968.

Bailey, Beth. *From Front Porch to Back Seat: Courtship in Twentieth-Century America*. Baltimore: Johns Hopkins University Press, 1988.

Barrows, Susanna, and Robin Room, eds. *Drinking: Behavior and Belief in Modern History*. Berkeley: University of California Press, 1991.

Baumohl, Jim. "Inebriate Institutions in North America, 1840–1920." *British Journal of Addiction* 85 (1990): 1187–1204.

Blocker, Jack S. *American Temperance Movements: Cycles of Reform*. Boston: Twayne, 1989.

———. "Did Prohibition Really Work? Alcohol Prohibition as Public Health Innovation." *American Journal of Public Health* 96 (February 2006): 233–243.

Blumberg, Leonard. "The American Association for the Study and Cure of Inebriety." *Alcoholism: Clinical and Experimental Research* 2, no. 3 (July 1978): 235–240.

Borden, Audrey. *The History of Gay People in Alcoholics Anonymous, from the Beginning*. New York: Haworth Press, 2007.

Bordin, Ruth. *Frances Willard: A Biography*. Chapel Hill: University of North Carolina Press, 1986.

———. *Woman and Temperance: The Quest for Power and Liberty, 1873–1900*. Philadelphia: Temple University Press, 1981.

Brandt, Allan M. *The Cigarette Century: The Rise, Fall, and Deadly Persistence of the Product that Defined America*. New York: Basic Books, 2007.

———. *No Magic Bullet: A Social History of Venereal Disease in the United States since 1880*. New York: Oxford University Press, 1985.

Braslow, Joel. *Mental Ills and Bodily Cures: Psychiatric Treatment in the First Half of the Twentieth Century*. Berkeley: University of California Press, 1997.

Brown, Edward M. "What Shall We Do with the Inebriate?: Asylum Treatment and the Disease Concept of Alcoholism in the Late Nineteenth Century." *Journal of the History of the Behavioral Sciences* 21 (January 1985): 48–59.

Brown, Sally, and David R. Brown. *Mrs. Marty Mann: The First Lady of Alcoholics Anonymous.* Center City, MN: Hazelden / Pittman Archives Press, 2001.

Brumberg, Joan Jacobs. *The Body Project: An Intimate History of American Girls.* New York: Random House, 1997.

———. *Fasting Girls: The Emergence of Anorexia Nervosa as a Modern Disease.* Cambridge, MA: Harvard University Press, 1988.

Buhle, Mari Jo. *Feminism and Its Discontents: A Century of Struggle with Psychoanalysis.* Cambridge, MA: Harvard University Press, 1998.

Burnham, John C. *Bad Habits: Drinking, Smoking, Taking Drugs, Gambling, Sexual Misbehavior, and Swearing in American History.* New York: New York University Press, 1993.

———. "New Perspectives on the Prohibition 'Experiment' of the 1920s." *Journal of Social History* 2, no. 1 (1968): 51–68.

Cahn, Susan K. *Coming on Strong: Gender and Sexuality in Twentieth-Century Women's Sport.* Cambridge, MA: Harvard University Press, 1994.

Campbell, Nancy D. *Using Women: Gender, Drug Policy, and Social Justice.* New York: Routledge, 2000.

Campbell, Nancy D., and Elizabeth Ettore, *Gendering Addiction: The Politics of Drug Treatment in a Neurochemical World.* Basingstoke: Palgrave Macmillan, 2011.

Cannon, Eion F. *The Saloon and the Mission: Addiction, Conversion, and the Politics of Redemption in American Culture.* Amherst: University of Massachusetts Press, 2013.

Cashman, Sean Dennis. *Prohibition: The Lie of the Land.* New York: Free Press, 1981.

Chafe, William H. *The American Woman: Her Changing Social, Economic, and Political Roles, 1920–1970.* London: Oxford University Press, 1972.

Chauncey, George. *Gay New York: Gender, Urban Culture, and the Making of the Gay Male World, 1890–1940.* New York: Basic Books, 1994.

Chavigny, Katherine A. "Reforming Drunkards in Nineteenth-Century America: Religion, Medicine, Therapy." In *Altering American Consciousness: The History of Alcohol and Drug Use in the United States, 1800–2000*, edited by Sarah W. Tracy and Caroline Acker, 108–123. Amherst: University of Massachusetts Press, 2004.

Clark, Adele E. "Women's Health: Life-Cycle Issues." In *Women, Health, and Medicine in America: A Historical Handbook*, edited by Rima D. Apple. New York: Garland Publishers, 1990.

Clark, Norman H. *The Dry Years: Prohibition and Social Change in Washington.* Seattle: University of Washington Press, 1965, rev. ed. 1988.

Cohen, Lizabeth. *A Consumer's Republic: The Politics of Mass Consumption in Postwar America.* New York: Alfred E. Knopf, 2003.

Cott, Nancy F. *The Bonds of Womanhood: "Woman's Sphere" in New England, 1780–1835.* New Haven, CT: Yale University Press, 1977.

Courtright, David T. *Dark Paradise: Opiate Addiction in America before 1940.* Cambridge, MA: Harvard University Press, 1982.

———. "The Female Opiate Addict in Nineteenth-Century America." *Essay in Arts and Sciences* 10, no. 2 (March 1982): 161–171.

———. *Forces of Habit: Drugs and the Making of the Modern World.* Cambridge, MA: Harvard University Press, 2001.

Crowley, John W., ed. *Drunkard's Progress: Narratives of Addiction, Despair, and Recovery.* Baltimore: Johns Hopkins University Press, 1999.

———. *The White Logic: Alcoholism and Gender in American Modernist Fiction.* Amherst: University of Massachusetts Press, 1994.

Darrah, Mary C. *Sister Ignatia: Angel of Alcoholics Anonymous.* Chicago: Loyola University Press, 1992.

Degler, Carl. *In Search of Human Nature: The Decline and Revival of Darwinism in American Social Thought.* New York: Oxford University Press, 1991.

D'Emilio, John. "The Homosexual Menace: The Politics of Sexuality in Cold War America." In *Passion and Power: Sexuality in History,* edited by Kathy Peiss and Christina Simmons. Philadelphia: Temple University Press, 1989.

D'Emilio, John, and Estelle B. Freedman. *Intimate Matters: A History of Sexuality in America.* New York: Harper & Row, 1988.

Dorris, Michael. *The Broken Cord.* New York: Harper & Row, 1989.

Dorsey, Bruce. *Reforming Men and Women: Gender in the Antebellum City.* Ithaca, NY: Cornell University Press, 2002.

Dr. Bob and the Good Oldtimers. New York: Alcoholics Anonymous World Services, 1980.

Duis, Perry R. *The Saloon: Public Drinking in Chicago and Boston, 1880–1920.* Urbana: University of Illinois Press, 1983.

Dumenil, Lynn. *The Modern Temper: American Culture and Society in the 1920s.* New York: Hill & Wang, 1995.

Ehrenreich, Barbara, and Deirdre English. *For Her Own Good: 150 Years of the Experts' Advice to Women.* New York: Anchor Books, 1978.

Enke, Anne. *Finding the Movement: Sexuality, Contested Space, and Feminist Activism.* Durham, NC: Duke University Press, 2007.

Faderman, Lillian. *Odd Girls and Twilight Lovers: A History of Lesbian Life in Twentieth-Century America.* New York: Columbia University Press, 1991.

Fass, Paula S. *The Damned and the Beautiful: American Youth in the 1920s.* Oxford: Oxford University Press, 1977.

Fee, Elizabeth. "Venereal Disease: The Wages of Sin?" In *Passion and Power: Sexuality in History,* edited by Kathy Peiss and Christina Simmons, 178–198. Philadelphia: Temple University Press, 1989.

Fillmore, Kaye Middleton. "The Epidemiology of Alcohol Use and Abuse among Women: A History of Science Approach." *Bulletin of the Society of Psychologists in Addictive Behaviors* 3, no. 3 (1984): 130–136.

———. "Issues in the Changing Drinking Patterns among Women in the Last Century." "Women and Alcohol: Health-Related Issues." Research monograph no. 16. National Institute on Alcohol Abuse and Alcoholism, National Institutes of Health, U.S. Department of Health and Human Services, 1986. Freedman, Estelle B. *Maternal Justice: Miriam Van Waters and the Female Reform Tradition.* Chicago: University of Chicago Press, 1996.

Giele, Janet Zollinger. *Two Paths to Women's Equality: Temperance, Suffrage, and the Origins of Modern Feminism.* New York: Twayne, 1995.

Glaser, Gabrielle. *Her Best-Kept Secret: Why Women Drink—and How They Can Regain Control.* New York: Simon & Schuster, 2013.

Golden, Janet. *Message in a Bottle: The Making of Fetal Alcohol Syndrome.* Cambridge, MA: Harvard University Press, 2005.

Gomberg, Edith S. Lisansky. "Historical and Political Perspectives: Women and Drug Use." *Journal of Social Issues* 38 (1982): 9–23.

Gordon, Linda. *Heroes of Their Own Lives: The Politics and History of Family Violence.* New York: Penguin Books, 1988.

Green, John Robert. *Betty Ford: Candor and Courage in the White House*. Lawrence: University Press of Kansas, 2004.
Groneman, Carol. *Nymphomania: A History*. New York: W. W. Norton, 2000.
Gutzke, David W. "'The Cry of the Children': The Edwardian Medical Campaign against Maternal Drinking." *British Journal of Addiction* 79 (1984): 71–84.
Hale, Nathan G., Jr. *The Rise and Crisis of Psychoanalysis in the United States: Freud and the Americans, 1917–1985*. New York: Oxford University Press, 1995.
Hallberg, Lillian Mae. "Rhetorical Dimensions of Institutional Language: A Case Study of Women Alcoholics." Ph.D. diss., University of Iowa, 1988.
Hamm, Richard F. *Shaping the Eighteenth Amendment: Temperance Reform, Legal Culture, and the Polity, 1880–1920*. Chapel Hill: University of North Carolina Press, 1995.
Hansen, Bert. "American Physicians' 'Discovery' of Homosexuals, 1880–1900: A New Diagnosis in a Changing Society." In *Framing Disease: Studies in Cultural History*, edited by Charles E. Rosenberg and Janet L. Golden, 104–133. New Brunswick, NJ: Rutgers University Press, 1992.
Hartmann, Susan M. *The Home Front and Beyond: American Women in the 1940s*. Boston: Twayne, 1982.
Harvey, Brett. *The Fifties: A Women's Oral History*. New York: HarperCollins, 1993.
Herman, Ellen. *The Romance of American Psychology: Political Culture in the Age of Experts*. Berkeley: University of California Press, 1995.
Herzberg, David. *Happy Pills in America: From Miltown to Prozac*. Baltimore: Johns Hopkins University Press, 2009.
Hessinger, Rodney. *Seduced, Abandoned, and Reborn: Visions of Youth in Middle-Class America, 1780–1850*. Philadelphia: University of Pennsylvania Press, 2005.
Hirshbein, Laura D. *American Melancholy: Constructions of Depression in the Twentieth Century*. New Brunswick, NJ: Rutgers University Press, 2009.
Hornik, Edith Lynn. *The Drinking Woman*. New York: Association Press, 1977.
Houck, Judith. *Hot and Bothered: Women, Medicine, and Menopause in Modern America*. Cambridge, MA: Harvard University Press, 2006.
Hyman, Merton M., comp. *Drinkers, Drinking, and Alcohol-Related Mortality and Hospitalizations*. New Brunswick, NJ: Center of Alcohol Studies, Rutgers University, 1980.
Jaffe, A. "Reform in American Medical Science: The Inebriety Movement and the Origins of the Psychological Disease Theory of Addiction, 1870–1920." *British Journal of Addiction* 73 (1978): 139–147.
Johnson, Bruce Holley. "The Alcoholism Movement in America: A Study in Cultural Innovation." Ph.D. diss., University of Illinois, 1973.
Johnson, Paul E. *A Shopkeeper's Millennium: Society and Revivals in Rochester, New York, 1815–1837*. New York: Hill & Wang, 1978.
Kandall, Stephen R. *Substance and Shadow: Women and Addiction in the United States*. With the assistance of Jennifer Petrillo. Cambridge, MA: Harvard University Press, 1996.
Kanner, Melinda. "Drinking Themselves to Life, or the Body in the Bottle." In *Reading the Social Body*, edited by Catherine B. Burroughs and Jeffrey David Ehrenreich, 156–184. Iowa City: University of Iowa Press, 1993.
Kelly, Joan. "Did Women Have a Renaissance?" In *Women, History and Theory*. Chicago: University of Chicago Press, 1984. Originally published 1977.
Kennedy, Elizabeth Lapovsky, and Madeline Davis. "The Reproduction of Butch-Fem Roles: A Social Constructionist Approach." In *Passion and Power: Sexuality in*

History, edited by Kathy Peiss and Christina Simmons. Philadelphia: Temple University Press, 1989.

Kline, Wendy. *Bodies of Knowledge: Sexuality, Reproduction, and Women's Health in the Second Wave*. Chicago: University of Chicago Press, 2010.

Krakauer, Jon. *Missoula: Rape and the Justice System in a College Town*. New York: Doubleday, 2015.

Kurtz, Ernest. *Not-God: A History of Alcoholics Anonymous*. Center City, MN: Hazelden Educational Services, 1979.

Kushner, H. I. "Taking Biology Seriously: The Next Task for Historians of Addiction?" *Bulletin of the History of Medicine* 80 (2006): 115–143.

Kyvig, David E. *Repealing National Prohibition*. 1979; rev. ed., Chicago: University of Chicago Press, 2000.

Leavitt, Judith Walzer. *Brought to Bed: Childbearing in America, 1750–1950*. New York: Oxford University Press, 1986.

———, ed. *Women and Health in America: Historical Readings*. Madison: University of Wisconsin Press, 1984.

Lender, Mark Edward. "Jellinek's Typology of Alcoholism: Some Historical Antecedents." *Journal of Studies on Alcohol* 40 (1979): 361–373.

———. "A Special Stigma: Women and Alcoholism in the Late 19th and Early 20th Centuries." In *Alcohol Interventions: Historical and Sociocultural Approaches*, edited by David L. Strug, S. Priyadarsini, and Merton M. Hyman, 41–57. New York: Hayworth Press, 1986.

———. "Women Alcoholics: Prevalence Estimates and Their Problems as Reflected in Turn-of-the-Century Institutional Data." *International Journal of the Addictions* 16, no. 3 (1981): 443–448.

Lender, Mark Edward, and James Kirby Martin. *Drinking in America: A History*. New York: Free Press, 1987.

Lerner, Barron H. *The Breast Cancer Wars: Faith, Hope, and the Pursuit of a Cure in Twentieth-Century America*. New York: Oxford University Press, 2001.

———. *One for the Road: Drunk Driving since 1900*. Baltimore: Johns Hopkins University Press, 2011.

———. *When Illness Goes Public: Celebrity Patients and How We Look at Medicine*. Baltimore: Johns Hopkins University Press, 2006.

Lerner, Michael A. *Dry Manhattan: Prohibition in New York City*. Cambridge, MA: Harvard University Press, 2007.

Levine, Harry Gene. "Demon of the Middle Class: Self-Control, Liquor, and the Ideology of Temperance in Nineteenth-Century America." Ph.D. diss., University of California, Berkeley, 1978.

———. "The Discovery of Addiction: Changing Conceptions of Habitual Drunkenness in America." *Journal of Studies on Alcohol* 39 (1978): 143–174.

Longo, Lawrence D. "The Rise and Fall of Battey's Operation: A Fashion in Surgery." In *Women and Health in America*, edited by Judith Walzer Leavitt, 270–284. Madison: University of Wisconsin Press, 1984.

Lunbeck, Elizabeth. *The Psychiatric Persuasion: Knowledge, Gender, and Power in Modern America*. Princeton, NJ: Princeton University Press, 1994.

Lurie, Nancy. "The World's Oldest Ongoing Protest Demonstration: North American Indian Drinking Patterns." *Pacific Historical Review* 40 (1971): 311–332.

Mancall, Peter. *Deadly Medicine: Indians and Alcohol in Early America*. Ithaca, NY: Cornell University Press, 1995.

Margolis, Maxine L. *Mothers and Such: Views of American Women and Why They Changed.* Berkeley: California University Press, 1984.

Martin, Scott C. *Devil of the Domestic Sphere: Temperance, Gender, and Middle-Class Ideology, 1800–1860.* DeKalb: Northern Illinois University Press, 2008.

May, Elaine Tyler. *Barren in the Promised Land: Childless Americans and the Pursuit of Happiness.* New York: Basic Books, 1995.

———. *Homeward Bound: American Families in the Cold War Era.* New York: Basic Books, 1988.

Meyerowitz, Joanne J. "Beyond the Feminine Mystique: A Reassessment of Postwar Mass Culture, 1946–1958." In *Not June Cleaver: Women and Gender in Postwar America*, edited by Joanne Meyerowitz, 229–262. Philadelphia: Temple University Press, 1994.

———. *How Sex Changed: A History of Transsexuality in the United States.* Cambridge, MA: Harvard University Press, 2002.

———, ed. *Not June Cleaver: Women and Gender in Postwar America, 1945–1960.* Philadelphia: Temple University Press, 1994.

———. *Women Adrift: Independent Wage Earners in Chicago, 1880–1930.* Chicago: University of Chicago Press, 1988.

Morantz-Sanchez, Regina. *Conduct Unbecoming a Woman: Medicine on Trial in Turn-of-the-Century Brooklyn.* New York: Oxford University Press, 1999.

Morgan, H. Wayne. *Drugs in America: A Social History, 1880–1980.* Syracuse, NY: Syracuse University Press, 1981.

Murdock, Catherine Gilbert. "Domesticating Drink: Women and Alcohol in Prohibition America." Ph.D. diss., University of Pennsylvania, 1995.

———. *Domesticating Drink: Women, Men, and Alcohol in America, 1870–1940.* Baltimore: Johns Hopkins University Press, 1998.

Murphy, Mary. "Bootlegging Mothers and Drinking Daughters: Gender and Prohibition in Butte, Montana." *American Quarterly* 46, no. 2 (1994): 174–194.

Musto, David F. *The American Disease: Origins of Narcotic Control.* New York: Oxford University Press, 1987. National Center on Addiction and Substance Abuse at Columbia University. *Women under the Influence.* Baltimore: Johns Hopkins University Press, 2006.

Newton, Esther. *Cherry Grove, Fire Island: Sixty Years in America's First Gay and Lesbian Town.* Boston: Beacon Press, 1993.

Nye, Robert A. "The Evolution of the Concept of Medicalization in the Late Twentieth Century." *Journal of History of the Behavioral Sciences* 39, no. 2 (Spring 2003): 115–129.

Odem, Mary E. *Delinquent Daughters: Protecting and Policing Adolescent Female Sexuality in the United States, 1885–1920.* Chapel Hill: University of North Carolina Press, 1995.

Okrent, Daniel. *Last Call: The Rise and Fall of Prohibition.* New York: Scribner, 2010.

Osborn, Matthew W. *Rum Maniacs: Alcoholic Insanity in the Early American Republic.* Chicago: University of Chicago Press, 2014.

Oudshoorn, Nancy. *Beyond the Natural Body: An Archaeology of Sex Hormones.* New York: Routledge, 1994.

Parsons, Elaine Frantz. *Manhood Lost: Fallen Drunkards and Redeeming Women in the Nineteenth-Century United States.* Baltimore: Johns Hopkins University Press, 2003.

Pass It On: The Story of Bill Wilson and How the AA Message Reached the World. New York: Alcoholics Anonymous World Services, 1984.

Pauly, Philip J. "How Did the Effects of Alcohol on Reproduction Become Scientifically Uninteresting?" *Journal of the History of Biology* 29 (1996): 1–28.

Peiss, Kathy. "'Charity Girls' and City Pleasures: Historical Notes on Working-Class Sexuality, 1880–1920." In *Passion and Power: Sexuality in History*, edited by Kathy Peiss and Christina Simmons, 57–69. Philadelphia: Temple University Press, 1989.

———. *Cheap Amusements: Working Women and Leisure in Turn-of-the-Century New York*. Philadelphia: Temple University Press, 1986.

———. *Hope in a Jar: The Making of America's Beauty Culture*. New York: Metropolitan Books, 1998.

Pennock, Pamela E. *Advertising Sin and Sickness: The Politics of Alcohol and Tobacco Marketing, 1950–1990*. DeKalb: Northern Illinois University Press, 2007.

Plant, Moira. *Women, Drinking, and Pregnancy*. London: Tavistock Publications, 1985.

Plant, Rebecca. *Mom: The Transformation of American Motherhood in Modern America*. Chicago: University of Chicago Press, 2010.

Powers, Madelon. *Faces along the Bar: Lore and Order in the Workingman's Saloon, 1870–1920*. Chicago: University of Chicago Press, 1998.

Robertson, Nan. *Getting Better: Inside Alcoholics Anonymous*. New York: William Morrow, 1988.

Roizen, Ronald. "The American Discovery of Alcoholism, 1933–1939." Ph.D. diss., University of California at Berkeley, 1991.

Room, Robin. "Alcoholism and Alcoholics Anonymous in U.S. Films, 1945–1962: The Party Ends for the 'Wet Generations.'" *Journal of Studies on Alcohol* 50 (1989): 368–383.

Rorabaugh, W. J. *The Alcoholic Republic: An American Tradition*. New York: Oxford University Press, 1979.

———. "Drinking in the 'Thin Man' Films, 1934–1947." *Social History of Alcohol and Drugs* 18 (2003): 51–68.

Rose, Kenneth D. *American Women and the Repeal of Prohibition*. New York: New York University Press, 1996.

Rosenberg, Charles E. *The Care of Strangers: The Rise of America's Hospital System*. New York: Basic Books, 1992.

———. "Framing Disease: Illness, Society, and History." In *Framing Disease: Studies in Cultural History*, edited by Charles E. Rosenberg and Janet Golden, xiii–xxiv. New Brunswick, NJ: Rutgers University Press, 1992.

Rosenzweig, Roy. *Eight Hours for What We Will: Workers and Leisure in an Industrial City, 1870–1920*. Cambridge: Cambridge University Press, 1983.

Rothman, Sheila M. *Living in the Shadow of Death: Tuberculosis and the Social Experience of Illness in American History*. Baltimore: Johns Hopkins University Press, 1994.

Rotskoff, Lori. *Love on the Rocks: Men, Women, and Alcohol in Post–World War II America*. Chapel Hill: University of North Carolina Press, 2002.

———. "Sober Husbands and Supportive Wives: Gendered Cultures of Drink and Sobriety in Twentieth-Century America, 1910–1965." Ph.D. diss., Yale University, 1999.

Rupp, Leila J. "Imagine My Surprise: Women's Relationships in Historical Perspective." *Frontiers* 5 (Fall 1980): 61–70.

Ryan, Mary P. *Cradle of the Middle Class: The Family in Oneida County, New York, 1790–1865*. Cambridge: Cambridge University Press, 1981.

Sandmaier, Marian. *The Invisible Alcoholics: Women and Alcohol Abuse in America*. New York: McGraw-Hill, 1980.

Schmidt, Laura, and Constance Weisner. "The Emergence of Problem-Drinking Women as a Special Population in Need of Treatment." In *Recent Developments in Alcoholism*, vol. 12, *Women and Alcohol*, edited by Mark Galanter, 309–334. New York: Plenum Press, 1995.

Sicherman, Barbara. "The Uses of a Diagnosis: Doctors, Patients, and Neurasthenia." *Journal of the History of Medicine and Allied Sciences* 32, no. 1 (1977): 33–54.

Sinclair, Andrew. *Prohibition: The Era of Excess*. Boston: Little, Brown, & Co., 1962.

Smith-Rosenberg, Carroll. "The Female World of Love and Ritual." In *Disorderly Conduct: Visions of Gender in Victorian America*, 53–76. New York: Oxford University Press, 1985.

———. "The Hysterical Woman: Sex Roles and Role Conflict in Nineteenth-Century America." In *Disorderly Conduct: Visions of Gender in Victorian America*, 197–216. New York: Oxford University Press, 1985.

———. "Puberty to Menopause: The Cycle of Femininity in Nineteenth-Century America." In *Disorderly Conduct: Visions of Gender in Victorian America*. New York: Oxford University Press, 1985.

Smith-Rosenberg, Carroll, and Charles Rosenberg. "The Female Animal: Medical and Biological Views of Woman and Her Role in Nineteenth-Century America." In *Women and Health in America*, edited by Judith Walzer Leavitt, 12–27. Madison: University of Wisconsin Press, 1984.

Stage, Sarah. *Female Complaints: Lydia Pinkham and the Business of Women's Medicine*. New York: W. W. Norton, 1979.

Starr, Paul. *The Social Transformation of American Medicine*. New York: Basic Books, 1982.

Tate, Cassandra. "Milady's Cigarette." Chapter 4 in *Cigarette Wars: The Triumph of the "Little White Slaver,"* 93–118. New York: Oxford University Press, 1999.

Tone, Andrea. *The Age of Anxiety: A History of America's Turbulent Affair with Tranquilizers*. New York: Basic Books, 2009.

Tracy, Sarah Whitney. *Alcoholism in America from Reconstruction to Prohibition*. Baltimore: Johns Hopkins University Press, 2005.

———. "The Foxborough Experiment: Medicalizing Inebriety at the Massachusetts Hospital for Dipsomaniacs and Inebriates." Ph.D. diss., University of Pennsylvania, 1992.

———. "The Paths of Fallen Angels." Paper presented at the College of Physicians, Philadelphia, March 7, 1996.

Tracy, Sarah Whitney, and Caroline Acker, eds. *Altering American Consciousness: The History of Alcohol and Drug Use in the United States, 1800–2000*. Amherst: University of Massachusetts Press, 2004.

Travis, Trysh. *The Language of the Heart: A Cultural History of the Recovery Movement from Alcoholics Anonymous to Oprah Winfrey*. Chapel Hill: University of North Carolina Press, 2009.

Tyrrell, Ian. "The U.S. Prohibition Experiment: Myths, History and Implications." *Addiction* 92 (November 1997): 1405–1409.

Valverde, Mariana. *Diseases of the Will: Alcohol and the Dilemmas of Freedom*. New York: Cambridge University Press, 1998.

Warsh, Cheryl Krasnick. "'Oh Lord, Pour a Cordial in Her Wounded Heart': The Drinking Woman in Victorian and Edwardian Canada." In *Drink in Canada*, edited by Cheryl Krasnick Warsh, 70–91. Montreal: McGill-Queen's University Press, 1993.

Welter, Barbara. "The Cult of True Womanhood, 1820–1860." *American Quarterly* 18 (Summer 1966): 151–174.

White, William L. *Slaying the Dragon: The History of Addiction Treatment and Recovery in America*. Bloomington, IL: Chestnut Hill Health Systems, 1998; 2nd ed., 2014.

Wilkerson, A. E., Jr. "A History of the Concept of Alcoholism as a Disease." D.S.W. diss., University of Pennsylvania, 1966.

Williams, Sarah E. "The Use of Beverage Alcohol as Medicine." *Journal of Studies on Alcohol* 41, no. 5 (1980): 543–566.

Wilsnack, Sharon C., and Linda J. Beckman, ed. *Alcohol Problems in Women: Antecedents, Consequences, and Intervention*. New York: Guilford Press, 1984.

Wood, Ann Douglas. "The 'Fashionable Diseases': Women's Complaints and Their Treatments in Nineteenth-Century America," 222–238, with response by Regina Markell Morantz, "The Perils of Feminist History," 239–245. In *Women and Health in America: Historical Readings*, edited by Judith Walzer Leavitt. Madison: University of Wisconsin Press, 1984.

Zeitz, Joshua. *Flapper: A Madcap Story of Sex, Style, Celebrity, and the Women Who Made America Modern*. New York: Crown Publishers, 2006.

Index

Abraham, Karl, 67–68, 137
abstinence: dry feminism, 21, 30, 60, 73; as extremism, 194n86; FAS and, 170; gender and, 154; Mann and, 139; motherhood and, 72, 132–133; necessity of, 18; physicians and, 148; psychiatrists and, 126, 140; Roth and, 152; in *The Smash-Up* (1947 film), 115–116; social status and, 7, 9; standards and, 11, 49–50, 57–58, 72, 104; temperance arguments and, 117; treatment and, 160–161; Washingtonian movement, 41; W. Wilson and, 141; wives and, 135
access: to alcohol, 21–22, 52, 57, 73, 138; control of, 4, 8–9; Mann and, 12, 104; to research, 111; social status and, 17; to treatment, 27, 44, 65, 133, 143–144, 146–147, 155, 163
addictions, 6; addiction medicine specialty, 108; comparison of, 11, 182n35, 209n32; definitions of, 8–9, 24; dependence issues, 24; FAS and, 171; Ford, Betty, 167–170, 212n14, 213n25; gender issues and, 173–174; iatrogenic addiction, 28; *Intervention* (2005 television show), 212n17; medicalization of, 13, 151; narcotics and opiates, 182n35; patent medicine and, 34; pharmaceuticals and, 152; psychiatrists and, 122–123; stigma and, 99, 166–169; Valium Panic, 169–170; wet feminism and, 21–22. *See also* Twelve Step program
African Americans, 16, 90–91
Al-Anon movement, 81, 144
alcohol-consumption patterns, 4–11, 191n35, 193n61, 194n70
alcoholic equalitarianism, 78–79, 96, 114, 166
Alcoholics Anonymous (AA): African American groups, 90–91; alcoholic equalitarianism, 166; anonymity and, 94, 97, 108, 196n5, 213n25; disease model and, 15, 96–97; female alcoholics, 79–83; female alcoholism, 17, 83–92; first woman in, 25, 93–94; gender comparisons in, 25, 75–97; genesis of, 77, 93; Mann and, 1, 26, 75–77; medicalization and, 4; and modern alcoholism movement, 14; Our Gal Group, 83–92; religious affiliation and, 91; Roth and, 88–89; sexuality issues, 26; sponsorship, 80, 83–92; women and, 25, 75–97. *See also* Twelve Step program
Alcoholics Anonymous: The Story of How Many More than One Hundred Men Have Recovered from Alcoholism (Alcoholics Anonymous, also known as "The Big Book"), 76–78, 86, 94, 105, 110
The Alcoholic Woman (Karpman), 127–128, 132, 138
alcoholism: defining of, 3, 108–114, 118; hitting bottom, 92–93; marriage and, 133–139; during Prohibition, 62–68; redefining of, 96; sexuality issues and, 133–139. *See also* gendered alcoholism
American Association for the Study and Cure of Inebriety, 24, 29, 32, 63
American Hospital Association, 148
American Medical Association (AMA), 26, 130–131, 147, 148
American Psychiatric Association, 122
Anti-Saloon League, 57, 107
Aristotle, 36
Atherton, Gertrude, 37, 42–43, 46, 56
at-home drinking, 5, 39, 51, 56, 58, 65, 68–73, 191n35

Banning, Margaret Culkin, 70, 72, 194n89
Belkin, Lisa, 165
"Beyond the Feminine Mystique" (Meyerowitz), 202n66
The Big Book. *See Alcoholics Anonymous: The Story of How Many More than One Hundred Men Have Recovered from Alcoholism* (Alcoholics Anonymous)

Bill W. *See* Wilson, Bill
Brill, A. A., 152
Brumberg, Joan Jacobs, 22
Burnham, John C., 191n39, 193n61

Campbell, Nancy, 174, 184n54
Chafetz, Morris, 212n11
Cohen, Elias, 208n26
"Confessions of a Female Inebriate" (Mrs. L.), 41–42
Council on Medical Education and Hospitals, 147
Crane, Stephen, 39–40, 51–52, 53, 55
Crothers, T. D., 34, 38, 43–44, 187n51

Daughter of the Vine (Atherton), 37, 42–43, 46, 56
The Days of Wine and Roses (1962 film), 25, 27, 95–96
Deex, Dorothy Jean, 159–163, 210n62, 211n67
delirium, 13, 63, 122, 193n66
dependency issues, 8, 13, 24, 32, 168
Diagnostic and Statistical Manual: Mental Disorders (DSM-I), 122–123, 155
disease definitions: defining alcoholism, 96–97, 108–114; gender differences and, 92–96; overview, 26, 98–118; *The Smash-Up* (1947 film), 114–118; social drinking and, 100–108; Travis disease model, 200n29
disease model of alcohol: advocates of, 14–17; anorexia nervosa comparisons, 22–23; Jellinek on, 201n48; Mann and, 107–108; medicinal drinking and, 47–48; tuberculosis comparisons and, 105–106; venereal disease comparisons, 63, 182n30
Dixon-Jones, Mary, 201n40
domesticity, 10, 31, 114, 120, 129, 132–133, 159
dosing: children and, 38; female problems and, 130; as folk custom, 185n8; gendered standards and, 7–8, 130, 185n8
Dr. Bob. *See* Smith, Bob
drinking customs: dosing, 7–8, 130, 185n8; gendered standards, 7–8; gender issues and, 7; Prohibition and, 180n19; WWII gender crisis and, 12

drinking mothers, 39, 72, 74, 133
drinking motivations: "female complaints" and, 8, 29–35, 42–43, 67, 120, 127, 129, 169; gendered differences in, 174; inebriate specialists and, 4, 40; judgment of, 5, 8, 10–11, 13, 16; of Lit Ladies, 70; psychological, 116; sexuality issues, 67; vanity as, 194n89
drug use: consumption patterns, 4; gendered control of, 46–47; narcotics, 9, 10, 34; National Council on Alcoholism and Drug Dependence, 199n6; National Institute on Drug Abuse, 166; omnipotence of drugs, 184n54; opium, 186n24; Pure Food and Drug Act of 1906, 9, 47, 62; Schuler case, 164; sedative use, 136, 152, 169, 209n32; social aspects of, 7
dry feminism, 21–22, 30, 60, 73, 104
Durfee, Charles H., 127

Eighteenth Amendment, 9, 50, 57, 61, 64, 66, 72, 73
eugenics, 72, 187n45
excesses, 5–6, 184n52, 194n86

fallen angel figure, 21, 31–32, 52
family issues: of alcoholics, 144; alcoholism and divorce, 49–50, 135–136; conventional marriage roles, 203n7; gender issues and, 204n34; marriage and drinking patterns, 42, 46, 49, 60–61, 70–72, 115, 131, 133–139, 160–161; reproduction and alcohol, 35–40; social workers and, 158–163, 206n56; treatment of female inebriates, 189n76
FAS (Fetal Alcohol Syndrome). *See* Fetal Alcohol Syndrome (FAS)
Fasting Girls (Brumberg), 22
Feldman, Paul E., 208n26
female alcoholics: AA wives and, 79–83; behavior of, 139–140; Chafetz on, 212n11; institutionalization, 155–158; medical treatment and, 151–154; overview, 118; sexuality issues and, 133–139; *The Smash-Up* (1947 film), 114–118
"The Female Alcoholic's Special Problems and Unmet Needs" (congressional hearings), 166

female alcoholism: definitions of, 5; hospital admissions rates, 208n26, 209n28
female inebriates: American view of, 186n32; family treatments for, 189n76; "female complaints" and, 7–8, 32–35, 130, 185n8; as Lit Ladies, 68–73; medicalization and, 184n2; overview, 24–25, 28–29; reproduction and, 35–40; temperance movement and, 29–30
femininity: alcoholism as failure of, 12, 127–133; biological diagnosis and, 5; definitions of, 4; medicinal reasons and idealized, 8, 33–34; motherhood and, 188n59
Fetal Alcohol Syndrome (FAS), 27, 170–172, 186n30, 213n36
Fitzgerald, Zelda, 58
flappers, 5, 22, 25, 50, 57–58, 60, 68–70, 103, 104, 192n41, 193n54
Ford, Betty, 167–170, 212n14, 213n25
Fort, Twila Florence, 111–113, 202n53
Freud, Sigmund, 67, 122

gendered alcoholism: conclusions, 27, 164–175, 212n9; femininity and, 20–23; history of, 6–12; medicalization and, 12–20; overview, 1–6, 24–27; term usage and, 23–24
gendered standards: diagnosis, 4; dosing and, 7–8, 130, 185n8; medicinal drinking, 7–8, 33–34; psychoanalytic treatment and, 5; recreational drinking, 4, 107; sex reformers and, 192n42
gender issues: Alcoholics Anonymous (AA) and, 25, 75–97; alcoholism and, 92; of consumption, 11; defining inebriety, 35; in disease definitions and the modern alcoholism movement, 26, 98–118; drug control and, 46–47; family members and, 204n34; gender convergence, 10; male alcoholism, 26, 119–140; masculinity crisis, 124–127; meanings of gender, 3; medicalization and, 20, 205n36; medical treatment and, 151–154; psychiatrists on, 206n55; psychoanalytic treatment and, 5; WWII gender crisis, 12, 98–99, 203n7
Glaser, Gabrielle, 174–175
Golden, Janet, 186n30

Gould, Katherine Clemmons, 49–50, 54, 56, 189n2
Grapevine (newsletter), 85, 89, 93, 108, 110
Great Depression, 73, 79, 124

Hall, Lucy M., 38
Harrison Narcotics Tax Act of 1914, 9, 47
Haymarket Square Relief Station, 146, 149, 150
Her Best-Kept Secret (Glaser), 174–175
heredity, 34–37, 130
Hirsh, Joseph, 206n46
Home Protection rhetoric, 10, 30, 51, 193n57
hospital admissions, 63–65, 146–151, 193n61, 194n70, 208n26, 209n26
Houck, Judith, 20
Hygeia (AMA periodical), 130

iatrogenic addiction, 28
Ignatia, Sister, 91, 94, 147
I'll Cry Tomorrow (Roth), 88, 151–152
incarceration, 54, 155–158, 163
inebriate (term), defining of, 10, 24
inebriate specialists: comparisons to, 93, 120, 123, 148, 152; explanations of, 32–33, 47, 50; medicalization and, 4, 43–46, 171; sympathetic treatment, 13, 35; temperance advocates and, 184n2
inebriety, 13, 15, 24, 32, 35–38, 40–46, 63, 65, 78, 108, 180n19
Intervention (2005 television show), 167, 212n17
The Invisible Alcoholics (Sandmaier), 170

Jellinek, E. M.: on alcoholism, 201n48; on children of alcoholics, 205n43; Mann and, 105; methodology of, 118, 201n50; "Phases in the Drinking History of Alcoholics," 110–113
Jolliffe, Norman, 64–65, 194n70
Jorgensen, Christine, 101, 200n25
journalists: depiction of women's drinking, 10, 59, 98–99, 137; female journalists, 73; investigative journalism, 46–47
Juvenile Protection Association of Chicago, 52–53

Karpman, Benjamin, 127–129, 132, 134, 138, 143, 206n60
Keeley Institute, 45, 66, 97, 151, 189n84
Kirkpatrick, Jean, 166
Knight, Robert, 124–125

League of Women Voters, 157
Lightner, Cindy, 171
Lit Ladies (term), 70, 74, 135
Long, Lois, 58
The Lost Weekend (1945 film), 114, 115
Lydia E. Pinkham's Vegetable Compound, 34, 47, 67, 130

Maggie (Crane), 39–40, 51–52, 53, 55
male alcoholism, 26, 79, 119–140, 205n37, 208n26, 209n28
Mann, Margaret "Marty": Alcoholics Anonymous (AA) and, 26, 76–77, 94, 197n32; anonymity and, 108, 196n5; attitude toward crisis and, 198n56; disease model and, 14, 16–17, 22; on drinking customs, 59; on families, 149; film depictions of alcoholism and, 114–117; *Grapevine* (newsletter) and, 108; hitting bottom, 92–93; image of, 197n36; Jellinek and, 105; Jorgensen comparison, 200n25; media coverage, 107; C. Nation and, 107; NCEA and, 88, 99, 104–105, 108; personal papers of, 21; *Primer on Alcoholism*, 113–114, 149, 151, 158; psychoanalytic language and, 204n22; public health campaign of, 26, 94, 99, 100–101; public health message, 201n44; public narrative of, 117–118, 138; *Reader's Digest* article on, 1–3, 27, 148–149; recovery, 107; sexual orientation of, 19, 84, 91–92, 139; sobriety of, 25, 133; sources, 195n1; sponsorship and, 83–85, 87–88; temperance advocates and, 106; Tiebout and, 75–76; tuberculosis comparisons and, 105–106; women's groups and, 90, 108; on women's magazines, 202n66
masculinity crisis, 124–127
May, Elaine Tyler, 206n47
media coverage, 73, 98; of AA, 109–110; *Intervention* (2005 television show), 212n17; on Mann, 107; on Sabin, 106. *See also* journalists; social commentators
medicalization: Alcoholics Anonymous (AA) and, 4, 78; changing theories, 4; dosing, 185n8; first wave of, 3–4; gendered alcoholism and, 12–20, 184n2; gendered treatments, 44–46, 151–154, 205n36; hospital admissions policies, 146–151, 193n61; institutionalization, 155–158; medical treatment, 146–151; mental health experts and, 4; new attitudes and, 144–146; overview, 12–15, 17–18, 141–144; physicians and, 26–27; during Prohibition, 62–68; public health advocates and, 4; scientific researchers and, 4; second wave of, 4, 5; social workers and, 158–163; stigma and, 144–146; temperance movement and, 43–46; therapeutic treatments, 8–9, 189n84; women's consumption patterns and, 6
medicinal drinking, 7–8, 33–34, 47–48
Menninger Clinic, 124–125, 204n22
methodology, 17
Meyerowitz, Joanne, 202n66, 205n36
middle class women, 7, 8, 9
modern alcoholism movement, 14, 26, 64–65, 98–100, 108–109, 114, 121–123, 158, 163, 212n11
Momism phenomenon, 125–128, 131
motherhood, 18; alcohol and, 18, 23; drinking and, 129–133; drinking mothers, 39, 72, 74, 133; family stability and, 71–72; FAS and, 27, 170–172, 186n30, 213n36; MADD and, 27, 170, 171–172; New Woman concept and, 55–56, 60–61; role-shift protocol and, 162; social dimensions of, 25, 29, 31
Mothers Against Drunk Drivers (MADD), 27, 170, 171–172
Murdock, Catherine Gilbert, 180n19, 191n35

Nation, Carry, 107, 194n86, 201n36
National Committee for Education on Alcoholism (NCEA), 2, 14, 21, 88, 99; AA and, 108; disease model and, 15; Mann and, 104–105; Parker and, 114. *See also* National Council on Alcoholism (NCA);

National Council on Alcoholism and Drug Dependence
National Council on Alcoholism (NCA), 2, 12, 156–157, 166
National Council on Alcoholism and Drug Dependence, 199n6
National Institute on Alcohol Abuse and Alcoholism (NIAAA), 166, 174, 212n11
National Institute on Drug Abuse, 166
NCEA. *See* National Committee for Education on Alcoholism (NCEA)
New England Home for Intemperate Women, 45–46
New Woman concept, 56–57
NIAAA (National Institute on Alcohol Abuse and Alcoholism), 166, 174, 212n11
Nicoll, Ione, 61
Noble, Douglas, 119–122, 124, 127, 129

Olson, Nancy, 166
Our Gal Group (Alcoholics Anonymous), 83–92
Oxford Group movement, 77

Parker, Dorothy, 114
patent medicine industry: as alternative, 34; gender issues and, 29; inebriate specialists and, 4, 15, 32; Lydia E. Pinkham's Vegetable Compound, 46–47, 67, 130; reformers and, 40–41
"Phases in the Drinking History of Alcoholics" (Jellinek), 110–111
physicians: dosing and, 7–8, 130, 185n8; on eugenic effect of alcohol, 187n45; medicalization and, 17, 184n2; sympathetic treatment, 8; temperance advocates and, 187n43; women's drinking and, 4
Pollock, Horatio M., 63–66
post-Repeal era, 166; gender issues in, 107–108; medicalization in, 142–143; research in, 108–109; treatment protocols during, 142–143
post-WWII era: changes during, 120–121; Momism phenomenon, 126–128, 131
pregnancy: dosing and, 8, 129; drinking and, 6, 33, 46, 120, 132, 186n30; effects of alcohol on, 23, 131, 187n45; Fetal Alcohol Syndrome, 170–171, 186n32

Primer on Alcoholism (Mann), 113–114, 149, 151
Progressive Era: eugenics, 72, 187n45; flappers, 57–62, 68–70, 103; New Woman concept and, 57–62; overview, 49–50; regulation in, 47; reversal of ideas of, 130; saloons, 57–62; women's drinking during, 25
Prohibition: establishment of, 9; evaluation of, 191n39, 193n61, 194n69, 201n36; legacy of, 7; overview, 49–50; post-Repeal beliefs, 184n54; as public health intervention, 62–63; repeal campaign, 73–74, 181n19, 193n57; repeal of, 4–5, 10, 15, 191n39; research on, 73; toward repeal, 73–74; Volstead Act, 50, 57, 72
Prohibition Era: alcohol-consumption patterns and, 4–5; at-home drinking during, 68–73; drinking customs and, 180n19; gender convergence in, 10, 101; medicine and alcoholism during, 62–68; women's drinking during, 25, 50, 57–60, 66–67
prostitution, 7, 37, 50–55, 60–61, 139, 155, 191n23
psychiatrists: alcoholic insanity, 194n69; alcoholism and, 26, 119–140, 203n7; American Psychiatric Association, 122; female alcoholics and, 127–133, 139, 206n55; Freud, Sigmund, 67, 122; masculinity crisis, 124–127; medicalization process and, 121–124; Momism phenomenon, 125–127, 131; nymphomania, 184n52, 191n32, 204n34; overview, 119–121; sexuality issues, 133–139, 206n55
psychoanalytic treatment, 5, 67–68, 126–127, 184n52, 204n22
public health movement: advocates of, 4, 8, 166; Mann and, 100–101; social drinking and creation of, 100–108
publicity and shame: binge drinking, 172–174; current issues, 174–175; date rape, 172–174; Fetal Alcohol Syndrome, 170–171; Ford, Betty, 167–169, 212n14, 213n25; Mothers Against Drunk Drivers (MADD), 27, 170, 171–172; overview, 164–165; Valium Panic, 169–170; women's alcoholism movement, 165–166

Pure Food and Drug Act of 1906, 9, 47, 62

rape, 172–174, 206n60
recreational drinking. *See* social drinking
Reformatory for Women (Framingham, MA), 155–158
research: on alcoholism, 104–105, 110–111, 166; post-Repeal era, 106, 137; on Prohibition, 73; scientific research, 4, 10, 14, 104–105, 114
Research Council on Problems of Alcohol, 104–105, 147
Rocky Meadows Farm, 127
Roosevelt, Eleanor, 61–62
Rose, Kenneth, 181n19
Roth, Lillian, 88, 136, 151–152, 207n69
Rotskoff, Lori, 203n7, 211n75
Rush, Benjamin, 13

Sabin, Pauline Morton, 61–62, 66, 73
saloons, 7, 51–57, 107, 190n14, 191n23, 191n35
Salvation Army, 66
Sandmaier, Marian, 170, 175
Schmidt, Laura, 21
Schuler, Diane, 164–165
Sears, Dr., 64–65
sexuality issues: AA and, 91; alcohol and, 9, 60, 67–68, 193n53; alcoholism and, 65–66, 95, 126, 133–139; attitudes on chastity, 11; dating customs, 9, 59, 192n46; female alcoholics and, 133–139; gendered standards, 192n42; nymphomania, 184n52, 191n32, 204n34; psychiatrists and, 133–139, 206n55; sexual orientation, 84, 91, 125, 137, 139
Shadel Sanitarium, 153
Sieberling, Henrietta, 77, 80
The Smash-Up (1947 film), 114–117
Smith, Anne, 80–81, 94
Smith, Bob, 77, 78, 80, 93, 147, 196n5
social commentators, depiction of women's drinking, 10, 59, 133–134, 137
social Darwinism, 35–36
social drinking: as counterpoint to alcoholism, 5, 10, 14–16, 104, 113, 121, 124, 146, 171; gendered standards, 4, 5, 107; implications of, 8–9; normalization of, 212n11; public health movement and, 100–108
social issues: social roles, 4; social sanctions differentiation, 8; social vulnerability, 4; social workers, 158–163, 206n56; socioeconomic classes, 10, 192n46
Sparks, Agnes, 35, 46
sponsorship, 83–92
sponsorship (Alcoholics Anonymous), 80
Strecker, Edward A., 126–128, 131

temperance advocates: criticisms of, 190n14; extremism among, 194n86; inebriate specialists and, 184n2; Mann and, 106; physicians and, 187n43; on prostitution, 191n25
temperance movement: attitudes and, 4; disease model of alcohol, 47–48; female complaints and, 29–35; gendered drug control, 46–47; individual treatment and medicalization, 40–46; legacy of, 4, 7; medicalization and, 43–48; and middle class women, 9; overview, 28–29; reproduction and, 35–40
temperance rhetoric, 7, 36
terminology use, 24
Their Mothers' Sons (Strecker), 126–128
They Call Them Camisoles (Wilson), 141–142
Thin Man films, 101
Tiebout, Henry, 1, 75–76, 77
Tracy, Sarah W., 18, 184n2
Travis, Trysh, 18, 200n29
treatments: access to, 27, 44, 65, 133, 143–144, 146–147, 155, 163; adrenal cortex extract injections, 209n39; Antabuse, 162–163; antihistamines, 209n39; aversion therapy, 152–154; conditioned reflex, 152–154; by family members, 189n76; hospitalization, 63–65, 146–151, 193n61, 194n70, 208n26, 209n26, 209n28; Keeley Cure, 45; non-alcoholic wives and, 189n85; professional resistance to, 144–146, 149; role-shift protocol and housewife role, 158–163; sterilization, 46; Washingtonian movement, 41–43, 97, 115, 159–162

Index

True Woman standard, 47
Turner, C. C., 153–154
Twelve Step program: anonymity and, 94; Betty Ford Center and, 213n25; film depictions of, 95; gender and, 79–81, 85, 92, 196n11; origin of, 77; self-diagnosis and, 78; women and, 83–92, 196n11. *See also* Alcoholics Anonymous (AA)
Twelve Traditions, 108
Twilight Sleep, 20

Valium Panic, 169–170
"The Victim of Excitement" (Hentz), 40
Volstead Act, 50, 57, 72

Wall, James H., 132, 154, 209n32
Warburton, Clark, 194n69
Washingtonian movement, 41–43, 97, 115, 159–162
Weisner, Constance, 21
wet feminism, 21, 58, 61, 73, 104
Wheeler, Wayne B., 57, 107
White, William L., 189n84
Wilson, Bill, 75–78, 80, 81, 83, 87, 88, 93, 94–95, 104, 107, 147, 188, 196n5
Wilson, Lois, 75–76, 77, 81, 99
Wilson, Wilma, 141, 148, 155

Woman's Christian Temperance Union (WCTU), 30, 57, 61–62, 106
Women for Sobriety, 166
women's alcoholism movement, 165–167
women's drinking: AA and, 25, 75–97, 196n11; at-home drinking, 10, 68–73; Chafetz on, 212n11; depiction of, 10; literature on, 6; medicine and alcoholism during Prohibition, 62–68; motivations, 10–11; New Woman concept, 55–57; during Progressive Era, 25, 29–74; during Prohibition, 25, 49–50, 57–62; promiscuity and, 52–55; research on, 11, 102, 173; saloons, 51–52. *See also* Mann, Margaret "Marty"
Women's Organization for National Prohibition Reform (WONPR), 61–62, 66, 73, 102, 106, 181n19, 193n57
WONPR (Woman's Organization for National Prohibition Reform). *See* Women's Organization for National Prohibition Reform (WONPR)
World Health Organization (WHO), 159–160
World War I, 64
World War II gender crisis, 12, 98–99, 102, 103, 203n7

Yale Center for Alcohol Studies, 14, 105, 109–110, 111, 157

About the Author

Michelle L. McClellan is a historian who lives and works in Michigan.

Available titles in the Critical Issues in Health and Medicine series:

Emily K. Abel, *Suffering in the Land of Sunshine: A Los Angeles Illness Narrative*

Emily K. Abel, *Tuberculosis and the Politics of Exclusion: A History of Public Health and Migration to Los Angeles*

Marilyn Aguirre-Molina, Luisa N. Borrell, and William Vega, eds. *Health Issues in Latino Males: A Social and Structural Approach*

Anne-Emanuelle Birn and Theodore M. Brown, eds., *Comrades in Health: U.S. Health Internationalists, Abroad and at Home*

Susan M. Chambré, *Fighting for Our Lives: New York's AIDS Community and the Politics of Disease*

James Colgrove, Gerald Markowitz, and David Rosner, eds., *The Contested Boundaries of American Public Health*

Cynthia A. Connolly, *Saving Sickly Children: The Tuberculosis Preventorium in American Life, 1909–1970*

Patricia D'Antonio, *Nursing with a Message: Public Health Demonstration Projects in New York City*

Tasha N. Dubriwny, *The Vulnerable Empowered Woman: Feminism, Postfeminism, and Women's Health*

Edward J. Eckenfels, *Doctors Serving People: Restoring Humanism to Medicine through Student Community Service*

Julie Fairman, *Making Room in the Clinic: Nurse Practitioners and the Evolution of Modern Health Care*

Jill A. Fisher, *Medical Research for Hire: The Political Economy of Pharmaceutical Clinical Trials*

Charlene Galarneau, *Communities of Health Care Justice*

Alyshia Gálvez, *Patient Citizens, Immigrant Mothers: Mexican Women, Public Prenatal Care and the Birth Weight Paradox*

Gerald N. Grob and Howard H. Goldman, *The Dilemma of Federal Mental Health Policy: Radical Reform or Incremental Change?*

Gerald N. Grob and Allan V. Horwitz, *Diagnosis, Therapy, and Evidence: Conundrums in Modern American Medicine*

Rachel Grob, *Testing Baby: The Transformation of Newborn Screening, Parenting, and Policymaking*

Mark A. Hall and Sara Rosenbaum, eds., *The Health Care "Safety Net" in a Post-Reform World*

Laura L. Heinemann, *Transplanting Care: Shifting Commitments in Health and Care in the United States*

Laura D. Hirshbein, *American Melancholy: Constructions of Depression in the Twentieth Century*

Laura D. Hirshbein, *Smoking Privileges: Psychiatry, the Mentally Ill, and the Tobacco Industry in America*

Timothy Hoff, *Practice under Pressure: Primary Care Physicians and Their Medicine in the Twenty-first Century*

Beatrix Hoffman, Nancy Tomes, Rachel N. Grob, and Mark Schlesinger, eds., *Patients as Policy Actors*

Ruth Horowitz, *Deciding the Public Interest: Medical Licensing and Discipline*

Powel Kazanjian, *Frederick Novy and the Development of Bacteriology in American Medicine*

Rebecca M. Kluchin, *Fit to Be Tied: Sterilization and Reproductive Rights in America, 1950–1980*

Jennifer Lisa Koslow, *Cultivating Health: Los Angeles Women and Public Health Reform*

Susan C. Lawrence, *Privacy and the Past: Research, Law, Archives, Ethics*

Bonnie Lefkowitz, *Community Health Centers: A Movement and the People Who Made It Happen*

Ellen Leopold, *Under the Radar: Cancer and the Cold War*

Barbara L. Ley, *From Pink to Green: Disease Prevention and the Environmental Breast Cancer Movement*

Sonja Mackenzie, *Structural Intimacies: Sexual Stories in the Black AIDS Epidemic*

Michelle L. McClellan, *Lady Lushes: Gender, Alcohol, and Medicine in Modern America*

David Mechanic, *The Truth about Health Care: Why Reform Is Not Working in America*

Richard A. Meckel, *Classrooms and Clinics: Urban Schools and the Protection and Promotion of Child Health, 1870–1930*

Alyssa Picard, *Making the American Mouth: Dentists and Public Health in the Twentieth Century*

Heather Munro Prescott, *The Morning After: A History of Emergency Contraception in the United States*

Andrew R. Ruis, *Eating to Learn, Learning to Eat: The Origins of School Lunch in the United States*

James A. Schafer Jr., *The Business of Private Medical Practice: Doctors, Specialization, and Urban Change in Philadelphia, 1900–1940*

David G. Schuster, *Neurasthenic Nation: America's Search for Health, Happiness, and Comfort, 1869–1920*

Karen Seccombe and Kim A. Hoffman, *Just Don't Get Sick: Access to Health Care in the Aftermath of Welfare Reform*

Leo B. Slater, *War and Disease: Biomedical Research on Malaria in the Twentieth Century*

Paige Hall Smith, Bernice L. Hausman, and Miriam Labbok, *Beyond Health, Beyond Choice: Breastfeeding Constraints and Realities*

Matthew Smith, *An Alternative History of Hyperactivity: Food Additives and the Feingold Diet*

Susan L. Smith, *Toxic Exposures: Mustard Gas and the Health Consequences of World War II in the United States*

Rosemary A. Stevens, Charles E. Rosenberg, and Lawton R. Burns, eds., *History and Health Policy in the United States: Putting the Past Back In*

Barbra Mann Wall, *American Catholic Hospitals: A Century of Changing Markets and Missions*

Frances Ward, *The Door of Last Resort: Memoirs of a Nurse Practitioner*

www.ingramcontent.com/pod-product-compliance
Lightning Source LLC
Jackson TN
JSHW020705110426
100738JS00003B/50